Exercises in Veterinary Radiology

Spinal Disease

Joe P. Morgan

Cleta Sue Bailey

Exercises in Veterinary Radiology - Spinal Disease

by
Joe P. Morgan, D.V.M.,Vet med dr. ACVR
Professor Emeritus
Department of Surgical and Radiological Sciences
School of Veterinary Medicine
University of California Davis
Davis, California 95616

and

Cleta Sue Bailey, D.V.M.,Ph.D.,ACVIM (Neurology)
Professor
Department of Surgical and Radiological Sciences
School of Veterinary Medicine
University of California Davis
Davis, California 95616

Venture Press
5 Skycrest Way
Napa, California 94558

Joe P. Morgan is a Diplomate of the American College of Veterinary Radiology and a Professor Emeritus in the Department of Surgical and Radiological Sciences, School of Veterinary Medicine, University of California Davis, Davis, California 95616.

Cleta Sue Bailey is a Diplomate of the American College of Veterinary Internal Medicine (Neurology) and a Professor in the Department of Surgical and Radiological Sciences, School of Veterinary Medicine, University of California Davis, Davis, California 95616

First edition, 2000

For information:

Venture Press
5 Skycrest Way, Napa, California 94558, USA

e-mail: jpmorgan@ucdavis.edu
www.ggweb.com/books/venturepress

Preface - Exercises in Diagnostic Radiology - Spinal Disease

Today it may be difficult for you to recall your bewilderment when first confronted with radiographs of the spine of the dog or cat. The apparently endless variety of shapes, sizes, and radiodensities did not help in your coming to understand how "normal" should appear. Hopefully, experience has led to the development of a technique of systematic analysis in the evaluation of radiographs, a sharpening of your powers of observation when searching for the abnormal on a radiograph, a development of a mental image of normal radiographic anatomy, and some knowledge of neurophysiology and neuropathology.

Still, the patients described in this text have 27 separate bones in the vertebral column plus the fused sacrum and endless caudal vertebrae. In addition. the cervical, thoracic, and lumbar vertebra have major differences in morphology and processes of varying shapes and sizes. Each vertebra articulates with those cranial and caudal through a unique type of joint, the intervertebral disc, plus the dorsally-located true vertebral joints. In addition, the ribs join the spine at the costovertebral joints through a diarthrodial joint.

The patterns of radiographic changes are similar to those found in the long bones except that the patterns are more difficult to identify because of the absence of a tubular bone with a prominent cortical shadow and medullary cavity.

Fortunately, it is possible to place a radiopaque contrast agent within the subarachnoid or extradural space resulting in the identification of mass lesions within the spinal canal not otherwise readily identified on noncontrast studies. Lesions identified on the myelogram can be conveniently divided into: (1) intramedullary, (2) intradural-extramedullary, and (3) extradural lesions and the classification of a lesion helps in the establishment of differential diagnosis. Epidurographic and discographic contrast studies are especially valuable for patients with lumbosacral lesions in which causes of canal stenosis are not identified on noncontrast studies.

The radiographic patterns that often cause errors in localization of the important spinal lesion are associated with frequently noted congenital lesions that cause prominent changes but do not result in spinal canal stenosis or cord compression. In addition, degenerative changes become frequent with advancing age causing lesions that may, or may not, result in canal stenosis and/or cord compression, but are such a slowly developing syndrome that they are not the cause of the myelopathy noted in the patient at this time. Another problem is the failure of the lesion to cause radiographic patterns seen on noncontrast studies and a failure to perform a contrast study that would have clearly identified both the location and type of the lesion.

Davis, California September, 2000

Contents - Cases

Contents - Textual Material

What This Book Contains and How To Use It

Contents

This book contains clinical descriptions with selected portions of radiographic studies of dogs and cats with spinal disorders. In addition, textual material covering major topics in clinical neurology and neuroradiology relevant to the cases is included. The cases are presented as they would be in a busy practice, without any particular order regarding the causes of the disorders. Most of the cases are organized into small groups with a common theme such as breed, an aspect of the clinical history, or a physical or neurologic abnormality. Certain cases are presented individually, usually with additional clinical or radiographic details. The cases are selected solely on the strength of the radiographic principle, with little regard to the incidence of the disorder represented. Therefore, some of the diseases shown are common, while others are rare. Additionally, the cases range from "classic" examples of illustrated diseases to unique presentations. All pathologic entities for which spinal radiographic studies are commonly of value are represented.

Cases

Each case description includes the animal's signalment, history, and physical and neurologic examination findings as recorded by the clinician at the time the animal was admitted to the UC Davis Veterinary Medical Teaching Hospital. Each case also includes the diagnosis and the author's comments. Many cases include information regarding the prognosis, treatment and outcome. Also scattered throughout are questions and answers about aspects of the cases.

The reader should remember the accuracy and completeness of a recorded history depends on the memory of the owner and the ability of the clinician to ask the appropriate questions. Also, the accuracy of the physical and neurological examination depends on several factors, including the presence of medication ameliorating clinical signs, the cooperation of the patient, the ability of the clinician to perform and interpret the examinations, and in some situations such as trauma, the necessity of limiting the neurologic exam. In some of the cases in this book the authors have edited the history and clinical findings in order to provide the reader the opportunity to construct an extensive list of differential diagnoses, and the opportunity to interpret the radiographs with less possibility of being "led' by this information. Although in most practices the same individual takes the history, performs the examinations and reads the radiographs, this approach can lead to bias in the radiographic interpretation. Ideally, a neurologist examines the animal and localizes the lesion, and a radiologist interprets the radiographic studies. We have attempted to approximate the ideal situation by including minimal clinical information for a number of the cases.

Radiographic studies

In an effort to bring the book into some sort of limit as to the number of pages, not all radiographs are included in each study. The limitation may be the portion of the vertebral column that is included or the limitation may be the number of views of an area of interest. You are advised in some descriptions that certain radiographs had no abnormal findings and are not shown. In other patients, oblique studies are included since they permit a better understanding of the nature of certain lesions, especially extradural masses.

Consistency is important in positioning of the radiographs on the view boxes. All lateral radiographs are positioned with the head of the patient on the left side of the radiograph. Dorsoventral and ventrodorsal radiographs are positioned as though the patient is suspended before the reader with its right to the reader's left in position to "shake hands" with the reader.

Often orientation on the radiograph is difficult. To assist the reader, specific vertebrae may be numbered, particularly in the mid-thoracic or mid-lumbar region. If the anatomic features are thought to be specific, such as found at a junction between major parts of the spine, labels may not be included and orientation may remain for the reader to determine. For patients with an abnormal number of vertebrae within a particular part of the spine, notation of the condition is made in the case description and/or the vertebrae are labeled.

Textual material

The book also includes summaries and short discussions of various aspects of clinical neurology and spinal radiography, e.g., the diagnostic approach to an animal with neck pain, and radiographic changes in disc disease. Introductory information regarding the neurologic examination, localization of neurologic lesions, and radiographic film-reading, is gathered at the beginning of the book. Additional material is dispersed throughout the book in association with relevant cases.

Table of contents and index

The Table of Contents is divided into two parts. The first part lists the cases by title and page number. The second part list the titles and page numbers for the textual topics. The Index lists only the diagnoses for all the disorders and diseases and the page numbers of the cases.

Suggestions for use

This book is intended for use by veterinary students in their clinical training years and by practitioners with an interest in spinal diseases of the dog and cat. As the cases are not specifically ordered, they and the accompanying textual material may simply be studied from the beginning of the book to the end. Readers interested in a particular disorder can consult the table of contents or the index and find the appropriate cases and textual material. Readers may also test themselves by attempting to interpret the radiographs without consulting the clinical history and signs. For the greatest value, we suggest reading the clinical information for each case, studying the radiographs, and then answering the questions before finally reading the diagnosis, answers to the questions, and additional comments.

Goals for students and clinicians using this book

The three major goals for those using this book are to learn how to:

1. Identify radiographic lesions of the vertebral column, vertebral canal, and spinal cord.
2. Use the clinical history and physical and neurologic examination findings to assess the clinical importance and currency of the lesions.
3. Recognize when diagnostic procedures other than noncontrast spinal radiographs are needed.

The authors believe these goals are best achieved by studying actual clinic cases.

These goals are the most difficult to achieve with older animals, which often have multiple sites of intervertebral disc degeneration or other degenerative disorders, and may have a second disorder as well. Animals with congenital vertebral column lesions also present particular problems in assessment of the clinical importance of the malformation. We have tried to include numerous examples of these common but problematic situations. We hope this book will help the students and clinicians using it become adept and comfortable in dealing with the diagnosis of spinal disorders.

Abbreviations

CT	Computed tomography
DV	Dorsoventral
Lat	Lateral (does not reflect right or left laterality)
LO	Left oblique (sternum to left of midline)*
LS	Lumbosacral junction of the vertebral column
Myel	Myelogram
MRI	Magnetic resonance imaging
NCR	Noncontrast radiograph(y)
RO	Right oblique (sternum to right of midline)*
TL	Thoracolumbar junction of the vertebral column
VD	Ventrodorsal

* Oblique views are taken with the animal in dorsal recumbency.

Summary of the Diagnostic Approach to Animals with Suspected Neurologic Disease

1. Note owner's complaint
2. Record animal's history (including verified vaccination and travel history)
3. Do complete physical examination

If historical or physical findings suggest neurologic disease is present, then…

4. Do complete neurological examination
5. Localize neurologic lesion(s) to neuroanatomical site(s)
6. Construct list of differential diagnoses
7. Outline ideal plan for diagnostic procedures
8. Discuss risks, cost, and alternatives to ideal diagnostic plan with owner

Summary of the Neurological Examination

1. Mentation
    a. level of consciousness
        1. obtunded
        2. stuporous
        3. comatose
    b. content of consciousness
        1. disoriented
        2. hysterical
        3. agressive
2. Posture
    a. general body position
    b. head position (roll, yaw)
3. Conformation, Muscularity
    a. conformation (skull, spine, limbs)
    b. muscularity
        1. atrophy
            a. focal
            b. regional
            c. generalized
        2. hypertrophy
            a. focal
            b. regional
            c. generalized
4. Movement
    a. gait pattern
    b. strength of voluntary movement
        1. paresis
            a. ambulatory
            b. nonambulatory
        2. paralysis
    c. coordination
    d. involuntary movements
5. Postural Reactions
    a. proprioceptive placing
    b. visual placing
    c. tactile placing
    d. hopping
    e. wheelbarrowing
    f. postural extensor thrust
    g. righting
6. Cranial Nerves
    a. olfactory
        1. response to non-irritating chemicals
        2. location of hidden food
    b. optic
        1. obstacle course
        2. menace response
        3. pupillary light reflexes
        4. visual placing
    c. oculomotor
        1. ptosis of upper eyelid
        2. spontaneous strabismus
        3. induced nystagmus
        4. pupillary light reflexes
    d. trochlear
        1. spontaneous strabismus
        2. position of dorsal retinal vein
    e. trigeminal
        1. ophthalmic
            a. autonomous zone – cornea. Corneal reflex. Aversion of head to corneal stimulation
        2. maxillary
            a. trigeminofacial reflex – eye blink in response to flick of maxillary vibrissae

b. cutaneous sensory testing – skin pinch at autonomous zone test site (skin of muzzle adjacent to upper canine tooth).
   3. maxillary and ophthalmic
     a. sensation in vestibule of nose
     b. blink reflex – tap at lateral or medial canthus of eye
   4. mandibular
     a. afferent
       1. cutaneous sensory testing – skin pinch at autonomous zone test site (skin of mandible adjacent to lower canine tooth)
     b. efferent
       1. masticatory muscle mass
       2. masticatory muscle function
f. abducent
   1. spontaneous strabismus
   2. induced nystagmus
   3. corneal reflex
g. facial
   1. afferent
     a. cutaneous sensory testing – skin pinch at autonomous zone test site (skin at mid-point of concave surface of pinna)
     b. taste test
   2. efferent:
     a. ear position and movement
     b. size of palpebral fissure
     c. blink reflex
     d. movement of external nares
     e. lip position and movement
     f. tear production
h. vestibulocochlear
   1. vestibular
     a. body position
     b. head position
     c. strabismus – check all head positions
     d. nystagmus – check all head positions
   2. cochlear
     a. response to sound
i. glossopharyngeal and vagus
   1. gag reflex
   2. swallow reflex
   3. cough reflex
   4. ability to swallow food or water
j. accessory
   1. mass of trapezius, omotransversarius, sternocephalicus, and cleidocephalicus muscles
k. hypoglossal
   1. mass of tongue
   2. movement of tongue
   3. ability to drink

7. Spinal Reflexes
  a. tendon reflexes
    1. patellar
    2. gastrocnemius
    3. biceps
    4. triceps
  b. withdrawal reflexes
  c. "abnormal" reflexes
    1. crossed extension
    2. spinal extensor thrust
  d. anal reflex
  e. cutaneus trunci reflex
  f. muscle tone
8. Somatosensation
  a. conscious proprioception (examined with placing reactions)
  b. mechanoreception, nociception (note increased or decreased sensitivity to stimuli)
    1. focal sensation
    2. cranio-caudal level of abnormality
    3. right-left symmetry
    4. general sensation
    5. superficial (skin). If absent, test…
    6. deep (subcutaneous tissue, periosteum)
9. Neuroanatomical Localization
  a. number of lesions
  b. primary localization
    1. brain
      a. medulla, pons, midbrain (with associated cranial nerves)
      b. cerebellum
      c. vestibular system
      d. hypothalamus
      e. thalamus
      f. basal nuclei
      g. cerebral cortex
      h. visual system
      i. limbic system, olfaction
    2. spinal cord
      a. C1-C5
      b. C6-T2
      c. T3-L3
      d. L4-L6
      e. L7-S3
      f. Cd 1—>
    3. peripheral nerve/muscle
      a. dorsal root and ganglia
      b. ventral root
      c. peripheral nerve
      d. neuromuscular junction
      e. muscle

Definition and Types of Myelopathies

A myelopathy is a disorder of the spinal cord. Myelopathies can be classified in two different ways as outlined below:

1. Origin of disorder
   a. Extrinsic myelopathy – caused by disorder originating outside the spinal cord. Example – compressive myelopathy caused by disc protrusion.
   b. Intrinsic myelopathy – caused by disorder originating within the spinal cord. Example – syringomyelia.
2. Extent of myelopathy
   a. Transverse – limited to one or a few segments of the spinal cord
      1. Partial – some neurologic function remains
      2. Complete – no neurologic function remains in area of the myelopathy
   b. Diffuse – affecting most or all of the spinal cord

Recognition of the type of myelopathy may suggest the cause. Hematomyelia, myelitis, and various degenerative and metabolic diseases usually produce disseminated myelopathies. Conversely, cord compression (whether due to disk herniation, vertebral fracture, or spinal tumor) usually produces a transverse myelopathy.

With the exception of the Schiff-Sherrington syndrome, the clinical signs of spinal cord lesions are seen in the part of the body caudal to the cranial limit of the spinal cord lesion. Although these signs may be unilateral early in the course of a disease, they are usually bilateral and may be asymmetrical. Their development may be sudden or gradual and is not necessarily indicative of the cause of the lesion, e.g., spinal tumors may result in acute paralysis. Often decreased proprioceptive placing and hyperesthesia are the first signs of spinal cord disease, followed by increasing degrees of motor loss, reflex abnormalities, changes in muscle tone, depressed pain perception, and, finally, absence of pain perception as the disease progresses.

Unfortunately, the clinical signs of spinal cord disease are not unique and may also occur with brain or peripheral nerve lesions. For example, quadriplegia can be caused by a brain lesion or a cervical spinal cord lesion; however, brain lesions nearly always produce additional signs of brain involvement. A peripheral nerve lesion may produce paralysis and anesthesia of a limb very similar to that caused by a spinal cord lesion. However, peripheral nerve lesions are usually unilateral, and the neurologic abnormalities are confined to the structures innervated by the diseased nerve. The examiner must also be aware of the possibility of multiple nervous system lesions, particularly with trauma or inflammatory disease.

Clinical Signs of Myelopathies

The clinical signs of spinal cord disease reflect loss of the neuronal functions mediated by the spinal cord, and include sensory dysfunction, loss of voluntary movement, spinal reflex abnormalities including changes in muscle tone and muscle atrophy.

Sensory dysfunction

Our ability to assess sensory function in animals is crude; we are limited essentially to conscious proprioception (the conscious perception of body position or movement) and nociception (the perception of stimuli that can potentially or actually cause tissue damage). Both are ultimately mediated by the cerebral cortex, and lesions anywhere along the neurologic route from the limb to the cerebral cortex can depress or obliterate these functions. Thus, sensory dysfunction alone may not be of value in localizing a lesion to the spinal cord, particularly if all four limbs are involved in the dysfunction. If only the pelvic limbs are involved, the lesion can be localized to the spinal cord caudal to T2.

Conscious proprioception is the afferent arm of the proprioceptive placing reaction. Loss of conscious proprioception is a sensitive indicator of neurologic disease, but because it depends on the cerebral cortex, conscious proprioception is subject to cortical influence and is very labile. Because a very frightened or pained animal may suppress its proprioceptive placing, depression of this reaction must be interpreted carefully.

The perception of pain may be exaggerated (hyperesthesia) or diminished (hypesthesia) or pain perception may be absent. Hyperesthesia is probably due to meningeal or nerve root irritation. Often it is localized to a focal area along the back, indicating the approximate location of a spinal cord lesion. If hypesthesia or anesthesia is present, the level of this abnormality along the back indicates the approximate cranial extent of the cord lesion. The assessment of pain perception is especially important in the prognosis of spinal cord disease; anesthesia always warrants a guarded prognosis for recovery.

Paresthesia and dysthesia are abnormalities of sensory perception that are often encountered in human medicine. Paresthesia is a perception of an external stimulus when there is none; dysthesia is the abnormal perception of a stimulus. Human patients often relate these sensations as burning, tingling or itching. Obviously our animal patients cannot communicate such information, but we can logically assume that these sensory abnormalities do occur in animals. A number of patients with neurologic disorders have a history and clinical signs of licking or chewing at parts of the body. Very possibly these animals are experiencing paresthesias or dysthesias.

Loss of voluntary movement

Voluntary movement must be differentiated from reflex movement by careful observation. Partial loss of voluntary movement is termed paresis; absence of voluntary movement is termed paralysis (combining form -plegia). Animals with deficits in voluntary movement may be described as follows:

Paretic – Weak voluntary movement
   Ambulatory – voluntary movement weak but effective (animal can walk)
   Non-ambulatory – voluntary movement weak but ineffective (animal cannot walk)
Paralyzed – Absent voluntary movement

Quadriparesis is paresis of all four legs, paraparesis is paresis of the pelvic limbs, and hemiparesis denotes that the weakness is limited to one side of the body and affects the pectoral and pelvic limb on that side.

Spinal reflex abnormalities

Spinal reflexes are reflexes that have their CNS components entirely within the spinal cord. Some reflexes such as the patellar reflex involve only a few segments of the cord, whereas others such as the cutaneus trunci reflex involve many segments. Depending on the location of the spinal cord lesion, these reflexes may be decreased or exaggerated. A decrease (or obliteration) occurs when the spinal cord segments containing the components of the reflex arc are damaged. Exaggeration of these reflexes occurs when spinal cord segments cranial to those mediating the reflexes are damaged.

Changes in muscle tone

Muscle tone is a spinal reflex phenomenon (the tonic muscle stretch reflex) and like other spinal reflexes, muscle tone may be decreased (hypotonia, atonia) or exaggerated (hypertonia), depending on the location of the cord lesion.

Muscle atrophy

Muscle atrophy subsequent to spinal cord disease is of two types: denervation atrophy and disuse atrophy. Denervation atrophy occurs when the alpha motor neuron (lower motor neuron) innervating a muscle is damaged and the trophic influence of the neuron upon the muscle is lost. Denervation atrophy occurs rapidly and is usually severe. Disuse atrophy occurs when a muscle is paralyzed by damage to neural structures proximal to the lower motor neuron. Disuse atrophy is slower in onset than denervation atrophy

Factors Determining Clinical Signs

The specific clinical signs of a myelopathies are determined by four major factors: (1) age of the patient, (2) the rate of onset of the disease or injury, (3) the nervous structures within the vertebral canal that are involved in the disease process, and (4) the cranio-caudal location of the lesion within the spinal cord.

Age

A deficit in part of the nervous system is often not apparent in a very young animal because that part of the nervous system is not yet operative. For example, syringomyelia in a puppy is usually not detected until the puppy begins to walk and run.

Rate of onset of disease

Acute spinal cord compression produces profound neurologic deficiency, whereas the same degree of compression applied over a long period of time results in more moderate neurologic signs. Ischemia, edema, hemorrhage, and the lack of time for development of compensatory neural mechanisms contribute to the incapacitating nature of acute neurologic injury.

Neural structures within the vertebral canal

The neural structures within the vertebral canal are the spinal nerves, the dorsal roots and dorsal root ganglia of the spinal nerves, the ventral roots of the spinal nerves, the meninges, and the spinal cord.

A spinal nerve is formed by dorsal and ventral spinal nerve roots, and carries both afferent and efferent fibers. A spinal nerve lesion causes sensory and motor dysfunction of the structures innervated by the diseased spinal nerve. Spinal nerves join or branch to form peripheral nerves; therefore, spinal nerve lesions are usually indistinguishable from peripheral nerve lesions.

The dorsal roots of the spinal nerves contain afferent fibers; therefore, lesions involving the dorsal roots and their ganglia (which contain the cell bodies of the dorsal root fibers) produce sensory abnormalities in the area of the body served by the involved dorsal roots. If the dorsal roots and their ganglia are irritated (as with inflammation), the perception of sensory stimuli may appear increased and be manifested clinically as pain (radicular pain or hyperesthesia) or the apparent presence of abnormal sensation (paresthesia) of the area innervated by the diseased roots. Radicular pain caused by disease of the dorsal roots innervating a limb may be expressed as lameness or reluctance to maintain weight on the limb. The recognition of lameness as a result of neurologic disease is very important for the diagnosis of several diseases, such as nerve

root tumors (Schwannomas), vertebral tumors, and disc disease. If the dorsal roots and their ganglia are severely damaged, sensation will be depressed (hypesthesia or anesthesia), proprioception will be diminished, and reflexes will be diminished or abolished because the afferent arm of the reflex arc is damaged.

The ventral roots carry motor fibers, and damage to them results in motor loss and a decrease or absence of reflexes because of destruction of the efferent side of the reflex arc. Polyradiculoneuritis (coonhound paralysis) is an example of ventral nerve root disease; characteristically, motor and reflex function is lost, but sensation is retained.

If both the dorsal and ventral roots of a spinal nerve are injured, the resultant clinical signs will be indistinguishable from those of a peripheral nerve or spinal nerve lesion. Because of the proximity of the structures within the vertebral canal, lesions of the nerve roots alone are rare, and the spinal cord and meninges are usually involved. An exception may be lesions of the cauda equina, such as those that occur with lumbosacral fractures. In such cases, however, the existence of deficits in several different areas of nerve supply (slack anus, atonic bladder, and flaccid, anesthetized tail) suggests a common, central location of the lesion rather than a peripheral site.

The meninges are well supplied with sensory endings; therefore, meningeal irritation or disease produces reflex muscle rigidity and pain in the area affected by the disease. Animals with cranial or cervical meningeal irritation exhibit cervical rigidity and pain upon movement of the neck. Animals with thoracolumbar meningeal irritation commonly have a painful, arched back and reluctance to move or walk. Severe or extensive meningeal irritation may produce opisthotonos. Meningeal signs may appear alone, particularly early in the course of a disease process, or in conjunction with signs of spinal cord disease, as exhibited commonly in intervertebral disk protrusion (i.e., pain and reluctance to move due to meningeal irritation, followed by paralysis due to spinal cord compression). Other causes of meningeal irritation and disease are meningitis and meningeal tumors. Clinically, these diseases may all appear the same, particularly early in their course.

The spinal cord is composed of many nerve fiber pathways with specific functions, and the clinical signs of spinal cord disease will reflect the pathways that are injured. Lesions of solitary tracts are rare. The marked intermingling of the fiber tracts makes the involvement of a single tract unlikely. Therefore, spinal cord disease usually presents signs indicating some degree of abnormality in most of the spinal cord functions, i.e., bilateral abnormalities in sensation, locomotion, reflexes, and muscle tone.

Cranio-caudal location of the lesion

The level of the spinal cord lesion determines the clinical signs because of the distribution of nerves to the forelimbs and hindquarters and the existence of two types of motor neurons, each with its own particular function. The nerve distribution allows the spinal cord to be divided into the following functional units:

Cervical (C1-C5 cord segments) - nerve fiber tracts ascending from thoracic limbs and hindquarters and descending from brain

Cervicothoracic (C6-T1 ± T2 cord segments) - origin of nerves to the thoracic limbs

Thoracolumbar (T3-L3 cord segments) - nerve fiber tracts ascending from hindquarters and descending from brain

Lumbosacral (L4-S3 cord segments) - origin of nerves to the pelvic limb, anus, bladder and perineum

Caudal (Cd1-Cd5 cord segments) - origin of nerves to the tail

Upper and Lower Motor Neurons

Motor neurons within the spinal cord are of two basic types, upper motor neurons and lower motor neurons. The functional difference between the two is used to localize cord lesions to the functional units of the spinal cord listed above.

The lower motor neurons to the thoracic limbs have their cell bodies in the spinal cord segments C6-T1 ± T2. The lower motor neurons to the pelvic limbs originate from cord segments L4-S2, and the lower motor neurons to the anal and urethral sphincters arise from S1-S3 segments.

Lower motor neurons

Lower motor neurons have their cell bodies in the spinal cord; their axons leave the cord via ventral nerve roots to become part of the peripheral nerves and terminate on a muscle. Lower motor neurons transmit reflex and volitional motor impulses to the muscle. An injury to a lower motor neuron (to its cell body in the spinal cord or its axon in the peripheral nerve) is called a lower motor neuron lesion and produces lower motor neuron signs. The lower motor neuron signs are:

Loss of voluntary motor activity in the muscle supplied by the neuron (paresis or paralysis)

Loss of reflex motor activity of the muscle (hyporeflexia or arreflexia)

Loss of muscle tone (hypotonia or atonia)

Denervation atrophy

Upper motor neurons

Upper motor neurons have their cell bodies in the brain. Their axons form the descending spinal tracts (e.g., rubrospinal tract) and terminate on interneurons that synapse with the lower motor neurons. Although upper motor neurons transmit both excitatory and inhibitory impulses to the lower motor neurons, an upper motor neuron lesion results in an increase in the excitatory state of the lower motor neurons due to mechanisms that are not clearly understood. The upper motor neurons signs are:

Loss of voluntary motor activity in the part of the body caudal to the lesion (paresis or paralysis)

Exaggerated reflex activity in that part of the body (hyperreflexia), including the appearance of "abnormal" reflexes

Increased muscle tone (hypertonia)

Disuse atrophy

Localization of Lesions within the Spinal Cord

The normal segmental spinal reflexes that are most commonly tested and the spinal cord segments from which they originate are:

Biceps tendon	C6-C8
Triceps tendon	C7-T1
Flexion (withdrawal)	C6-T1, L6-S1
Patellar (knee jerk)	L4-L6
Anal	S1-S3

These reflexes may be exaggerated with upper motor neuron lesions, or decreased or absent with lower motor neuron lesions.

The "abnormal" spinal reflexes that may appear with upper motor neuron lesions and the spinal cord segments mediating them in the thoracic limbs and the pelvic limbs are:

Crossed extension	C6-T1, L4-S1
Spinal extensor thrust	C6-T1, L4-S1

These reflexes are not strictly abnormal. They occur in the normal dog and are important in postural, supporting, and walking mechanisms, but they are difficult or impossible to elicit with standard examination techniques.

The postural reactions (proprioceptive placing,, visual and tactile placing, hopping and extensor postural thrust) are also used for the assessment of spinal cord damage. The expression of these reflexes is dependent upon ascending and descending pathways and input from the brain; thus, their localizing value is limited. Examination of these reactions is important, however, because their depression or absence indicates neurological damage that might be located in the spinal cord. The relationship between the site of a spinal cord lesion and the resultant motor neuron signs can be summarized as follows:

Cervical lesion – upper motor neuron (UMN) signs to all four legs and sphincters.

Cervical enlargement – lower motor neuron (LMN) signs to the thoracic limbs, upper motor neuron (UMN) signs to the pelvic limbs and sphincters.

Thoracolumbar lesion - upper motor neuron (UMN) signs to the pelvic limbs, and sphincters.

Lumbosacral lesion - lower motor neuron (LMN) signs to pelvic limbs and sphincters.

In certain conditions, the patellar reflex may appear exaggerated when in fact it is neurologically normal. This "pseudoexaggeration" occurs when there is a sciatic nerve lesion producing a lower motor neuron lesion of the stifle flexor muscles. The loss of tone and reflexes in these flexors allows the quadriceps to contract without opposition in response to the patellar tendon tap. Therefore, the patellar reflex occurs very briskly, has a greater excursion, and may even be pendulous. Pseudoexaggeration occurs commonly in cauda equina lesions and is a common cause of confusion in localizing spinal cord lesions.

Vertebrae Versus Spinal Cord Segments

Radiography of the vertebral column is probably the diagnostic procedure most commonly used to diagnose myelopathies. However, there is not a one-to-one relationship between the vertebrae and the spinal cord segments they contain In general, the spinal cord is foreshortened and ends at the L6 level, producing the following correlation:

C1-C5 cord segments lie within C1-C4 vertebrae

C6-T1 cord segments lie within C5-C7

T3-L3 cord segments lie within T1-L2

L4-L7 cord segments lie within L3 and L4

S1-S3 cord segments lie within L5

Cauda equina, within the vertebral canal from L5 caudally

There is some variability in this correlation, particularly in the vertebral level at which the spinal cord ends. Chondrodystrophoid breeds have shorter vertebral bodies and therefore the spinal cord terminates further caudally. Termination of the spinal cord is frequently at L7 or within the sacrum in these breeds.

Diagnostic Approach to Spinal Cord Lesions

Despite the numerous causes of myelopathies, the nervous system can respond in only a limited number of ways, producing a few distinct syndromes, that is, transverse or disseminated myelopathies with upper or lower motor neuron signs, meningeal signs, and dorsal or ventral root signs. Thus, the possible causes of any one myelopathy are numerous, and the clinician must use a diagnostic procedure that will detect these causes. A systematic approach ensures that the less common causes of myelopathies will not be misdiagnosed and mistreated.

A complete, accurate vaccination, medical and surgical history, and a thorough physical examination are the first steps in the diagnosis of any neurologic problem. The physical examination is often difficult to perform because the patient may be paretic or paralysed. Certain limitations may be imposed on the clinician. Whereas manipulation of a fracture or luxation within a limb is an acceptable method of causing a diagnostic crepitus or abnormal movement, in spinal disease this maneuver could cause additional severe spinal cord injury and therefore is contraindicated. It is possible, even in the paretic or paralysed dog, to carefully palpate the spinous processes for determination of their spacing or alignment and thus determine possible vertebral fracture-luxation. This is difficult or impossible to do in obese patients. Examination for soft tissue injury may indicate the site of trauma or the presence of a draining fistulous tract may be indicative of the site of an infectious lesion. Either of these findings are helpful, but require further examination to definitively diagnose or provide a prognosis for the lesion.

A complete, unbiased neurologic examination is necessary to accurately localize the spinal cord lesion (or lesions). Localization is essential for establishing the correct neuroanatomic diagnosis, e.g., cervical transverse myelopathy or thoracolumbar meningopathy. Misdiagnosis commonly occurs when only the major area of neural deficit is examined and the more subtle changes in other parts of the nervous system are overlooked. A common example is the young dog with an apparently uncomplicated transverse myelopathy of unknown origin in which patient a complete neurologic examination would have revealed vestibular and cerebellar signs, encephalomyelopathy, most likely due to canine distemper.

Several diagnostic procedures follow the neurologic examination in determining the cause of a myelopathy and localizing the lesion precisely. The rule of starting with the least risky procedure should be followed. The recommended basic procedures for diagnosing myelopathies are: (1) noncontrast spinal radiography, (2) cerebrospinal fluid (CSF) analysis, and (3) myelography. Additional procedures such as CT, MRI, or electromyographic (EMG) testing may also be necessary. Ultimately, diagnosis may require biopsy or surgical exploration.

Radiographs must include the area of the spine that could be involved in producing the clinical signs and are best made of the entire spine. Correct technique and positioning are vital for achieving radiographs of good diagnostic quality. Comparison studies made weeks or months apart can be useful in diagnosing chronic intervertebral disc disease, vertebral infections, or vertebral tumors.

If the noncontrast radiographs are not diagnostic or are equivocal, CSF analysis is performed. The fluid should be collected from the cerebellomedullary cistern for suspect cervical cord disease or from the lumbar subarachnoid space for suspect thoracolumbar cord disease. CSF analysis will often detect bacterial, fungal, and viral diseases, central nervous system tumors, and unsuspected trauma. CSF analysis should not be performed in cases of known trauma, since the diagnosis is already known and if brain edema and increased intracranial pressure are present, cerebral and cerebellar herniation may occur at the time of the CSF puncture.

If noncontrast radiographs and CSF analysis are not diagnostic, myelography should be performed. CSF analysis is usually done prior to myelography to rule out the presence of infectious myelitis. The injection of the contrast media into the infected spinal cord or meninges may disseminate or aggravate the original infection.

Occasionally, a vertebral lesion palpated or identified radiographically cannot be definitely diagnosed as post-traumatic, congenital, infectious, or neoplastic, and a bone biopsy may be necessary. The biopsy can be achieved with a biopsy needle using fluoroscopic assistance or by surgical cutdown.

Needle electromyographic (EMG) examination of the paraspinal and limb musculature may also be useful in localizing spinal cord lesions but its value is somewhat limited. The EMG will be abnormal only if the lower motor neuron is damaged; that is, the cell body of the lower motor neuron in the gray matter or the axon of the lower motor neuron in the ventral root. The EMG may be normal in disorders affecting primarily the white matter. Additionally, the EMG does not yield specific information regarding the cause of the disorder. Electrodiagnostic testing is of value in ruling out the presence of neuromuscular disease in quadriparetic or paraparetic animals. On the horizon is electrophysiological evaluation of spinal cord function by recording cerebral somatosensory evoked potentials and spinal cord evoked potentials. These techniques are currently being used in human medicine, but are just being developed in veterinary medicine. Potentially, these techniques provide noninvasive ways of localizing a cord lesion, determining its severity, formulating a prognosis, and even evaluating the response to therapy.

"Klaus" Has a Sore Neck

Case Description

"Klaus" is a 4-year-old male Rottweiler with a history of being unable to bend his neck to eat or drink for 5 days. The owners fed him from an elevated position. Quickly a right forelimb lameness developed, the dog could not rise on the pelvic limbs, and at admission he is unable to rise. Weak voluntary movement is present in all 4 limbs, proprioception is absent, and spinal reflexes are present. The lesion is localized to the cervical spinal cord; despite the lack of lower motor neuron signs, the forelimb lameness suggests cervical myelopathy/radiculopathy.

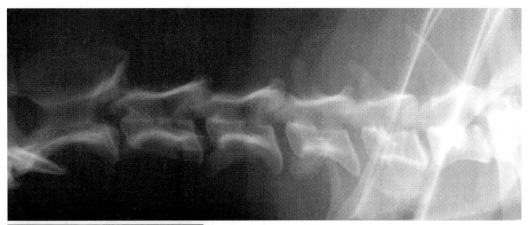

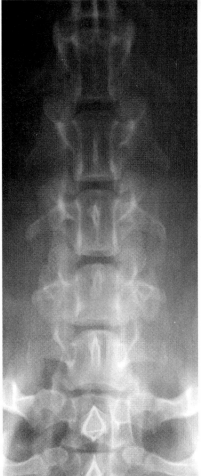

Radiographic Findings

Collapse of the C6-7 interspace without end plate sclerosis, spondylosis, or any disc calcification is noted on the noncontrast radiographs.

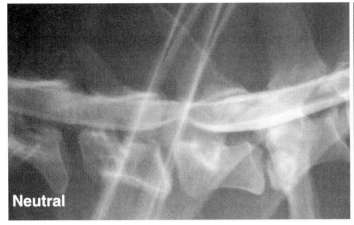

Neutral

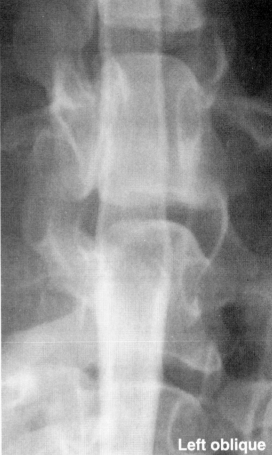

Left oblique

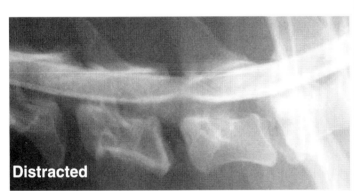

Distracted

Myelographic Findings

A ventral, extradural mass at C6-7 causes marked elevation of the ventral contrast column, thinning of the dorsal contrast column, and narrowing of the spinal cord. The cord is widened at this site on the VD oblique projection with narrowing of the lateral contrast columns. The pooling of the contrast agent caudal to the lesion is indicated by the increase in the density and width of the contrast columns and is the result of the compression of the subarachnoid space by the mass preventing a free flow of the contrast agent. The diagnosis is an extradural mass most likely a disc herniation.

Note the marked difference in the size of the extradural mass when comparing the radiograph made with neutral positioning of the neck with the distracted view made by pulling longitudinally on the neck. The dynamics of the disc disease is easily identified offering the surgeon information of value in deciding the nature of treatment.

Comment

A ventral slot procedure was performed and a large amount of extruded, fibrous disc material was removed from the floor of the vertebral canal. The postoperative recovery was stormy with frequent seizures. This is common in larger dogs especially if the myelogram is followed immediately by surgery with dependent positioning of the head that permits increased flow of the contrast agent into the head. Marked pain was noted following surgery suggesting entrapment of the C6 nerve root. Despite these problems, "Klaus" was discharged 3 days after admission able to move the head without pain and without the forelimb lameness.

Unfortunately, a discospondylitis developed at the surgical site postoperatively resulting in collapse of the adjacent vertebrae. Fortunately, only minimal vertebral malalignment occurred. "Klaus" returned 6 months later with progressive pelvic limb lameness/ataxia. An LS epidurogram identified a dorsal protruding LS disc that was thought to be of clinical importance. This patient's course demonstrates the multicentric nature of disc disease.

A Painful, Older Dog

Case Description

"Prince" is a 10-year-old male cocker spaniel with both neck and back pain.

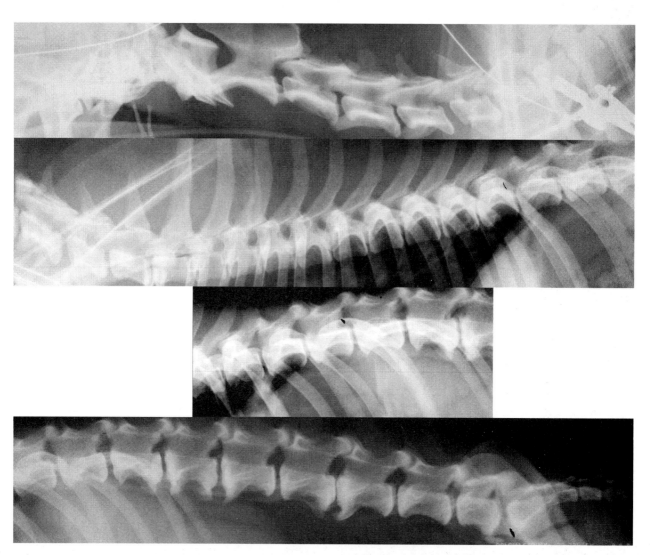

Radiographic Findings

The noncontrast radiographs shown on this page indicate collapse of C3-4, C4-5, L1-2, L2-3, and L4-5 disc spaces indicating "Prince" has generalized disc disease. Most of the changes appears chronic because of the end plate sclerosis and spondylosis deformans. A contrast study is required to determine the lesion of greatest importance.

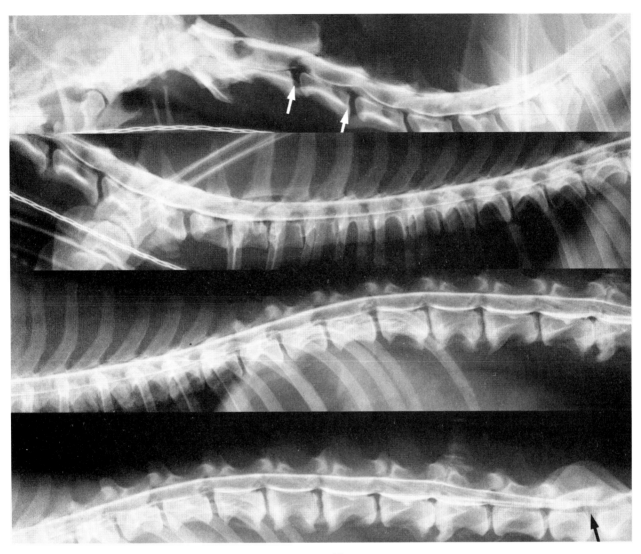

Myelographic Findings

The views from the myelogram are shown above and suggest a large disc herniation at C3-4 (white arrow) with a smaller disc herniation at C2-3 (white arrow). C4-5, C6-7, and L1-5 also have small disc herniations. A large disc herniation also involves the LS disc (black arrow).

Comments

Older dogs often have a number of degenerative changes in the spine, complicating determination of which change is the most important clinically. In this dog, the larger disc herniation at C3-4 is probably the cause of the acute onset of clinical signs.

If sufficient contrast agent is utilized for the myelogram, the lumbosacral subarachnoid space fills and the character of the LS disc can be evaluated. In "Prince", the absence of any primary vertebral canal stenosis provides sufficient space for the LS disc to protrude without causing clinical signs.

Note how contrast agent leaks backward along the needle tract following injection because of the excessive amount of contrast agent used and/or the rapid rate of injection.

Because of his breed, "Prince" is not calcifying his discs, making radiographic identification of herniated discs more difficult and necessitating the use of myelography.

Disc Disease in a Doberman

The original descriptions of disc disease by Hansen separated the nature of disc degeneration by type of skeletal maturation - Type I (chondroid degeneration) occurring in chondrodystrophoid breeds, and Type II (fibroid degeneration) occurring in nonchondrodystrophoid breeds. However, Type I disc disease can occur in nonchondrodystrophoid breeds. This example in a Doberman Pinscher will help to explain this nature of disc disease.

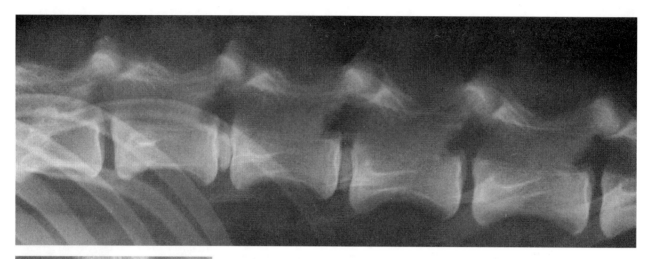

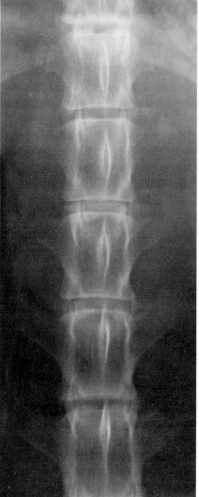

Case Description

"**Blue**" is a 5-year-old male Doberman Pinscher who presented with a history that he had cried out while rising from a recumbent position 8 days previously and had been favoring his right pelvic limb since that time. Now 'ie is paraplegic after acute loss of function of the pelvic limbs this morning. On physical examination "Blue" has pelvic limb paralysis with deep pain sensation. Proprioceptive placing is absent bilaterally in the pelvic limbs. Spinal reflexes are present. The cutaneus trunci reflex is depressed caudal to L3.

The tentative rule-out diseases include: (1) Type I disc disease, (2) ischemic myelopathy, (3) neoplasia, and (4) spinal trauma.

Radiographic Findings

Noncontrast radiographs on this page show several calcified discs with a suggestion of minimal protrusion of the L2-3 disc.

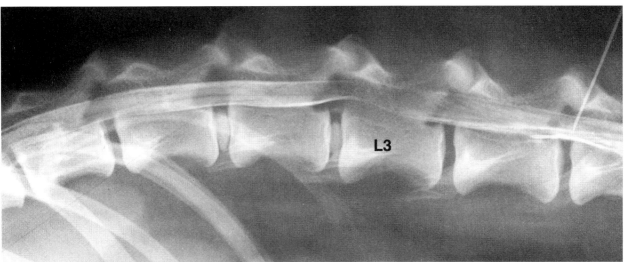

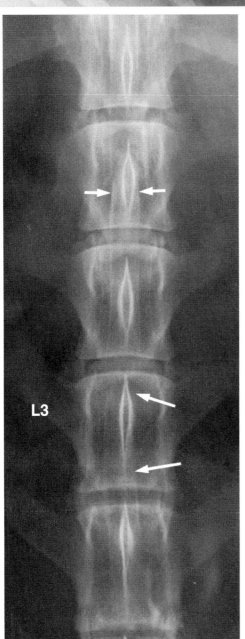

Myelographic Findings

The myelogram seen on this page clearly shows an extradural mass from L2 to the midbody of L3 that is ventral and left sided causing displacement of the spinal cord and narrowing of the subarachnoid columns (arrows). Cord swelling is not present. The myelogram also shows a constricting lesion at L1 as seen only on the ventrodorsal view (arrows).

Comments

The size of the extradural mass seems to be massive for a disc protrusion especially when a large amount of calcified tissue remains in the L2-3 disc space. Also, the width of the L2-3 disc space is near normal which would be unusual for a disc that has herniated.

A left sided hemilaminectomy was performed and a mass of disc tissue was removed surgically. Adjacent calcified discs were all fenestrated. The L1 lesion was not surgically explored which is probably an error in case management since the lesion is probably a second disc herniation. The loss of the cutaneus trunci reflex caudal to L3 is more likely caused by the L1 lesion than the L2-3 lesion.

Localization Errors

Mistakes can be made in localizing and assessing spinal cord disease. The most common error is failure to assess diagnostically the entire spinal area that might be affected in a particular case. For example, if an animal has both a T3-L3 myelopathy and an L4-S3 myelopathy, only lower motor neuron signs will be present in the pelvic limbs. The neural pathways through which the upper motor neuron signs are expressed are destroyed by the lower motor lesion, and upper motor neuron signs do not develop. Therefore, if an animal has lower motor neuron signs in the pelvic limbs, the spinal cord from T2 caudally must be examined. If an animal shows lower motor neuron signs in the forelimbs, the cord from C1 to T1 must be examined. In addition, an animal with two or three lesions in the same cord area may be clinically indistinguishable from an animal with only one such lesion. These complex cases are especially characteristic of degenerative intervertebral disc disease, trauma, and systemic infections.

Another problem is a disparity between the neuroanatomical localization and the radiographic findings. If an animal has a radiographic lesion in an upper motor neuron area but is showing lower motor neuron signs, then either the radiographic lesion is not clinically significant (i.e., it may be a congenital abnormality or healed lesion) or the radiographic lesion has initiated a diffuse myelopathy(i.e., progressive myelomalacia subsequent to acute, severe disc herniation, or microbial myelitis associated with discospondylitis). Since progressive myelomalacia and microbial myelitis can be fatal, the clinician need to be alert for clinical-radiographic disparity.

The Schiff-Sherrington syndrome is opisthotonus of the neck and extensor rigidity of the thoracic limbs caused by an acute, severe spinal cord lesion caudal to T2. The examiner may mistake this syndrome for quadriplegia and begin looking for a cervical cord lesion, rather than a lesion caudal to T2.

Spinal shock is the condition of spinal areflexia that occurs following an acute, very severe, spinal cord lesion. In people, this condition is severe and can persist for weeks. In non-primates, spinal shock is very transient, lasting only a few minutes in most instances. Therefore, an animal with lower motor neuron signs most likely has an actual lower motor neuron lesion, not spinal shock. The localization of its lesion and assessment of its prognosis should be done with this fact in mind, and the animal should not hastily be regarded as having no chance for recovery.

A common and very serious error is mistaking the withdrawal reflex for pain perception. Since the examiner falsely assumes pain perception is present, the owner may be given a good prognosis when, in fact, recovery is very unlikely . An animal with a completely transected spinal cord may still have a flexion reflex, but it certainly cannot perceive a noxious stimulus applied caudal to the transection, and it certainly is not going to walk again. Clinicians must look diligently for evidence of cerebral perception of noxious stimuli, such as turning the head toward the stimulus and licking or biting, arousal, anxiety and attempts to get away, and vocalizing.

Prognosis Based on Clinical Signs

The clinical signs of spinal cord damage have prognostic value, particularly for traumatic lesions. In general, the more depressed the sensation, the more severe the lesion and the more guarded the prognosis for recovery of neural function. Anesthesia is a grave sign, especially if present for more than a few hours. The degree of motor loss is also directly related to the severity of the lesion. However, paralysis can occur with sensation remaining nearly normal (as well as can be clinically ascertained). Therefore, paralysis does not warrant as grave a prognosis as does anesthesia.

With upper motor neuron lesions, the patellar and flexor reflexes are the first to become exaggerated. As the lesion increases in severity, the crossed extension reflex becomes apparent, and then the spinal extensor thrust appears. Crossed extension usually takes about a week to develop completely, but it may appear sooner if the lesion is very severe. Spinal extensor thrust takes even longer to develop. Animals with morphologically or functionally transected spinal cords may eventually develop spinal walking (a.k.a. reflex walking). These animals are have an irreversible lesion and are, of course, paralyzed and anesthetic in the affected part of the body. Unfortunately, the development of spinal walking is often mistaken for the recovery of voluntary movement.

Different Causes for Cauda Equina Syndrome

Cauda equine syndrome is a specific clinical entity in which the neurological signs are somewhat predictable. The cause is frequently a protruding degenerated LS disc whose rate of degeneration is often associated with a transitional LS vertebral segment. The clinical progression is based on the degree of resulting canal stenosis. These three cases demonstrate different causes for cauda equina syndrome and several of the radiographic techniques that can be used in diagnosis.

Case Description

"Kayla" is a 7-year-old female Labrador retriever with progressive back pain.

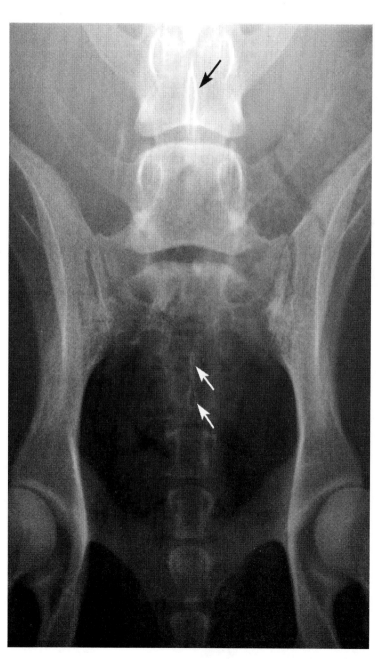

Radiographic Findings

The lateral views of the noncontrast radiographs of the spine were normal. An abnormality was identified in the arch of L7 and the sacrum that was seen best on the VD view. The change is characterized by an absence of spinous processes. The normal processes are identified for comparison (arrows). The lesion has the appearance of a congenital lesion such as a spina bifida, which has an absence of bone tissue in the arch. The lesion could also be destructive, as with a tumor such as a chondrosarcoma. No evidence of malalignment or instability at the LS junction was noted. Contrast studies were performed.

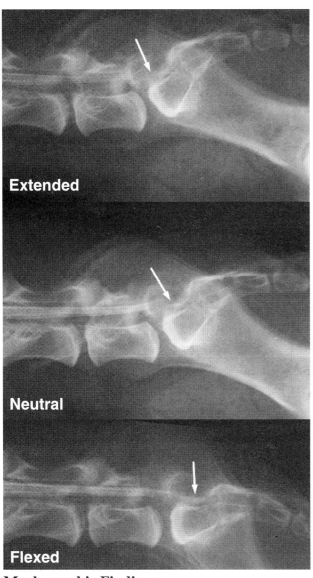

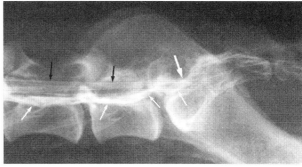

Epidurographic Findings

A lateral view from an epidurogram (above) identifies a dorsally herniating LS disc (small white arrows) as well as the dorsal mass (large white arrow). The contrast agent in the subarachnoid space is residual from the myelographic study (black arrows). Epidural contrast agent is identified (white arrows).

Myelographic Findings

The myelogram includes neutral, flexed, and extended positioning (above) and shows elevation of the lumbar subarachnoid space with marked blunting of the contrast columns over the sacrum. A dorsal mass displaces the lumbar subarachnoid space ventrally (arrows).

Comments

At surgery, a dorsally protruding LS disc was evident in addition to a ventrally protruding mass consisting of hypertrophied interarcuate ligament. A lumbosacral spina bifida was evident with an absence of spinous processes indicating a congenital lesion. The spina bifida may have contributed to an accentuation of the lumbosacral disc motion and encouraged disc degeneration.

Case Description

"**Wilt**" is a 5-year-old male Airedale terrier with a history of progressive LS pain of several months duration. Original radiographs were made of "Wilt's" spine 2 years ago. At that time, early LS disc degeneration was evident. On today's physical examination, the pain was clearly evident; however, no neurologic deficits were detected. The entire spine was radiographed with only minimal narrowing of the C6-7 disc space with end plate sclerosis and spondylosis deformans noted at T10-11. The major changes were noted at the LS junction.

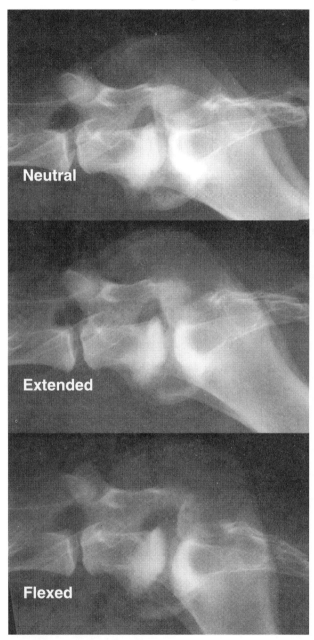
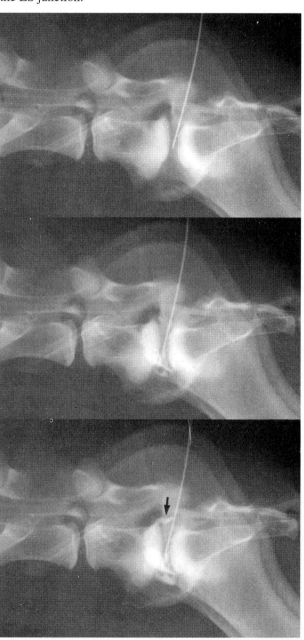

Radiographic Findings

The noncontrast studies (above) show marked end plate sclerosis and spondylosis deformans. Malalignment and instability are evident on stress radiographs.

Discographic Findings

In the discographic studies (above) a needle was placed in the LS disc space and an injection of contrast agent was made slowly using 0.2 cc aliquots as is seen in the progressive views. Some contrast agent is visible within the region of the protruded dorsal anulus (arrow). Subarachnoid contrast media remains from the myelogram (not shown).

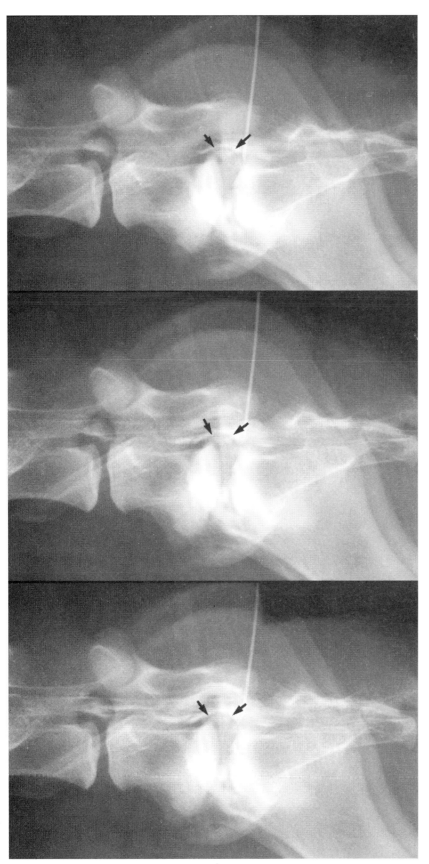

Epidurographic Findings

The needle was withdrawn slightly and contrast agent injected for an epidurogram that further outlined the protruding dorsal anulus (arrows). This injection was made in 1.0 cc aliquots.

The protruding disc plus the ventral slippage of the sacrum caused vertebral canal stenosis that was compressing the conus and causing pain.

Comments

"Wilt" had a decompressive dorsal laminectomy at the LS junction. Unfortunately a bronchopneumonia developed postsurgically that complicated his recovery. The pneumonia had cleared on radiographs made 2 weeks later at the time of release from the clinic. Pain was not present following surgery.

Case Description

"Echo" is a 9-year-old female Labrador retriever who has a history of progressive paraparesis and pain in the LS region for the past 2 years. She has been tentatively diagnosed as having LS disc disease.

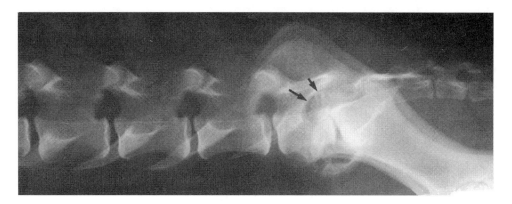

Radiographic Findings

A noncontrast radiograph of the spine (above) shows collapse and wedging of the LS disc space with a moderate amount of spondylosis deformans. Marked enlargement of the intervertebral foramina at the LS disc space accompanies the suggestion of destruction of the articular facets (black arrows). Special procedures are necessary to confirm the tentative diagnosis.

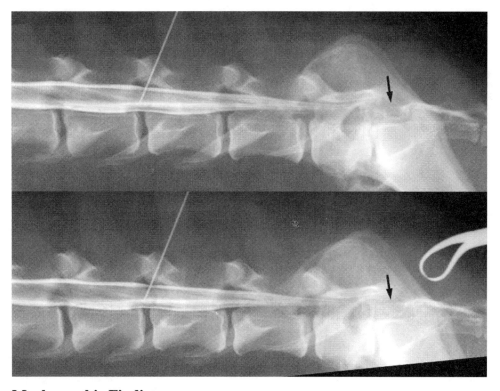

Myelographic Findings

Two views from the myelogram (above) with the spinal needle remaining in position, have good filling of the lumbar subarachnoid space; however, the filling terminates within the vertebral canal at the level of L7. Dorsal tethering is marked making it difficult to determine the presence of an extradural mass lying on the floor of the canal. However, a large dorsal mass appears to cause a depression of the contrast column (black arrows).

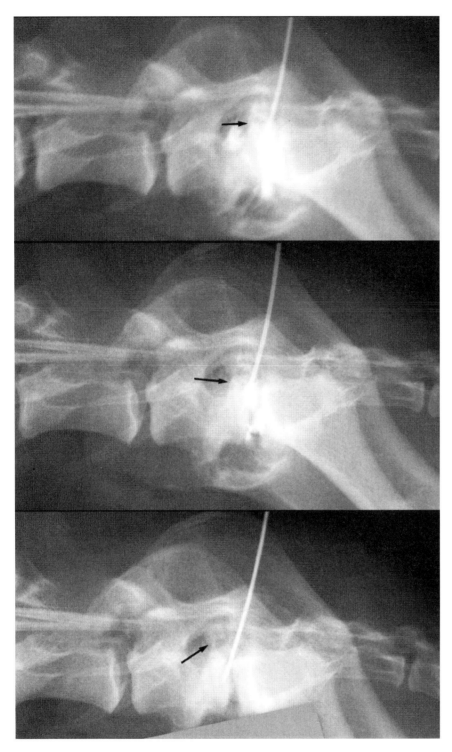

Disco-epidurographic Findings

Three views from the disco-epidurogram (above) delineate the destruction of the LS disc. The abnormally located contrast agent that normally would remain within the nuclear region of the disc is seen within the vertebral canal where it delineates a large, ventrally located, extradural mass of discal tissue at the LS junction (arrows). Malalignment and vertebral instability are difficult to determine.

Comments

"Echo" had a dorsal decompressive laminectomy. A dorsally protruding LS disc was found in combination with a ventrally protruding mass associated with an apparent congenital anomaly in the roof of the sacrum. Stabilization of the LS region was thought necessary and was achieved by placement of pins in L7 and the sacrum and embedding the dorsal pin ends in methylmethacrylate.

Cauda Equina Syndrome

The cauda equina is the bundle of nerve roots within the lumbosacral vertebral canal caudal to the spinal cord. This bundle is composed of the L7, sacral, and caudal nerve roots. Cauda equina syndrome is a cluster of clinical signs caused by a lesion of the cauda equina. The characteristic neurologic deficits associated with cauda equina syndrome are a combination of lower motor neuron signs of the muscles innervated by L7 (primarily the sciatic nerve), the bladder, the anus, and/or the tail. These deficits are evident clinically as pelvic limb weakness with toe scuffing and leg crossing when walking, urinary and fecal incontinence, and weakened tail carriage and wagging. Pain upon lumbosacral palpation or movement may be present depending on the specific cause of the syndrome. Individual dogs often have only 2 or 3 of the clinical signs.

Causes

1. Anomalies
   a. spina bifida/myelomeningocele complex
   b. primary lumbar or sacral vertebral stenosis
   c. sacral osteochondrosis
2. Metabolic disease
   a. pathologic fracture secondary to metabolic bone disease
3. Tumor
   a. primary bone tumor
   b. metastatic tumor to bone
   c. primary neural tumor of cord, meninges, or nerve roots
   d. hematogenous metastatic tumor to cord, meninges, or nerve roots
   e. invasive extraspinal primary soft tissue tumor to spinal tissues
   f. invasive extraspinal hematogenous metastatic soft tissue tumor to spinal tissues
4. Noninfectious Inflammatory
   a. meningeal and/or nerve root inflammation caused by herniated disc material
5. Infectious Inflammatory
   a. spondylitis
   b. discitis
   c. discospondylitis
   d. soft tissue infection
6. Trauma/Compression
   a. spinal fracture-luxation
   b. traumatic disc protrusion
7. Degenerative disease
   a. degenerative disc disease
   b. synovial cyst formation
   c. ligamentum flavum hypertrophy
   d. vertebral joint capsule hypertrophy
   e. stenosis associated with
      1. segmental malalignment
      2. segmental instability

Diagnostic procedures

Because of the variety of diseases that may cause cauda equina syndromes and the number of anatomical structures and tissues that may be involved, determining the cause of a cauda equina syndrome often requires several diagnostic procedures. These procedures commonly include:

1. Noncontrast spinal radiographs of the entire spine help to identify additional spinal lesions
   a. conventional views (lateral and ventrodorsal)
   b. stress views (lateral views of lumbosacral region with the hips in neutral, fully flexed, and fully extended positions)
2. Analysis of lumbar subarachnoid CSF
3. Myelography of the entire spinal column (lateral and ventrodorsal views)
   myelography rarely illuminates the lumbosacral vertebral canal or its contents adequately, but it helps to rule out the presence of additional spinal lesions further cranially, whose clinical signs could be masked by the cauda equina syndrome
4. L7-S1 discography (lateral and ventrodorsal views)
5. Lumbosacral epidurography (lateral conventional and stress views)
6. Electromyography, and nerve conduction velocity studies (motor and sensory)
7. Computed tomography
8. Magnetic resonance imaging

Magnetic resonance imaging (MRI) may soon replace discography and epidurography. MRI should not replace myelography or electro-physiologic testing, however. Myelography examines the entire spinal cord. Many animals with cauda equina syndrome and/or lumbosacral pain have degenerative disease (e.g., intervertebral disc degeneration) or vertebral malformations, which may be present at multiple sites. Animals with cauda equina syndrome may have a second or third lesion in the T3-L3 spinal cord that is being masked by the lower motor neuron signs. Therefore, assessing the spinal cord, particularly the T3-L3 area, is necessary in order to detect these lesions and form an accurate prognosis and appropriate treatment plan.

Change in Size or Shape of Vertebral Body

Normally, the body of the vertebra is rectangular in conformation and similar in appearance to the vertebrae cranial and caudal. Changes in size and shape of the vertebral body occur with: (1) a compression fracture or a healing fracture, (2) a pathologic fracture of the vertebra, secondary to tumor, infectious process, or metabolic disease, (3) shortening associated with discospondylitis, (4) certain congenital anomalies such as hemivertebra ("butterfly" vertebra), transitional vertebrae, or block vertebra, (5) developmental lesions such as those seen in cervical spondylopathy and sacral osteochondrosis, and (6) certain normally shorter vertebrae (L7).

Congenital lesions are the most common cause of malformation of the vertebral body and its processes and while the bone organ is abnormal, the bone tissue remains normal. Thus, the density of the trabecular bone, the width of the cortical bone, and smoothness of the periosteal surface remain normal in appearance regardless of the severity of change in the size or shape of the bone. Since the lesions are congenital, adjacent vertebral vertebrae assume abnormal shapes as they attempt to compensate for the deficiencies of the primary lesion. This pattern of compensation occurs at the time of skeletal maturation. Congenital abnormalities do not cause clinical signs unless there is malalignment of vertebra or instability with the resulting canal stenosis causing a cord compression.

A single example of a developmental lesion fits into a pattern similar to that seen in osteochondrosis of the appendicular skeleton and is one of the causes of cervical spondylopathy. At a young age a part of the vertebral body, often the cranial aspect of the body of C7, fails to develop normally into osseous tissue. While causing no clinical signs, the malformed vertebrae often become malaligned, unstable, and provokes disc degeneration that leads to spinal cord compression. A similar lesion can occur in the dorsal aspect of the cranial end plate of the sacrum where it can be associated with a cauda equina syndrome.

Trauma is a common cause of altered size and shape of a vertebral body. In the immature patient, compression with shortening occurs often with preservation of the end plates. Fracture lines are usually not identified. However, in the mature patient, fracture lines are prominent with separation of the multiple fragments. With healing, regardless of age, the vertebral body appears malformed but with uniform density as the fracture lines fills with callus.

Inflammatory processes within the vertebral body can cause sufficient destruction so that a shortening of the body and a change in shape occurs. Usually destruction of the vertebral cortex or end plate provides distinguishing characteristics if these lesions are compared with those that are congenital or developmental. Determination of whether these lesions are acute or chronic may be difficult and is usually based on maturity of surrounding reactive bone. Determination of whether the lesion contains viable micro-organisms is not possible radiographically. These lesions do not usually cause clinical signs due to cord compression, however meningitis and/or myelitis may uncommonly occur. Usually, the clinical signs are due to the osteomyelitis alone.

Tumors are often destructive in nature and compression pathologic fracture may occur and may resemble traumatic fractures. The degree of bony response associated with the pathologic fracture is usually minimal. Clinical signs may be only those of pain from the fracture or may also include those of a transverse myelopathy because of vertebral instability and cord injury or compression.

Pathological fractures can result from dietary problems associated with a low calcium diet leading to a nutritional secondary hyperparathyroidism. Only rarely is there spinal cord injury or compression associated with this type of fracture.

Change in the size or shape of the vertebral body is a major diagnostic finding in radiography of the spine. In the determination of an abnormality, comparison with adjacent vertebrae is commonly done. This will be satisfactory except in the atlanto-axial region where the morphology of C1 and C2 varies markedly and in the caudal lumbar region where the body of L7 is appreciably shorter than the body of L6.

Causes

1. Congenital lesion
    a. hemivertebra
    b. "butterfly" vertebra
    c. transitional vertebra
    d. block vertebra
2. Developmental lesion
    a. cervical spondylopathy
    b. sacral osteochondrosis,
3. Traumatic lesion
    a. compression fracture
    b. healing fracture
4. Inflammatory lesion
    a. discospondylitis
    b. pathologic fracture
5. Neoplastic lesion
    a. primary bone tumor with pathologic fracture
6. Degenerative lesion
    a. pathologic fracture in osteopenic bone
    b. modeling associated with chronic disc disease (especially at the cervicothoracic and TL junction)

More Than One Radiographic Study

More than one radiographic study is often needed to make a diagnosis. The temporal aspect of spinal disease is especially evident in disc degeneration in which the progression of the disease can be noted on successive radiographic studies. This case is typical of the episodic nature of many cases of disc disease.

Case Description

"**Ming Toi**" is a 6-year-old female Pekingese who has had two episodes of spinal problems. At the time of the first admission, she was paraparetic with upper motor neuron signs in the pelvic limbs and an area of hyperesthesia at the TL junction. Disc disease was diagnosed and a TL fenestration was performed at that time. The clinical signs subsequently resolved.

Seventeen months later, she became acutely quadriplegic with upper motor neuron signs in all four limbs. Examine the two sets of radiographs; note the abnormalities in each and the differences between the two.

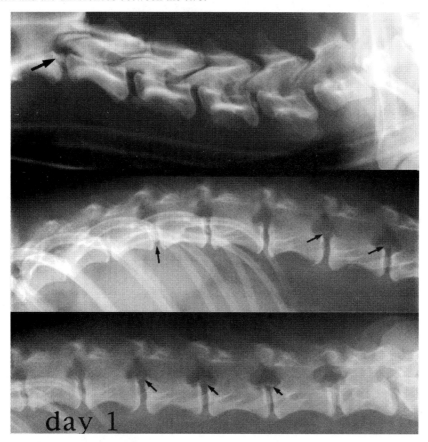

Radiographic Findings (first study)

Radiographs from the first study (above) show a series of degenerative changes including:

1. a calcified disc at C2-3 (arrow)
2. a minimally narrowed disc space at C5-6 with a calcified nucleus
3. a narrowed disc space between the last thoracic vertebrae (arrow)
4. dorsal protrusion of calcified disc tissue from L2-5 (arrows)
5. calcified discs at L5-6 and L6-7.
6. only 6 lumbar-type vertebrae

The thoracolumbar discs were fenestrated, however, the cervical discs were not treated.

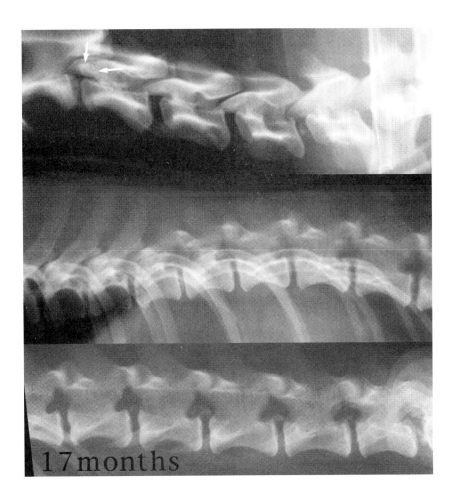

17months

Second Radiographic Findings (17 months later)

Views from the second radiographic study (above) made 17 months following surgery at the time of the second admission show the following series of changes:

1. a herniated disc at C2-3 with a large calcified mass in the vertebral canal (arrows)
2. the narrowed disc space at C5-6 with a calcified nucleus remains as before
3. the discs in the TL region have been fenestrated and all disc spaces are empty
4. the post-fenestrated discs at L2-6 are protruding into the vertebral canal more prominently than before

Comment

The first pattern of disc disease was most prominent at the TL region and those discs were fenestrated. The calcified disc at C2-3 was not treated at that time even though it had the potential for subsequent herniation.

The caudal lumbar discs remain a potential problem in the future. A stenosis at the site of a LS transitional segment was noted on both studies and is always a potential problem. The LS disc was heavily calcified and the transitional segment was associated with 2 fused sacral vertebrae. The height of the vertebral canal at the transitional segment was one-half the height of the canal at the last lumbar type vertebra.

Four Dogs with Suspected Spinal Tumors

Spinal tumors are uncommon and can produce various clinical syndromes, dependent on if they originate in soft tissues or bone. The soft tissue tumors can affect the vertebrae or neural tissue, and can be primary or metastatic. The bone tumors can also be primary or metastatic. Because the incidence of spinal tumors is low, the average clinician has difficulty gaining an appreciation for the "typical" clinical signs or radiographic features of these tumors. This group of dogs includes those with soft tissue tumors as well as bone tumors—two dogs with neural tumors affecting the spine secondarily, one dog with a soft tissue tumor invading a joint, and one dog with a primary bone tumor.

The general pattern of radiographic changes in both primary and secondary vertebral tumors is that of a destructive lesion with cortical destruction and adjacent disc space collapse. Pathologic fractures may be present. Some primary and secondary tumors have productive new bone as the major radiographic pattern, or have a mixed pattern of bony destruction and production. A soft tissue paravertebral mass is frequently associated with intrapelvic tumors which metastasize to the lumbar vertebra.

The portion of the vertebra involved by the tumor varies. The vertebral body is often involved, however, the vertebral arch is involved alone or in conjunction with the body in many cases. The spinous processes and the transverse processes are less commonly involved. Radiographic diagnosis of spinal tumors is difficult.

Soft tissue tumors may occur without changes to the vertebrae and are only detected through the use of a contrast study such as myelography.

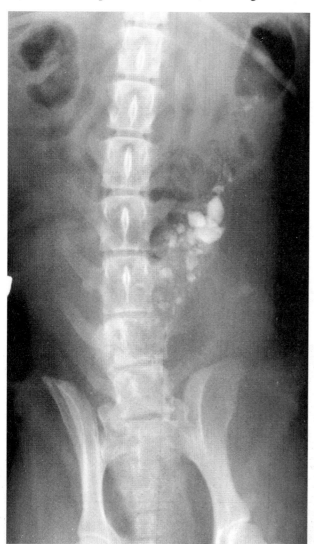

Case Description

"**Max**" is a 9-year-old female shepherd with paraparesis for 2 months with little response to drug treatment. The soft tissue mass over the lumbar region was not appreciated at first because of fat accumulation. Spinal radiographs were made.

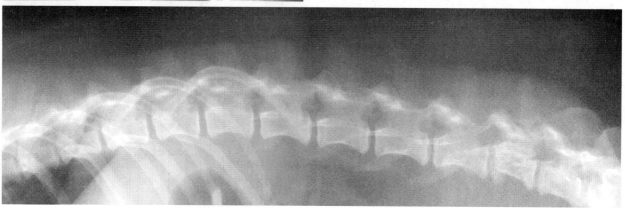

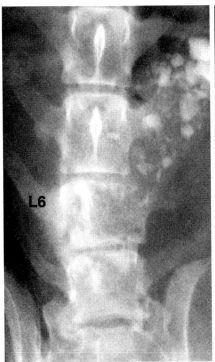

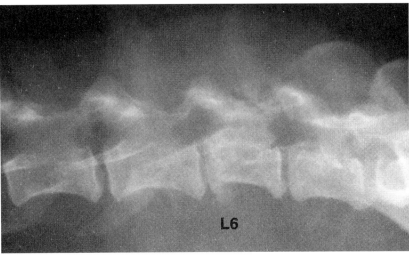

Radiographic Findings

All of the views are made with noncontrast technique and show a pathologic fracture of L6 involving both the body and the arch with compression of the fragments. Destruction of the cranial end plate is a prominent feature. A marked increase in the size of the intervertebral foramina at L5-6 and L6-7 is more difficult to visualize and is thought to be the effect of the expanding lesion. Examination of the VD radiograph shows destruction of the transverse processes on the left side of the affected vertebrae. The scoliosis centering at L5-6 probably represents the collapse of the vertebral fracture being greater on the left (see the detailed views above).

Comments

Destructive vertebral lesions that result in end plate destruction and a compression fracture in an adult patient are usually the result of malignant lesions. This lesion is somewhat unusual because it appears to involve several adjacent vertebrae. A Schwannoma was diagnosed at necropsy.

The debris in the descending colon causes difficulty in evaluation of the vertebral destruction on the VD view.

The 10 mm metastatic nodule superimposed over the trachea is the most easily identified of the metastatic pulmonary nodules.

A differential diagnosis can be often based on the following features:

Soft tissue tumor expanding into bone
1. several adjacent vertebrae are affected
2. any portion of the vertebrae is affected
3. bone destruction is prominent
4. a perivertebral soft tissue mass is identified
   Primary bone tumor
1. a single vertebra is affected
2. the body is most likely affected
3. bone destruction is prominent
4. no perivertebral soft tissue mass is identified
   Tumor metastatic to bone by hematogenous route
1. several adjacent or noncontiguous vertebrae are affected
2. any portion of a vertebra is affected
3. bone destruction is prominent
4. no perivertebral soft tissue mass is identified

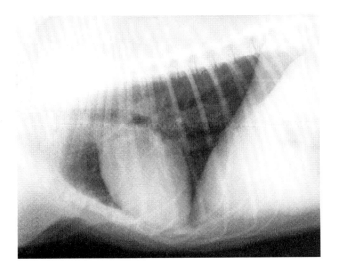

Case Description

"**Reimas**" is a 13-year-old male hound mix who has a hard mass on the left side of the lumbar spine that is not painful on palpation. He is ataxic in the pelvic limbs and does not have proprioceptive placing reactions in those limbs. Abdominal radiographs were made.

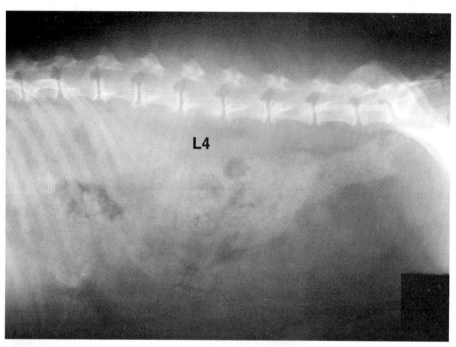

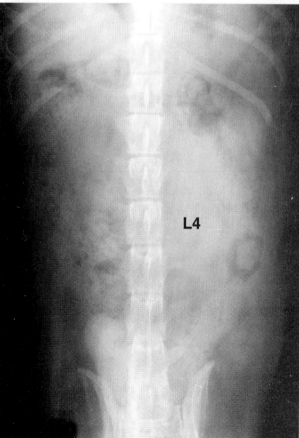

Radiographic Findings

Abdominal radiographs show: (1) destruction of the left transverse processes of L3, L4, and L5, (2) destruction of the spinous process of L3, and (3) possibly decreased bone density in body of L4 and L5. These features are all strongly suggestive of a malignant process. Inflammatory processes usually stimulate a more prominent periosteal new bone formation.

The histopathologic diagnosis was a tumor, probably a neurofibroma, originating in the paravertebral soft tissues with secondary involvement of the spine.

Question #1

What is the meaning of the loss of proprioception in the pelvic limbs?

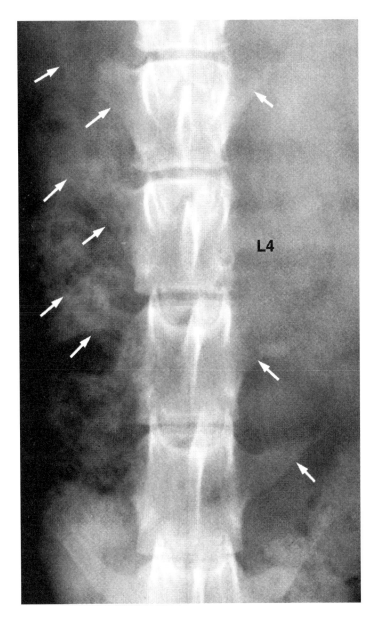

Comment

The enlarged view above makes it easier to appreciate the features of the tumor expansion. Identification of the normal transverse processes of the right (arrows) and the near normal transverse processes on the left (arrows) makes it possible to determine the absence of the process on the left of L4.

The detection of bony destruction is difficult in this patient because of the overlying soft tissue shadows on the VD view caused by bowel contents on the right and because of the difficulty in finding a normal vertebra with which to compare. Probably all of the lumbar vertebrae have areas of destruction.

Note the incidental findings of 8 lumbar-type vertebrae without a transitional segment at the LS junction, and a solitary cystic calculus. A radiographic study of the thorax was radiographically normal.

Answer #1

Proprioception (position sense) is conveyed in the spinal cord by large diameter nerve fibers that are more susceptible to pressure (compression) than smaller diameter fibers; therefore, deficits in proprioception (placing reactions) are often the first sign of spinal cord compression.

Case Description

"**Helen**" is a 5-year-old female retriever who has been lame on the right pelvic limb for 2 months. She has muscle atrophy in the right pelvic limb. Survey radiographic studies were made of the spine and pelvis. The spinal radiographs were normal. The pelvic radiographs are shown.

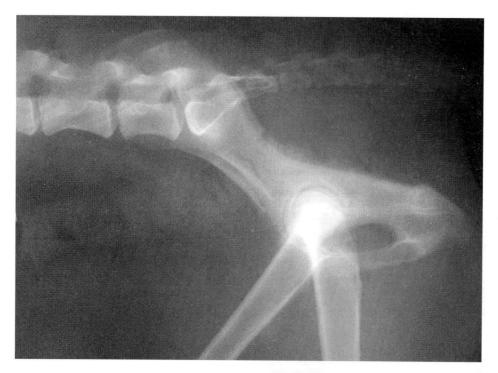

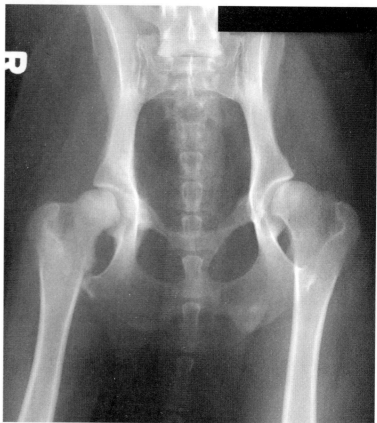

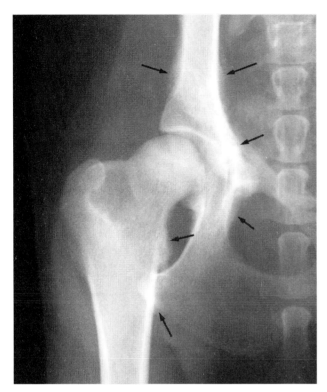 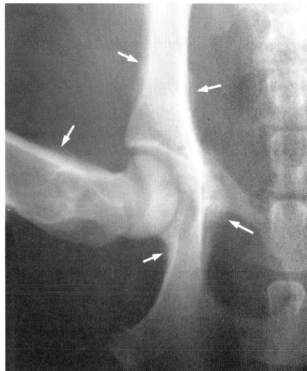

Radiographic Findings

The pelvic radiographs show a productive/destructive lesion adjacent to the right acetabulum with a periosteal response.

The detail views above include the view with the hind limb extended and the view with the hind limb flexed. The trabecular bone cranial to the affected acetabulum is missing and the subchondral bone of the affected hip joint is less dense. Both views permits detection of periosteal new bone on the pelvis (arrows) plus the reactive new bone near the lesser trochanter (arrows).

"Helen" has chronic arthrosis and femoral head subluxation in both hip joints, probably secondary to hip dysplasia and it is necessary to separate the radiographic changes of the arthrosis from those of the bone lesion.

Because of the chronic appearance of the bone lesion, its productive nature, and the involvement of more than one bone, the most likely radiographic diagnosis is a bone infection. Detection of involvement of the joint is not possible. It was assumed that the inflammatory lesion was probably hematogenous or perhaps had spread from an adjacent soft tissue site. Because of the predominately productive nature of the lesion, a fungal etiology was strongly considered. A metastatic bone tumor was considered less likely because of the productive nature of the lesion. Metastatic spread from an adjacent soft tissue tumor was thought possible. A primary bone tumor was not thought likely because of involvement of more than one bone (pelvis and femur).

The pathologic diagnosis was a sarcoma—either an anaplastic lymphoid tumor such as a reticulum cell sarcoma, or a soft tissue spindle cell sarcoma of synovial origin. Involvement of bone on both sides of a joint closely matches the expected picture of a synovial cell sarcoma. These tumors mimic an inflammatory lesion in their early stages before the destructive pattern develops.

Comments

"Helen" has a difficult lesion to diagnosis because the changes of osteoarthrosis secondary to hip dysplasia need to be separated from the features of the tumor. While uncommon, the periosteal new bone on the proximal femur could possibly be related to the joint instability associated to the arthrosis. The absence of trabecular bone within the ilium could be due to disuse of the limb. The soft tissue atrophy only helps to age the lesion but not to distinguish the etiology of the lesion. The spine has no radiographic lesions and the thorax was radiographically normal. A lesion of this type requires evaluation of bone and/or soft tissues to confirm a diagnosis.

Case Description

"**Tara**" is a 6-year-old female shepherd who has a chronic, left pelvic limb lameness and muscle atrophy, which has been tentatively diagnosed as due to arthrosis secondary to hip dysplasia. Radiographs were made of the pelvis.

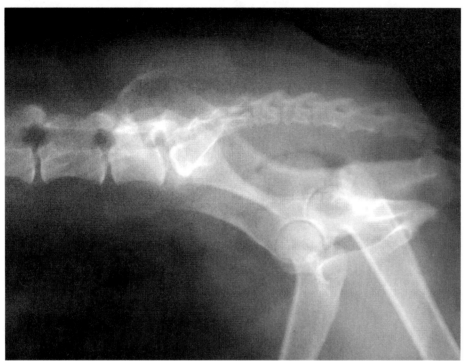

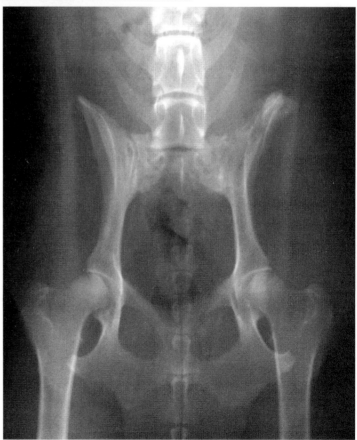

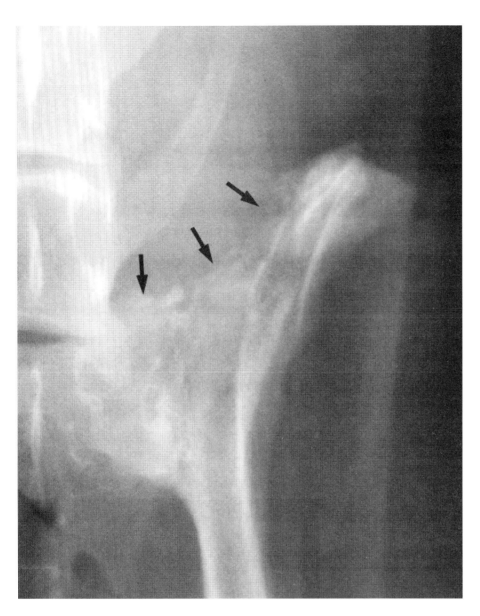

Radiographic Findings

A destructive lesion is present in the left ilium (arrows, see detailed view above). The lesion is seen more clearly on the lateral view because the positioning is slightly oblique. The lesion appears to invade the sacrum as indicated by the change in appearance of the sacroiliac joint.

A malignant bone tumor was the principle diagnosis because of the destructive nature of the lesion. An inflammatory process is less likely because of the absence of a strong periosteal response. The sacroiliac joint is unique in that both neoplastic and inflammatory lesions may cross it following fibro-osseous ankylosis..

The biopsy diagnosis was an osteosarcoma.

Comments

Cases such as "Helen" and "Tara" illustrate that an axial skeletal tumor may produce clinical signs suggestive of either orthopedic or neurologic disease. Lameness may be caused by musculoskeletal disease or by meningeal, nerve root, or peripheral nerve disease.

Muscle atrophy can also be caused by lesions in any of these tissues. A lesion of non-neural tissue would produce disuse atrophy; whereas, a lesion of nerve cell bodies or nerve fibers would produce denervation atrophy. Generalized atrophy of a lame limb suggests disuse atrophy. Atrophy of a single muscle or a group of muscles innervated by one nerve is suggestive of denervation atrophy. Differentiating the two types of atrophy on the basis of clinical signs is often difficult, however. Electromyographic examination or biopsy of the atrophied muscles should yield a definitive characterization of the atrophy.

Spinal Tumors in the Dog

Early diagnosis of tumors affecting the spine of the dog is particularly desirable because immediate treatment is required to avoid a potentially devastating result. Therapy is difficult at best and has the greatest chance of success when applied early. The incidence of tumors affecting the spine of the dog is low when compared with tumors in the appendicular skeleton, but they are often included in the differential diagnosis of certain myelopathies.

Types of Tumors

Tumors affecting the spine of the dog may be classified by cell type and origin. Tumors may affect the vertebra and either be primary bone tumors or metastatic tumors.

A primary malignant bone tumor may arise from any tissue normally present in bone (bone organ), e.g., bone, cartilage, fibroblasts, blood vessels, adipose connective tissue, bone marrow, and nervous tissue. Malignant tumors arising in connective tissue components are variously classified according to the cell of origin, e.g., osteosarcoma, chondrosarcoma, fibrosarcoma, hemangiosarcoma, etc. Tumors more commonly arise in mesenchymal precursors of osseous or cartilaginous tissue and less frequently arise from fibrous connective and vascular tissue of bone. Osteosarcomas and chondrosarcomas are the most frequently identified primary vertebral tumor.

The median age of dogs with primary vertebral tumors is between 6 and 8 years. Males are reported to be more frequently involved than females. Only rarely do the dogs with vertebral tumors fall below the 40-pound critical weight that has been established as a level below which primary bone tumors rarely occur.

Tumors are classified as secondary if they are metastatic, i.e., of a cell type not normally present in the vertebra. Tumors metastatic to the vertebra can include any cell type and reach the spine: (1) through a hematogenous route, (2) by direct spread from an adjacent soft tissue tumor, or (3) via the systemic circulation following earlier localization in the lung. However, in some cases, tumor emboli may pass directly through the pulmonary capillary bed and continue until they reach vascular beds in bone where they lodge and grow with the absence of pulmonary metastases. Generally metastatic tumors affect more than a single vertebrae and often are not contiguous.

Spinal tumors may also be primary in the spinal cord, meninges, and nerve roots or may be metastatic to these organs. In addition, either primary or metastatic tumors may affect any of the tissues contained within the epidural space.

Clinical Signs

A tumor usually produces its effect on the spinal cord or nerve roots by direct pressure on the neural elements and by interference with circulation. However, this varies widely dependent on the location of the tumor, in surrounding bone or within the cord. Eventually, the tumor causes a transverse myelopathy and, therefore, the clinician must include tumors in the differential diagnosis of a transverse myelopathy. As with transverse myelopathies in general, the signs are usually bilateral and may be asymmetric. However, unilateral signs may appear early in the course of the disorder. The rate of progression is usually slow, but occasionally clinical signs appear and progress so rapidly that they resemble severe infectious myelopathies or even traumatic myelopathies.

Often, animals with spinal cord or spinal column tumors show only pain for weeks or even months prior to the development of neurologic deficit. When spinal roots of nerves to the limbs are involved, the animal may have radicular pain that is often demonstrated as a lameness, without neurologic deficit. This fact must be remembered when an orthopedic cause for lameness cannot be discovered. Other early signs such as weight loss, anorexia, and lethargy are also common. Occasionally a palpable mass is noted on careful examination. The clinician should be suspicious of tumor in any mature animal presenting with this clinical picture

Diagnosis

Spinal tumors are diagnosed in the same manner as other causes of transverse myelopathies: (1) localization of the level of the lesion, (2) evaluation of noncontrast radiographs, (3) spinal fluid analysis, and (4) evaluation of the myelogram. Noncontrast radiographs reveal tumors that have caused bony changes. If noncontrast radiographs are not diagnostic, CSF from the appropriate puncture site (cerebellomedullary cistern for cervical lesions and lumbar subarachnoid space for thoracic and lumbar lesions) can be analyzed; it may aid in ruling out meningitis and myelitis and may actually be suggestive of a tumor. The classic "tumor spinal fluid" has a normal or near-normal white cell count with an elevated total protein level; however, tumor cells are rarely seen.

If noncontrast radiography and CSF analysis are not diagnostic and if surgery is indicated, i.e., the animal is not helplessly paralyzed or dangerously debilitated, a myelogram should be performed. This procedure may localize the tumor with respect to the level of the spinal cord involved as well as with respect to dura (extradural, intradural-extramedullary, or intramedullary).

Radiographic changes in primary and secondary tumors to bone

A radiographic feature of both primary and secondary tumors to bone is that of a destructive lesion with cortical destruction, end plate destruction, and adjacent disc space collapse. Pathologic fractures are noted. A smaller group of tumors, both primary and secondary, have productive new bone as the major radiographic pattern, or have a mixed pattern of bony destruction and production.

If a myelogram is performed, all of these bone tumors

have an extradural location. Contrary to the common mass associated with disc degeneration, tumor masses are not related to the disc space, may be multiple, and may be associated with surrounding destructive or productive patterns in the bone.

Intra- or parapelvic tumors that spread to the lumbar, sacral, and pelvic bones cause an aggressive periosteal response. These tumors include bladder and urethral transitional cell carcinomas, prostatic adenocarcinomas, and perianal gland carcinomas. Typically, multiple adjacent vertebrae are involved. Ventral paravertebral soft tissue masses are identified in almost all cases.

Differential diagnoses based on the radiographic findings include bacterial or fungal spondylitis or discospondylitis, which can be primarily hematogenous, secondary to external puncture wound, postsurgical, or associated with a foreign body or grass lawn migration. Bone infection may cause a more productive radiographic pattern than either primary or secondary tumors. Involvement of multiple vertebrae cannot be used to exclude either of these diagnoses.

Radiographic changes in primary and secondary soft tissue tumors

A more meaningful classification of tumors affecting the cord, meninges, and nerve roots is one based on the location of the lesion with respect to the dura mater and the spinal cord. This approach is appropriate because benign or malignant clinical behavior of tumors affecting the nervous system is more often determined by the location and size of the tumor than by its cell type; the location of a tumor also often suggests its cell type. The groups in this classification are extradural tumors, intradural-extramedullary tumors, and intramedullary tumors. Extradural tumors are most common.

Radiographic changes on noncontrast studies
1. Primary bone tumors
   a. radiographic features in bone
      1. destructive: productive: mixed - 2:1:1
      2. broken cortex
      3. may lack aggressive features
      4. single lesion
   b. radiographic features in soft tissues
      1. paravertebral mass
      2. uncommonly mineralization
   c. differential diagnosis
      1. secondary tumor
      2. spondylitis
      3. healing vertebral fracture
2. Secondary bone tumors
   a. radiographic features in bone

1. destructive: productive: mixed - 3:2:1
      2. broken cortex
      3. end plate destruction
      4. may lack aggressive features
      5. collapsed disc space
      6. multiple skip lesions
   b. radiographic features in soft tissues
      1. paravertebral mass
      2. stimulate periosteal response
      3. uncommonly mineralization is present
   c. differential diagnosis
      1. primary tumor
      2. spondylitis
3. Metastatic to vertebrae from pelvic region
   a. radiographic characteristics in bone
      1. paravertebral mass
      2. extracortical new bone
      3. multiple lesions
         a. pelvis
         b. sacrum
         c. lumbar vertebrae
   b. radiographic features in soft tissues
      1. paravertebral mass
      2. uncommonly mineralization is present
      3. increased size of lymph nodes
   c. differential diagnosis
      1. spondylitis
      2. discospondylitis
4. Soft tissue tumor
   a. enlargement of spinal canal
   b. enlargement of intervertebral foramina

Abdominal Studies in the Dog

The pain that the clinician detects on abdominal palpation may originate in the abdomen or may be the result of movement or pressure on the lumbar vertebrae. Fortunately, the lumbar spine is clearly seen on most abdominal studies. These studies may therefore provide useful information even in cases of spinal disease. Examine the abdominal studies of these patients and see if you can identify the spinal lesions. In each case, what do you think is the clinical importance of the spinal lesions you identify? What would you recommend to the owner as the next step in handling each dog?

Case Description

"Barney" is a 15-year-old female beagle who is being evaluated because of hepatomegaly and suspect pulmonary metastases from surgically removed malignant mammary tumors.

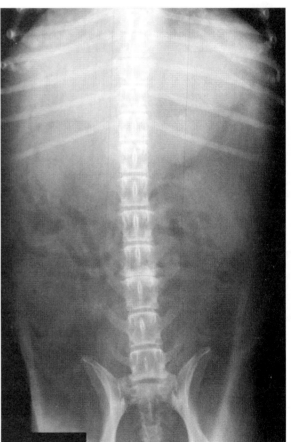

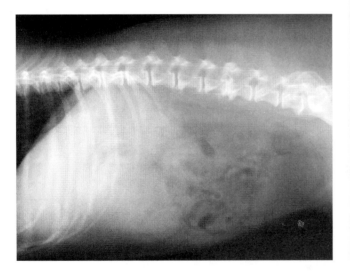

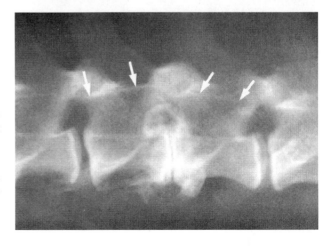

Abdominal Radiographic Findings

The abdominal radiographs (above) permit the detection of hepatomegaly and a chronic, calcified, herniated disc at L4-5 with a collapsed disc space, end plate sclerosis, spondylosis deformans, and vertebral canal enlargement.

The vertebral canal enlargement is more easily seen on the detail view to the right (arrows). Note the ring-like calcification of the herniated discal tissue.

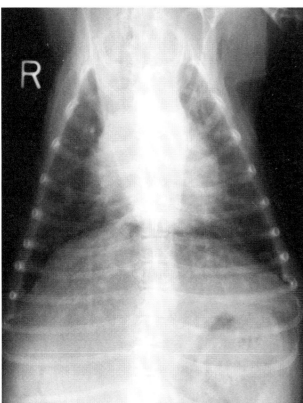

Thoracic Radiographic Findings

"Barney's" thoracic radiographs show multiple pulmonary nodules probably representing pulmonary metastatic disease.

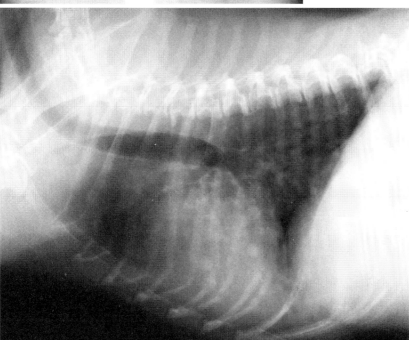

Comments

A slowly enlarging mass, such as a herniating disc, may cause the vertebral canal contents to be displaced dorsally and the roof of the vertebral canal to shift dorsally to accommodate the new mass. It is interesting that a mass of this dimension within the vertebral canal was not showing clinically evident paresis/paralysis probably influenced by the slow increase in size of the mass.

Question #1

What should the clinician recommend for such a disc lesion in "Barney" who is not showing clinical signs related to the spinal lesion?

Case Description

"**Jake**" is a 3-year-old male pointer with a 6-week history of a painful abdomen, stranguria, and dyschezia. Abdominal radiographs were made.

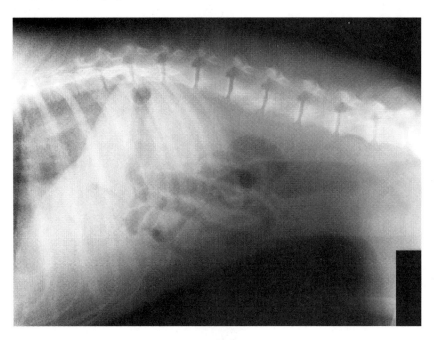

Abdominal Radiographic Findings

The abdominal radiographs show new bone formation on L2-L4 and a ventrally located paravertebral soft tissue mass. These features are more clearly seen on the detail view below and are diagnostic of a spondylitis secondary to migrating grass awn (seed head).

Question #2

What should be done next?

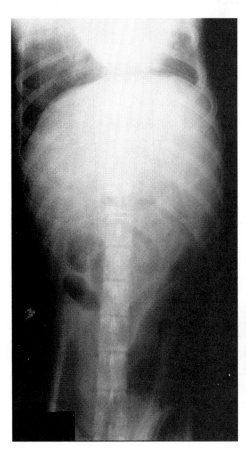

Comment

Radiographs made 6 weeks later showed the new bone formation on L2-L4 to remain essentially unchanged. However, with antibiotic treatment, the clinical signs had resolved.

Spondylitis often causes clinical signs suggesting abdominal pain. Note that it is not possible to determine the stage of activity of the spondylitis from the radiographic changes.

You note the abnormal location of the left hemidiaphragm and ask the owner of possible earlier disease. On questioning, the owner reports a total left lung resection.

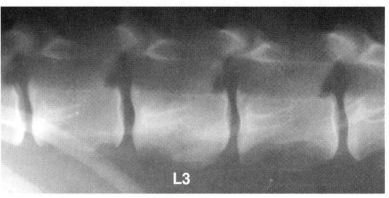

Case Description

"**Dollie**" is a mature female Boxer who has delivered 3 puppies and is being radiographed to determine if additional pups remain. Abdominal radiographs were made.

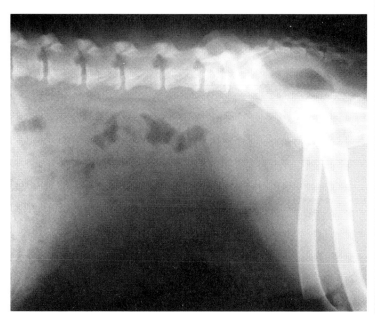
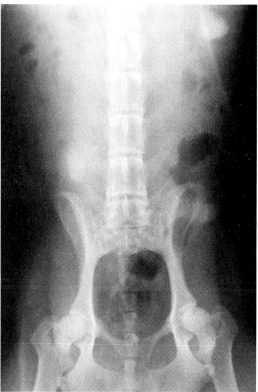

Abdominal Radiographic Findings

The abdominal radiographs fail to show any fetal skeletons; however, the enlarged postpartum uterus is visible. Examination of the lumbar spine shows a shortened body of L7 seen more clearly on the detailed view below with a diminished height (stenosis) of the lumbar vertebral canal (arrows) and marked stenosis of the sacral vertebral canal (arrows).

Subluxation of both femoral heads is noted without radiographic evidence of changes typical of secondary arthrosis. The radiographic diagnosis is a postpartum uterus without evidence of additional fetuses with LS canal stenosis.

Comments

Because of the stenosis, "Dolly's" vertebral canal has less space than normal. Therefore, she is at risk for developing cauda equina compression secondary to an acquired lesion that might be inconsequential to a dog with a canal of normal height. Although she does not appear to have disc disease now, degeneration and herniation of the LS disc is very common in older, large breed dogs. "Dolly" is particularly vulnerable to developing a cauda equina syndrome caused by a protruding LS disc later in her life.

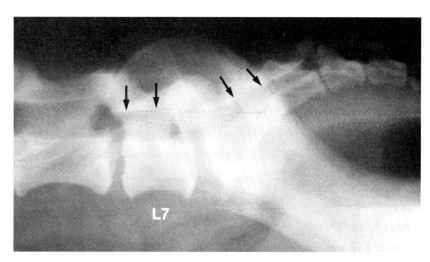

Case Description

"**Wheezer**" is a 5-year-old female shepherd that had an abdominal radiographic study because of a suspected enlarged uterus. The breeding history was uncertain. Abdominal radiographs were made.

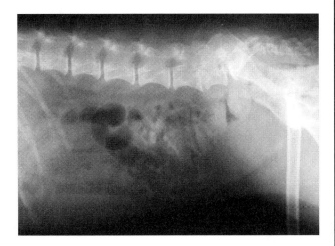

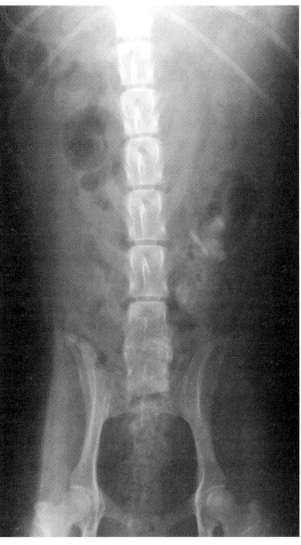

Abdominal Radiographic Findings

The abdominal radiographs show a normal abdomen except for:
1. Splenomegaly
2. A congenital lesion at L6-7 characterized by
   a. a block vertebra
   b. a thin disc space
   c. hypoplastic spinous processes
   d. failure of the vertebral joints to form normally
3. No evidence of
   a. vertebral canal stenosis
   b. instability or malalignment of the vertebrae

In the absence of canal stenosis or associated vertebral instability or malalignment, this form of congenital anomaly is probably without clinical importance.

Comments

Lesions such as this are often thought of as a post-traumatic lesion or a lesion following a discospondylitis or fenestration. The absence of any reactive bone around the affected vertebrae and the smooth nature of the cortical surfaces strongly suggest a congenital anomaly. The hypoplastic spinous processes are certainly a congenital anomaly and suggest that the entire lesion is congenital (see the enlarged view).

Examine the detail view of the LS region. Did you notice the old fracture of the last sacral segment (arrow)? When the owner was quizzed, she admitted that "Wheezer" had been in an automobile accident 3 weeks ago.

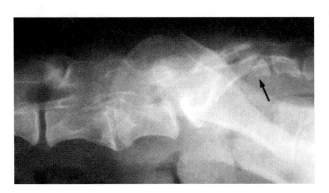

Question #3

What should be done next with regard to the congenital spinal lesion?

Answer #1

Although "Barney" does not have a history of clinical signs related to his disc disease, the enlargement of the vertebral canal suggests the presence of an expanding mass within the canal. An argument could be made to do a CSF analysis and a myelogram. Unfortunately, "Barney" also has a serious problem with the pulmonary metastases.

Answer #2

Microbial culture and antibiotic sensitivity tests should be done on "Jake's" urine and blood. If any draining tracts develop, the exudate should also be cultured. If these tests do not identify a causative microorganism, the choice of antibiotics should be based upon the organisms most likely to be associated with this problem in your geographical area.

Answer #3

Because "Wheezer" does not have any clinical signs indicating a neurologic problem at L6-7, nothing further needs to be done with regard to the congenital anomaly at this time. She may be at increased risk for degeneration of the discs adjacent to the block because the malformation alters the normal distribution of stress and movement among these discs.

Dynamic Radiography

Dynamic radiography of the vertebral column is the careful use of flexion and extension views in both noncontrast radiography as well as in myelography to gain information about a suspect area of vertebral instability and is used in the following situations: (1) suspect occipito-atlanto-axial instability (OAA congenital anomaly); (2) malalignment of the caudal cervical spine (C4-7) with dorsoventral or lateral change in the dorsal vertebral arch which results in narrowing of wedging of the vertebral canal (cervical spondylopathy); or (3) L-S instability (cauda equina syndrome associated with instability).

Vertebral Canal Stenosis in the Dog

Vertebral canal stenosis is a narrowing of the vertebral canal or nerve root canals that may be local, segmental, or generalized. The stenosis can be primary, being associated with a congenital or developmental lesion that creates a canal of less than normal dimensions. The lesion may be associated with spinal dysraphism, congenital vertebral block, or hemivertebra. Secondary or acquired canal stenosis implies that the vertebral canal developed normally and the narrowing is secondary to a soft tissue or bony mass. This type of canal stenosis results most frequently from degenerative changes resulting in protrusion of discal tissue into the canal or from degenerative or traumatic changes that result in malalignment of the vertebrae resulting in a stenotic site. The stenosis may be focal or more extensive.

The concept of absolute versus relative stenosis is important. Absolute stenosis indicates a midsagittal vertebral diameter that is small enough to result in direct neural compression. Relative stenosis is not a pathological condition but represents a variation within the normal range of measurements of vertebral canals and thus implies a diameter that is less than normal but asymptomatic. Relative stenosis carries a risk of becoming symptomatic following the development of space-occupying lesions of the vertebral canal, such as disc protrusion, that would otherwise be clinically unimportant. Most dogs develop clinical signs associated with a relative stenosis in adult life.

Congenital stenoses may have normal vertebral height but with pedicles that tend to be short and laminae that are massive, or they may have a trefoil-shaped canal instead of the more normal oval shape. On noncontrast radiography or myelography only estimates of the midsaggital and interpedicular diameters can be made. With the advent of computerized tomography, much more accurate measurements can be made and a canal that has normal midsaggital and interpedicular diameters may be found to have a trefoil shape and diminished cross-sectional area.

Pathophysiology

The pathophysiology of clinical symptoms resulting from canal stenosis is complex and poorly understood. Pressure on the arteries, capillaries, and veins, as well as compression of the nerve roots occurs. The arterial obstruction, venous hypertension, and pressure or traction on the sinuvertebral nerves (of Luschka) and the primary rami are all believed to be important in causing symptoms of spinal stenosis.

Classification

1. Primary canal stenosis caused by the bony arch
    a. congenital stenosis caused by
        1. hypertrophic articular processes
        2. a congenital vertebral block
        3. a congenital hemivertebra (wedge)
            a. with normal articular processes
            b. with hypotrophic articular processes
        4. a butterfly vertebrae
        5. transitional vertebral vertebrae
            a. with normal articular processes
            b. with hypertrophic articular processes
        6. a primary kyphosis, lordosis, or scoliosis
        7. vertebral malalignment
            a. at the OAA region
            b. with cervical spondylopathy
            c. at the LS junction
        8. vertebral instability
            a. with congenital absence of dens
            b. with cervical spondylopathy
        9. idiopathic stenosis at T4-5 in the Doberman Pinscher
        10. intervertebral foraminal stenosis
    b. developmental canal stenosis caused by inborn errors of skeletal growth
        1. achondroplasia
        2. hereditary multiple exostosis (multiple osteochondromatosis)
        3. Disseminated Idiopathic Skeletal Hyperostosis (DISH)
        4. mucopolysaccharidosis (VII)
        5. malalignment caused by cervical osteochondrosis
        6. overnutrition
        7. osteochondrosis of
            a. cervical articular processes
            b. sacrum
        8. multiple epiphyseal dysplasia
        9. prenatal and perinatal malnutrition
    c. idiopathic canal stenosis
        1. with conjoining cord lesion (benign tumors)
        2. without conjoining cord lesion
            a. thoracic vertebral stenosis in the Doberman Pinscher
2. Primary canal stenosis caused by nonosseous components
    a. periarticular cysts
    b. soft tissue developmental tumor (teratoma)
3. Secondary canal stenosis caused by
    a. degenerated disc
    b. abscess
    c. tumor mass
    d. malalignment
        1. post-traumatic
        2. postsurgical
        3. post-inflammatory

"Mollie's" Problems

The more explosive is the protrusion of the disc nucleus, the more severe is the injury to the cord. Examine "Mollie's" radiographs and determine the nature of the cord injury. Both noncontrast radiographs (NCR) and views from the myelogram (Myel) are included.

Case Description

"Mollie" is a 6-year-old dachshund with paraplegia for 5 days. Both a noncontrast radiographic study and a myelogram are shown.

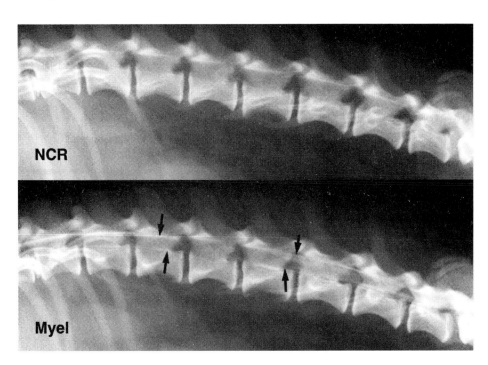

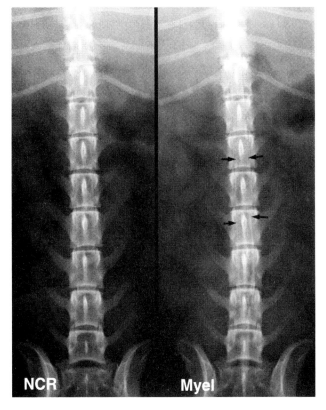

Radiographic Findings

The noncontrast radiographs show a narrowing of the disc space at L3-4 and calcified tissue within the vertebral canal dorsal to that disc space. Multiple calcified discs are seen from T11 to T13.

Myelographic Findings

The myelogram shows a ventral and left-sided extradural mass with spinal cord swelling that has compressed the subarachnoid space (arrows). This pattern is typical for an acute, Type 1 disc disease.

Comment

A typical, acute, Type 1 disc protrusion in a chondrodystrophic breed causes cord swelling that compresses the adjacent subarachnoid space. The compressed space does not fill completely with contrast agent; consequently, the extradural nuclear tissue may not be well outlined and may be difficult to identify.

Hindquarter/Pelvic Limb Pain

In dogs, hindquarter pain or pelvic limb pain resulting in reluctance to move and lameness (limping, decreased weight-bearing on the limbs) is most commonly due to musculoskeletal disease. This is particularly true if neurologic deficits are absent. On the other hand, neurologic disease can cause regional pain and lameness, and do so without causing neurologic deficits. Of the neurologic diseases, disc disease is most commonly blamed in this situation. However, many other neurologic diseases and diseases involving the vertebral column can cause pain and lameness, and many of these diseases require more aggressive, specific therapy than the rest and confinement often recommended for dogs with early disc disease. None of the dogs in this group had disc disease.

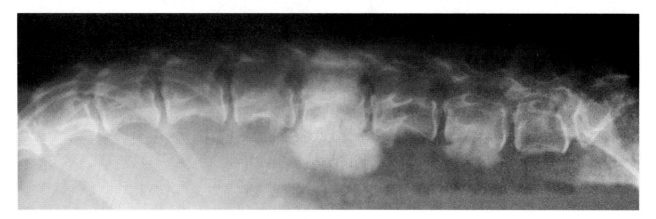

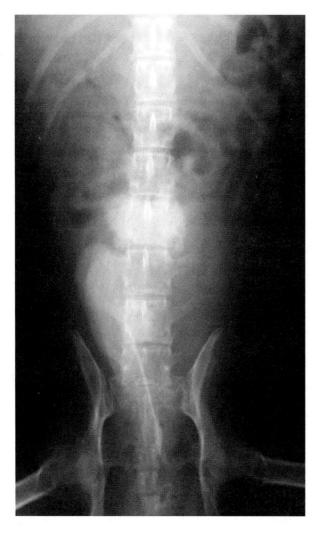

Case Description

"Lopey" is a 13-year-old male Dachshund with reluctance to move, pain in the caudal lumbar area, and paraparesis progressing to paraplegia over the past 3 to 4 weeks. He also had weight loss over the past 2 months. On examination, he had lower motor neuron signs in the hindquarters, specifically hypotonia of the pelvic limbs and an atonic/areflexic anal sphincter.

Radiographic Findings

Noncontrast radiographs show a productive lesion that is aggressive in appearance affecting the vertebrae L2 to L7. The width of disc spaces is preserved and the end plates are normal in density and thickness. The spine has minimal osteoporosis, probably age dependent, and it is difficult to know if any of the loss of density represents a destructive component of the disease.

Because of the productive nature of the lesions and the irregular involvement of the lumbar vertebrae, the diagnosis is metastatic tumor, probably associated with an intrapelvic primary tumor. Differential diagnosis could include a form of chronic spondylitis that is hematogenous and probably fungal.

Necropsy identified the lesion as a metastatic transitional cell carcinoma of the urinary bladder. The deep iliac, lumbar, cranial mediastinal and bronchial lymph nodes were all enlarged and contained tumor cells. "Lopey's" neurologic signs appeared to be due to involvement of peripheral nerves by the tumor.

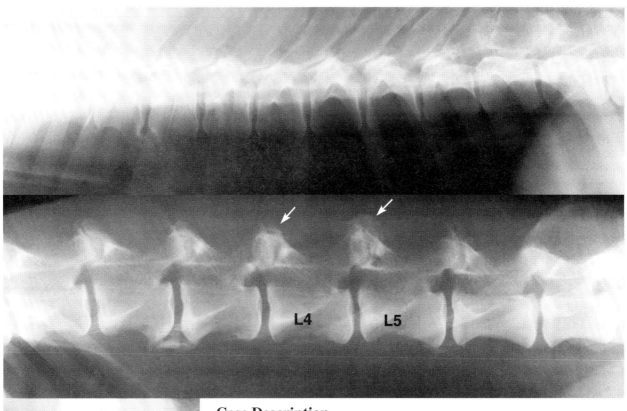

Case Description

"**Faron**" is an 8-year-old male Great Dane who was brought to the clinic for the problems of reluctance to rise, apparent hindquarter pain, paraparesis and fecal incontinence of 9-months duration. The dysfunction had been gradually progressive. Proprioceptive placing was decreased in the pelvic limbs, but spinal reflexes were normal. The lesion was localized to T3-L3.

Radiographic Findings

The noncontrast radiographs show periarticular changes around the vertebral joints throughout the spine (arrows). The changes are especially prominent at L4-5 on the lateral view. Determination of the importance of these lesions is difficult. Myelography or magnetic resonance imaging would be necessary to examine the vertebral canal and the spinal cord.

A diagnosis is equivocal. Arthrosis of the true vertebral joints is thought to be painful, but need not cause neurological signs. Necropsy failed to identify a lesion in the nervous system. Minimal dural ossification was noted, but this is usually an incidental finding without clinical importance. Degenerative myelopathy or some other intrinsic myelopathy may have been present and would not be detected on necropsy unless the spinal cord is carefully examined histologically.

Case Description

"**Briar**" is a 2-year-old male Doberman Pinscher who had a survey lateral spinal radiographic series made because of mild pain in the hindquarters. A ventrodorsal view was added because of a suspect thoracolumbar lesion.

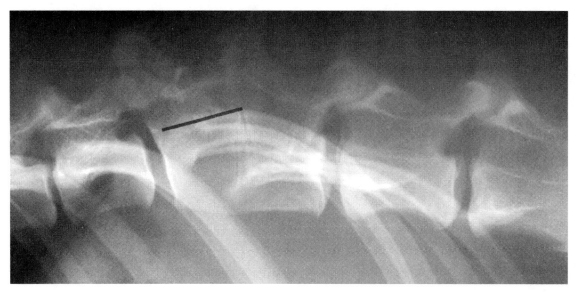

Radiographic Findings

The noncontrast radiographs show the vertebral bodies of T12 and T13 are shorter than normal and malaligned, resulting in sharp kyphosis. The T12-13 disc space is incompletely formed, the vertebral arches are incompletely formed and have failed to separate, the vertebral joints are poorly developed, and costovertebral joints of the 13th ribs are malformed.

The diagnosis is a congenital block vertebra affecting both the vertebral bodies and the vertebral arches, with an associated vertebral canal stenosis (line marks the floor of the canal).

The vertebral malalignment suggests post-traumatic lesion. The young age of the patient and absence of any clinical history of trauma is supportive of the lesion being congenital.

A myelogram is necessary to assess the degree of vertebral canal stenosis and determine if the lesion is compressing the spinal cord. The owners declined further diagnostic tests or treatment.

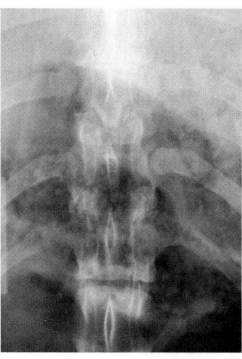

Comment

No reactive bone is noted except the smooth plate of new bone ventrally, suggesting repair of vertebral instability.

"Briar" had 6 lumbar-type vertebrae and a transitional LS vertebra. Identification of one congenital lesion always makes it tempting to interpret all suspect lesions as congenital, especially since congenital lesions are common in the dog.

The VD view is difficult to interpret because of gastric contents.

Case Description

"**Beast**" is a 2-year-old male Great Dane who has a history of neck pain that progressed to include pelvic limb pain. The hip joints are painful on flexion. He was thought to be neurologically normal.

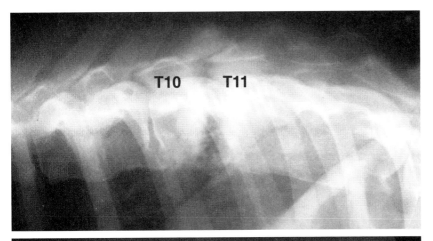

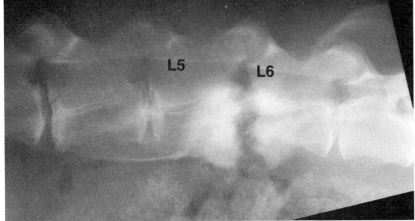

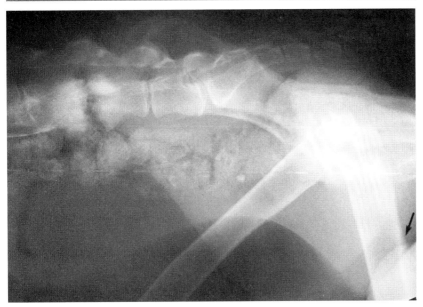

Radiographic Findings

The noncontrast vertebral radiographs show disc space widening with end plate destruction at T10-11 and L5-6. New bone has fused the true vertebral joints at T11-12 and T12-13 and the vertebral bodies of T8-T10, T11-T13, and L4-5. Thus, both acute/chronic destructive/productive patterns seem to be present.

The diagnosis is hematogenous discospondylitis and infectious joint disease in the vertebral joints. The bony fusion is thought to be secondary to chronic infection.

Staphylococcus aureus was cultured from an aspirate of a lumbar disc space. Because of the destructive changes at the disc spaces, histologic examination of biopsy cores from those sites was noninformative.

Comments

Neither primary nor metastatic tumors in the spine center on disc spaces or result in eventual fusion of the vertebrae. The presence of separated lesions, so-called "skip" lesions, is strongly supportive of the diagnosis of hematogenous discospondylitis.

Did you spot the periosteal new bone on the caudal aspect of the left femur as seen on the lateral view of the pelvis (black arrow)? This lesion probably represents an additional hematogenous inflammatory lesion.

"Beast" has perivertebral new bone typical of that found in patients with DISH.

Case Description

"**Dutchess**" is a 9-year-old female shepherd with pelvic limb lameness for 3 weeks. Neurologically, she appeared normal.

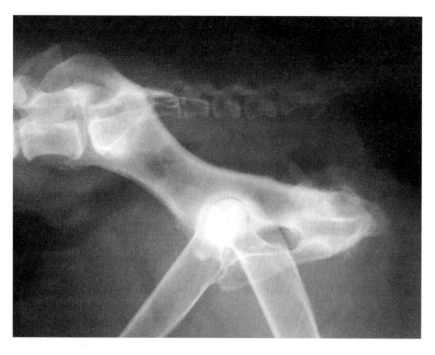

Radiographic Findings

The noncontrast radiographs of the pelvis show a large productive lesion in the right ischium with a reactive border that generates a rather long zone of transition. The lesion appears to originate from the bone and might be caused by hematogenous osteomyelitis or a primary or metastatic bone tumor. The aggressive nature of the margin, underlying cortical destruction, and the long zone of transition suggest a primary bone tumor. The soft tissue atrophy in the right hind limb supports the clinical history of lameness.

The lesion is seen more clearly on the enlarged view (below) made with the hindlimbs in a flexed position.

The diagnosis on biopsy was a primary anaplastic sarcoma of bone. Thoracic radiographs were radiographically normal.

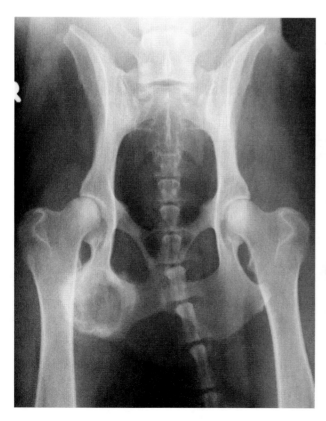

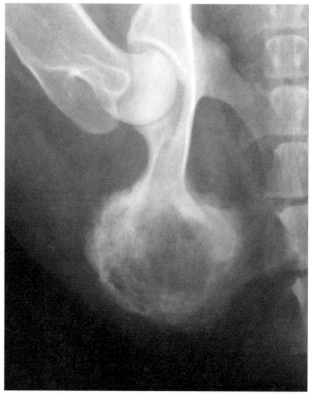

Question #1

What soft tissues in the vertebral canal have pain receptors, and if diseased, could be the source of pain?

Question #2

A disease of which of these would classically NOT cause neurologic signs?

Question #3

Can you name a peripheral nerve lesion that typically causes lameness without neurologic deficits? (Neurologic deficits may appear late in the course of this disorder).

Answer #1
Nerve roots, meninges.

Answer #2
Meninges.

Answer #3
Peripheral nerve sheath tumor.

Rules for Good Radiography of the Spine

The following rules help to assure quality radiographs of good diagnostic quality which may permit the obtaining of a diagnosis without having to resort to myelography.

1. Make the following views in the survey spinal study.
   a. in large dogs, lateral views of the cervical, thoracic, and lumbar spine.
   b. in small dogs and cats, a single lateral view of the spine
2. Make the following views in a spinal study with the patient anesthetized or heavily sedated.
   a. in large dogs, a separate ventrodorsal and lateral radiograph of the cervical, cervicothoracic, thoracic, thoracolumbar, and lumbar regions
   b. in small dogs and cats, a separate ventrodorsal and lateral radiograph of the cervical, thoracic, and lumbar regions
   c. oblique view of the cervical spine to visualize the odontoid process
   d. oblique views of the cervical spine if any suspect lesions are detected
3. If in doubt concerning a radiographic change, make a coned-down view that is centered over the suspected region.
4. In obese patients, a compression band can be used to improve radiographic quality.
5. Radiolucent sponges can be used to alter the position of the patient so that the vertebral column is parallel to the table top.
6. Avoid rotation of the patient by placing wedges under the sternum and abdomen.
7. The neck can be stretched by gentle traction to permit identification of an area of vertebral instability.
8. Stress views are helpful in the demonstration of instability in the cervical and LS regions.
9. Use a relatively high range of kVp settings.
10. Use of a grid is helpful if the thickness of the patient is over 14 cm.
11. A compression spoon can be used to shift the position of soft tissue organs overlying an area of interest.

Changes in Width of Disc Space

The width of the disc space can be judged from both lateral and ventrodorsal radiographs with the accuracy of the evaluation dependent on patient positioning and x-ray beam direction. Diseases that result in a narrowing or collapse of the disc space include: (1) congenital vertebral anomaly such as block vertebrae, (2) acute nuclear prolapse or herniation, (3) chronic degenerative disc disease, (4) traumatic fracture-luxation, (5) discitis, or (6) following surgical fenestration. Often the narrowing of the disc is not uniform but is in the form of a wedge suggesting that the dorsal support for the disc in the form of the interarcuate ligament or ligamentum flavum and vertebral joints are still intact, while the disc has lost its ventral support. Thus, the collapse is ventral with maintenance of width dorsally. This might occur with acute disc herniation or following trauma or surgical fenestration and result in a minimal kyphosis. A wedge-shaped disc with collapse dorsally is uncommon and probably post-traumatic.

Recognition of the disc as a type of joint makes it easier to understand the changes that take place in both the disc space and the adjacent vertebral end plates. Thus, the appearance of the end plates tells much about the condition of the associated intervertebral disc. A series of patterns can be noted with the passage of time in the end plates adjacent to a slowly degenerative disc. First, the end plates increase in thickness and density. Eventually they come into contact at which time they become polished and eburnated. A destructive pattern associated with the final stage of disc disease results in almost complete disappearance of the end plate and a type of fibrotic ankylosis. The sclerotic appearance of the end plates is not present with an acute disc rupture, traumatic herniation, or fracture-luxation.

Another pattern identified in the end plates associated with chronic disc disease is the formation of vertebral osteophytes that form around the periphery of the end plate and are often referred to as spondylosis deformans or vertebral osteophytes.

A pattern indicative of a more acute destructive change in the end plate is associated with disc space collapse secondary to inflammatory disease and is referred to as a spondylitis that may be primary or may occur secondary to a primary discitis.

The contents of the disc also reflect the nature of the ongoing disease. Calcification within the disc informs the clinician of the status of disc degeneration.

A final change to the disc space occurs at the time of bony fusion following fracture-luxation, fenestration, or discitis. The nature of the injury determines the amount of reactive new bone surrounding the disc space. The more stable the vertebrae, the less the reactive bone required in the healing process. Segmental fusion can be confused radiographically with block vertebra in which a disc space failed to form. Often the degree of modeling present assists in this determination. The less modeling, the more likely the lesion is congenital, the more modeling, the more likely the fusion is secondary.

Causes

1. Absent disc space
   a. primary
      1. congenital block vertebrae
      2. hemivertebra
      3. transitional vertebra
   b. secondary
      1. healed fracture
      2. healed discitis
      3. collapsed pathologic fracture
2. Narrow disc space
   a. primary
      1. congenital block vertebrae
      2. hemivertebra
      3. "butterfly" vertebrae
   b. secondary
      1. degenerating disc
      2. fracture-luxation
      3. adjacent primary vertebral tumor
      4. discitis
3. Collapsed disc space
   a. primary
      1. congenital block vertebrae
      2. hemivertebra
      3. "butterfly" vertebrae
   b. secondary
      1. compression fracture
      2. spondylitis/discitis
      3. post-fenestration
      4. degenerating disc
      5. pathologic fracture
4. Disc space fusion
   a. block vertebrae
   b. healed fracture
   c. healed spondylitis/discitis
   d. healed post-fenestration
   e. aging change cervical spine or TL junction
5. Unique conditions
   a. OAA congenital anomalies
   b. LS degenerative lesions
   c. rigid spine associated with DISH
   d. transitional vertebral vertebrae

Why Myelography?

Often the features on the noncontrast radiographic study of the spine do not allow an unequivocal diagnosis. In that situation, it is appropriate to use another diagnostic technique to confirm the suspect diagnosis. If CSF analysis does not provide a diagnosis, myelography is the most often used technique in spinal studies. An exception occurs in patients with a suspect lumbosacral lesion where discography or epidurography may be the special study of choice. The following cases required use of myelography to establish the diagnosis.

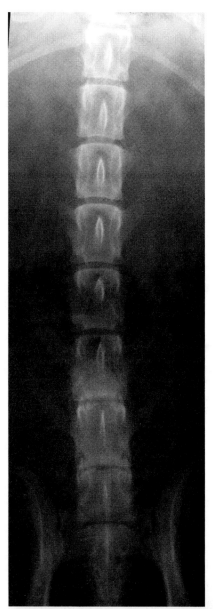

Case Description

"Ollie" is a 3-year-old male cocker spaniel with increased patellar reflexes and decreased proprioceptive placing bilaterally in the pelvic limbs.

Radiographic Findings

The noncontrast studies on this page have a "cloudy" shadow just dorsal to the L3-4 disc space with a minimal amount of calcified tissue remaining within the disc. The disc space is thought to be of normal width and the end plates are not sclerotic. Scoliosis with concavity to the left is probably related to muscle spasm. This is not a breed that frequently has degenerative disc disease and it was thought that a myelogram might be helpful in diagnosis. The suspected location of the lesion just cranial to the lumbar enlargement would be expected to produce upper motor neuron signs in the pelvic limbs. It was thought better to make the injection for the myelogram at L5-6.

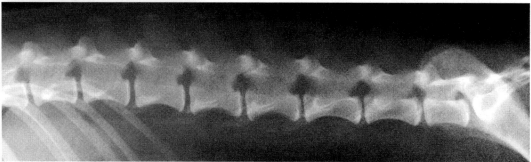

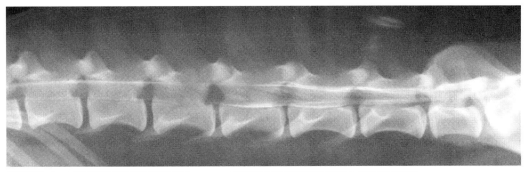

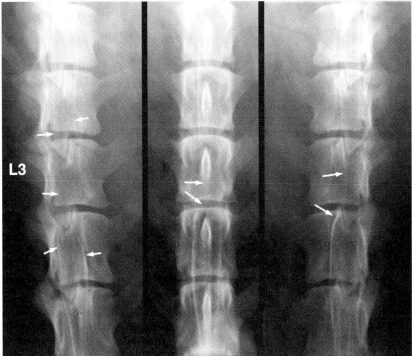

Myelographic Findings (enlarged views)

The myelographic studies show a large right-sided extradural mass over L3-4. Note on the lateral view that the cord appears swollen and the subarachnoid columns are narrowed. However, on the ventrodorsal and oblique views the mass is extradural, large, right-sided, and ventral (arrows). The diagnosis is a Type 1 nuclear protrusion resulting in a right sided extradural mass. The trauma of the protrusion caused cord edema/ hemorrhage.

Comments

With an obstructive lesion, the contrast medium injected in the lumbar area tends to remain in that area because of the compressed subarachnoid spaces. Note also the contrast agent leaking out of the subarachnoid space into the needle tract because of increased pressure within the subarachnoid space.

The myelogram confirms the noncontrast radiographic findings, but in addition demonstrates the exact size and location of the extradural mass. Because of the degree of cord swelling (edema/hemorrhage), the myelogram also suggests that the protrusion is acute and/or developing quickly. The findings on the noncontrast and myelographic studies and the age of the patient are all supportive of the diagnosis of a herniated disc, placing that diagnosis first on the list of differential diagnosis. However, an extradural tumor or abscess could also cause these myelographic features. Whatever the cause of the extradural mass, a surgical exploration is recommended to decompress the spinal cord and accurately identify the mass. "Ollie's" surgery confirmed that the extradural mass was a herniated disc.

The manner in which the caudally projecting articular facets fit between the cranially projecting articular facets create what has incorrectly been described as a "joint space". This is in fact, the lateral portion of the interarcuate space. Note on the lateral views, the narrowing in width of this "space" cranial to L4-5 and the larger, more normal appearing spaces at L4-5 and caudally. The variation in the manner in which these facets articulate may be the result of perivertebral muscle spasm that is secondary to radicular or meningeal irritation or inflammation. The narrowing of the crescent shaped lucency is a prominent radiographic feature often described with acute disc protrusion. Actually, the width of the crescent may be influenced by many spinal lesions.

Case Description

"**Willimina**" is a 4-year-old female Labrador retriever with a 3-month history of progressive quadriparesis/ataxia, and loss of proprioceptive placing in all four limbs.

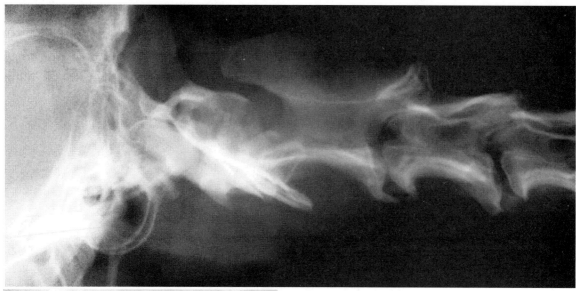

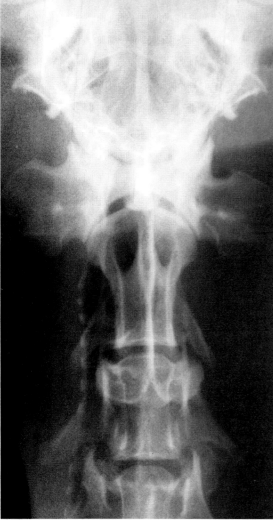

Radiographic Findings

The noncontrast radiographs seen on this page are equivocal, at best. Some thought there was a destructive lesion in the arch of C1. Others even thought there were well marginated, calcific densities associated with this destructive lesion. Everyone agreed that spondylosis deformans was evident in the cervical region. The other point on which every one agreed was that a myelogram would be helpful.

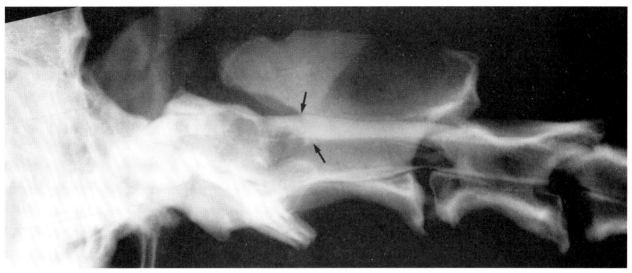

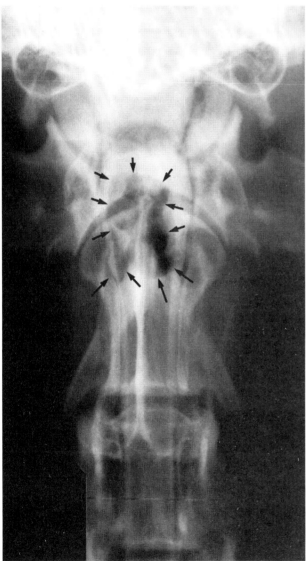

Myelographic Findings

A myelogram using a cerebellomedullary cistern injection clearly shows a filling defect in the dorsal subarachnoid space at C1 The lesion appears as an intramedullary type of lesion, but also suggests a "tee" sign that is diagnostic of an intradural-extramedullary mass (arrows). The ventral contrast column is displaced ventrally suggesting that the lesion may occupy a portion of the cord. The contour of the mass is lobulated and forms a margin with the contrast pool (arrows).

The size and lobular shape of the lesion and the possibility of it containing calcified nodules suggests the diagnosis of a chondrosarcoma. The lesion seems to involve both the cord and meninges. It appears to originate in the meninges and then expands causing resorptive changes in the bony arch of C1.

"Willimina's" mass was identified histopathologically as a chondrosarcoma and was thought to be a primary bone tumor.

Question #1

Can you name two other tumors that occur more commonly than chondrosarcomas as intradural-extramedullary masses?

Case Description

"Keena" is a 7-year-old female dachshund with progressive paraparesis over the last 10 days. She has been paraplegic for the past 2 days. She has deep pain perception in the hindquarters, however the cutaneus trunci reflex is absent caudal to L1. Examine the noncontrast studies and decide if you would make a positive diagnosis.

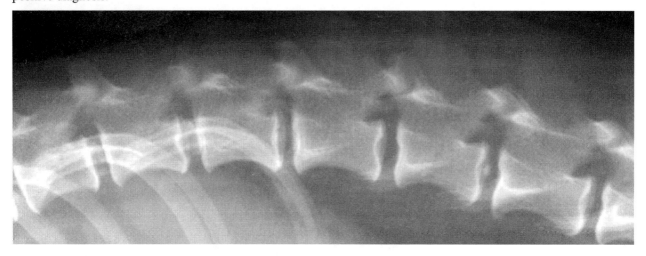

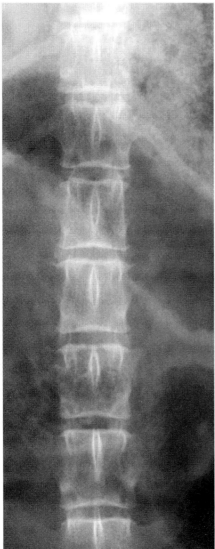

Radiographic Findings

In "Keena", the noncontrast radiographs, seen on this page, show a suspect calcified mass within the vertebral canal that is overshadowed by the pedicles of L1. A shell of calcified nucleus is present within the L1-2 disc space. The adjacent cranially positioned discs are heavily calcified. None of the disc spaces are narrowed and no evidence of secondary changes such as spondylosis deformans or end plate sclerosis is identified.

Question #2

What is the importance of the presence or absence of deep pain perception in assessing the severity of a myelopathy?

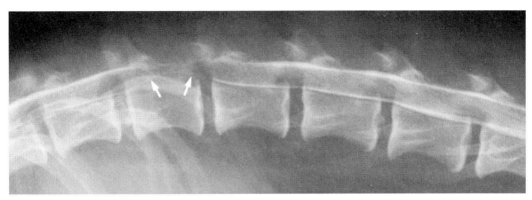

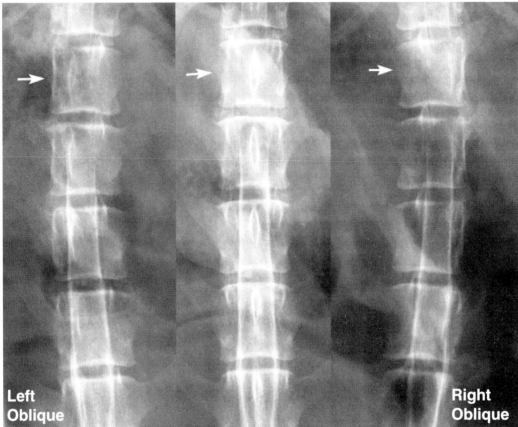

Left
Oblique

Right
Oblique

Myelographic Findings

The myelogram confirms an extradural mass at L1 with marked cord elevation, cord compression, and compression of the subarachnoid spaces (arrows). Oblique views can be compared with the VD view and are often of assistance in making a determination of the laterality of an extradural mass. In "Keena", the mass appears on the midline. Note that if the cord is compressed by the extradural mass as seen on the lateral view, it may appear widened on the ventrodorsal view.

The diagnosis is a Type 1 disc protrusion at L1-2 that was confirmed surgically.

Comments

Additional information can usually be gained from the myelogram. The accumulation of contrast agent in the lumbar subarachnoid space is greater than expected and results from the tendency of the fluid to pool caudally at the time of injection.

An important myelographic feature is the limited degree of cord swelling, which suggests a slowly developing mass. This is typical of disc protrusion in an older dog in which the nucleus has become partially desiccated. The slow extrusion of the nucleus explains the rather minimal neurological deficits when compared with the massive size of the extradural mass.

Case Description

"Lexa" is an 8-year-old female shepherd with a caudal ataxia for the past 2 weeks. She has proprioceptive deficits; however, her spinal reflexes are normal.

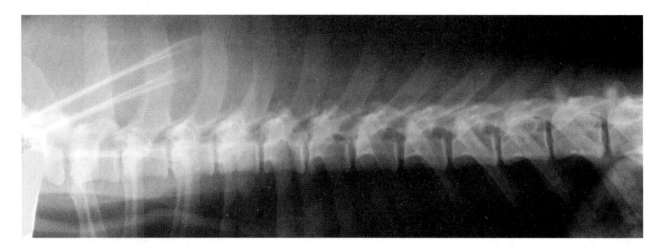

Radiographic Findings

Examination of her noncontrast radiographs seen above fails to indicate any abnormality.

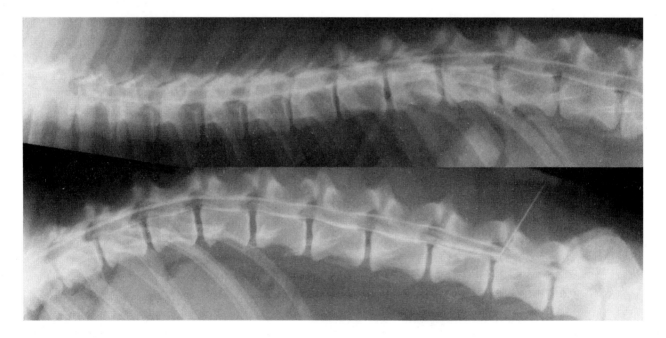

Myelographic Findings

The myelogram is not completely satisfactory because contrast agent leaks into the epidural space. However, the contrast columns flow cranial to the level of T4-5 where elevation and narrowing of the spinal cord is identified just over the disc space (arrows on detail view on next page). The dorsal contrast column is collapsed. The findings are interpreted as indicating an extradural mass at T4-5.

"Lexa's" owner refused surgery and she was treated conservatively and lost to follow-up.

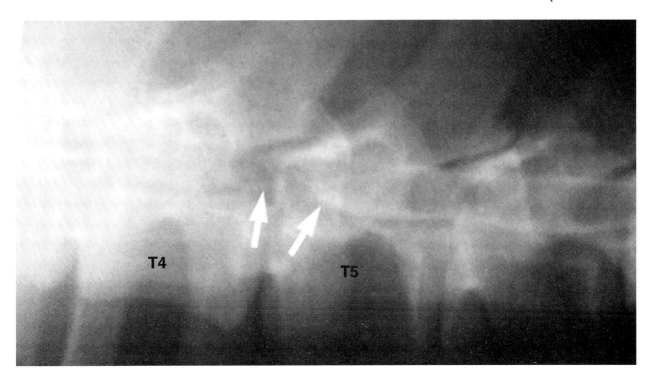

Comment

The extradural mass is assumed to be a protruding disc. The location is unusual and the case is an excellent example of the requirement of examining the entire spine. The cranial thoracic spinal cord is particularly difficult to evaluate on the myelogram because of the increase in tissue thickness associated with the shoulders. If a defect in the contrast columns is suspected, the making of additional radiographs that are centered over the areas of suspicion are often helpful in confirming what was only a suspect diagnosis.

Question #3

List 10 different causes of the extradural mass pattern on a myelogram

Answer #1

Schwannoma and meningioma

Answer #2

Determining the presence of nociception (pain perception) is important is assessing the severity of a myelopathy (particularly compressive myelopathies) because this function is one of the last functions to be lost as the severity of a myelopathy increases. Proprioception is generally affected first, then voluntary movement, then pain perception. With increasing severity of the myelopathy, the perception of superficial painful stimuli (pinch applied to the skin) is generally lost before the perception of painful stimuli applied to deep structures (e.g., bone). Therefore, the loss of deep pain perception (which is usually accompanied by complete loss of proprioception and paralysis) indicates a very severe myelopathy. Recovery is not hopeless, but appropriate therapy must be instituted immediately.

Answer #3

1. Herniated disc
2. Tumor
3. Foreign body (e.g. bullet)
4. Abscess
5. Granuloma
6. Hemorrhage/hematoma
7. Bone fragment associated with a fracture
8. Synovial cyst
9. Hyperplastic tissue (ligaments, joint capsule, bone)
10. Vertebral malformation (vertebral stenosis, hemivertebra)

Two Patients with Thoracic Limb Abnormalities

In some patients, we have provided a more detailed commentary concerning the clinical signs, especially those noted on the neurological examination. "Chabot" and "Ladd" are two interesting cases with similar presentation.

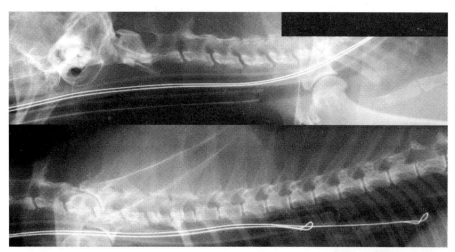

Case Description

"**Chabot**" is a 7-year-old male domestic, short-haired cat with a chief complaint of lethargy, weakness, unsteady gait and decreased appetite of 3 weeks duration. He was presented to the medicine clinic where he was noted to be depressed with slight dehydration, but also appeared ataxic with a stiff left pelvic limb when ambulatory. "Chabot" also had decreased proprioceptive placing in the left forelimb.

Because of these observations, a complete neurological examination was performed. The findings included left hemiparesis and decreased proprioceptive placing of the left limbs. Spinal reflexes were normal except for the presence of crossed extension of the left pelvic limb when the right pelvic limb was stimulated. The left biceps reflex also seemed less prominent than the right one. The neuroanatomic localization was a left-sided C6-7 myelopathy. Differential diagnoses included cervical neoplasia, inflammatory disease, trauma, cervical disc disease, and fibrocartilagenous emboli.

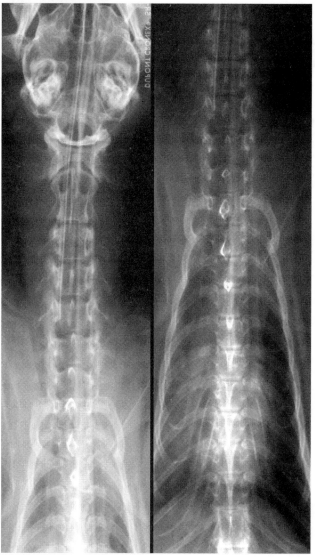

Radiographic Findings

The noncontrast spinal radiographs seen on this page show only minimal degenerative changes throughout the spine. Analysis of CSF aspirated from the cerebellomedullary cistern showed no abnormalities. "Chabot" was scheduled for a myelogram.

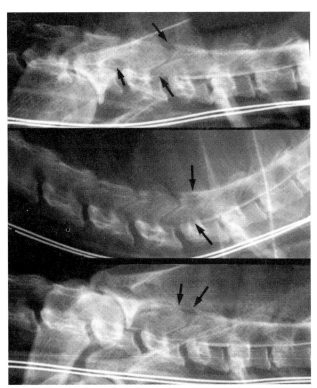

Myelographic Findings

Marked widening of the spinal cord at the level of C6-7 is seen on both lateral (black arrows) and VD views (white arrow) with a thinning of the subarachnoid spaces. A golf "tee" sign is present dorsally on the lateral views (black arrows).

These features are diagnostic of an intradural-extramedullary mass and because "Chabot" is a cat, lymphosarcoma is a most likely diagnosis, followed by meningioma.

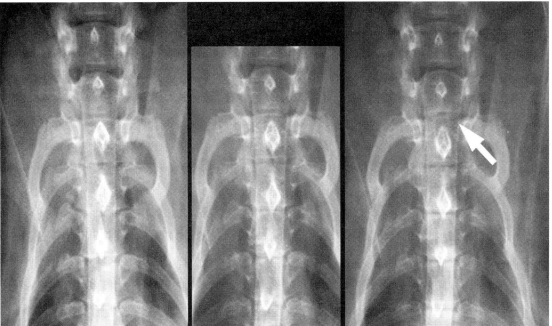

Comments

"Chabot" was taken to surgery and a dorsal laminectomy was performed at C5-6-7. An approximately 1 x 0.5 x 0.5 cm light brown, very friable mass was found on the left side of the spinal cord at the level of C6. The mass appeared to compress the cord but did not invade it. Complete removal of the mass was not possible. The histopathologic diagnosis of the tissue removed was that of a meningioma.

Review of the noncontrast radiographs shows that the positioning of the thoracic limbs is not adequate and the shoulders are superimposed over the site of the tumor. Reevaluation of the height of the cervical vertebral canal suggests that it is possible that the expanding tumor mass had increased the height, however, the cervical enlargement causes a normal expansion at this site.

Because "Chabot" was presented with lethargy and weakness, thoracic radiographs were made. Cardiomegaly with evidence of biventricular failure was noted. No metastatic nodules were detected.

Case Description

"**Ladd**" is a 4-year-old male shepherd mix who was referred to the clinic with a tentative diagnosis of brachial paralysis because he was dragging a forelimb. The owner reported a progressive right forelimb paralysis that had been noted for 3 months, as well as cervical pain for the past week. Muscle atrophy of both shoulders was evident on physical examination. On neurological examination, proprioceptive placing was decreased in all 4 limbs. An exaggerated patellar reflex was noted bilaterally. The lesion was localized to C1-C5. Spinal radiographs were made.

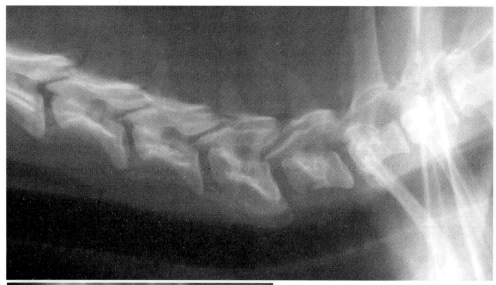

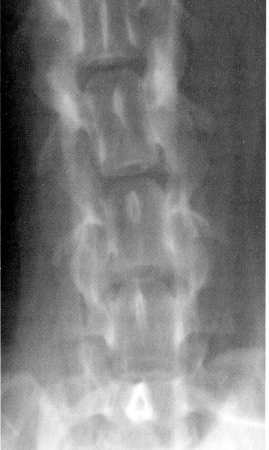

Radiographic Findings

The noncontrast radiographic studies of the spine were normal. Only the cervicothoracic region is shown. A myelogram was scheduled.

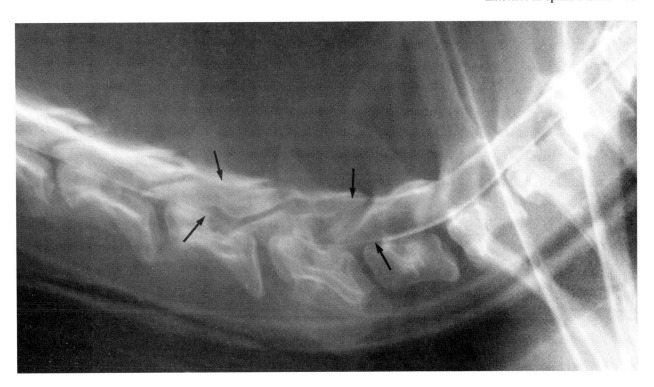

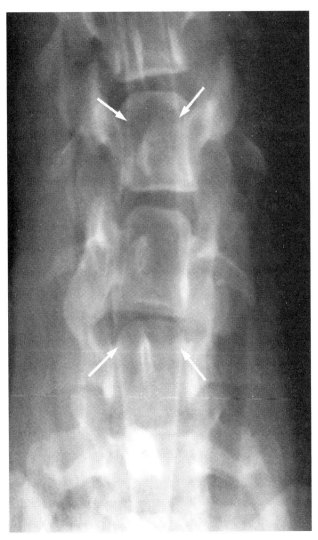

Myelographic Findings

The spinal cord widens abruptly at C5-6 with narrowing of the subarachnoid contrast columns seen on both views (arrows). The classification of the lesion is an intramedullary mass, and a primary spinal cord tumor is considered most likely. Other lesions on the differential list include metastatic tumor especially lymphosarcoma.

A 4.0 x 1.0 x 1.0 cm astrocytoma was diagnosed at necropsy.

Comments

Because "Ladd" weighed 30 kg, 13.5 cc of contrast agent were injected in the lumbar region (0.45 cc/kg body weight), providing a good flow of contrast agent into the cervical region. It is important that sufficient contrast agent be used to permit identification of both cranial and caudal limits of the suspected tumor mass.

Ladd's lesion was localized to C1-5 because his brain and cranial nerve function were normal, and because he had deficits in placing reactions in all 4 limbs in conjunction with upper motor neuron signs (normal or increased spinal reflexes). The exaggeration of the normal tendon reflexes, such as the patellar reflex, is often the first upper motor neuron abnormality to appear in a developing myelopathy.

Four Male Dogs with Lumbosacral Pain

Noncontrast radiographs of dogs with lumbosacral pain may be diagnostic. Commonly, however, additional radiographic studies are necessary. Secondary bony changes around the LS disc often complicate the radiographic interpretation. Note the differences in these studies.

Case Description

"**Ox**" is an 8-year-old male Rottweiler who has neurological signs of a cauda equina syndrome.

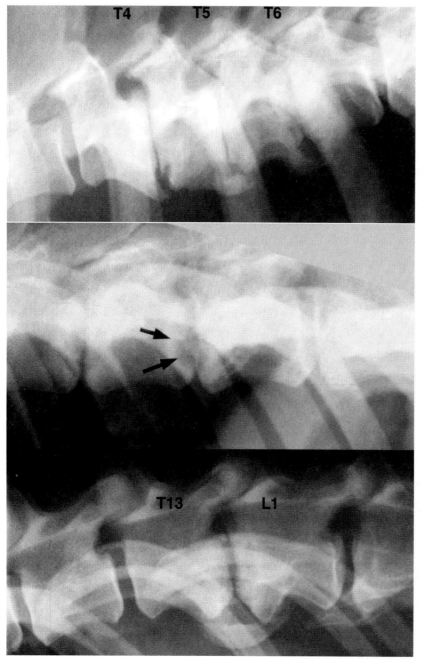

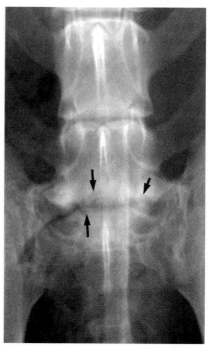

Radiographic Findings

The noncontrast radiographs show disc space collapse with end plate destruction at the T4-7, T9-11 (arrows), T13-L1, and LS discs (arrows). There is shortening of the bodies of T4-7. Secondary vertebral osteophyte formation is seen at the T4-7, T13-L1, and LS discs. The diagnosis is a hematogenous discospondylitis with the LS lesion probably the most important clinically.

Comment

The midthoracic lesions appear to be both acute and chronic and possibly superimposed upon chronic disc disease that has resulted in disc space collapse.

Hematogenous discospondylitis often develops at the site of degenerated discs.

"Ox" is somewhat unique because one of the less radiographically extensive lesions (LS) appears to be causing the more obvious clinical signs. It would have been helpful to perform stress studies, epidurography, electrodiagnostic studies, and perhaps CT or MRI to further characterize the LS lesion.

Case Description

"**Bootek**" is a 4-year-old male shepherd who had pain on palpation of the LS region for the past 2 months. Pelvic limb muscle atrophy was noted on physical examination.

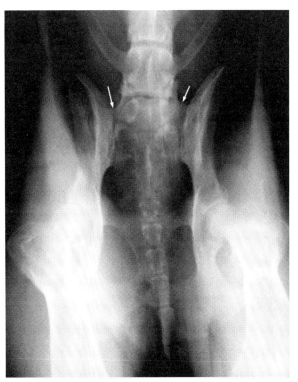

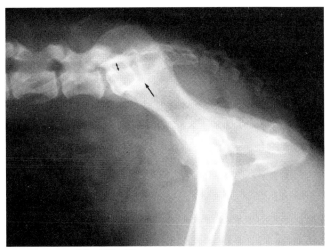

Radiographic Findings

The noncontrast radiographs show a transitional LS vertebra separated from the sacrum (black arrow) with symmetrical transverse processes (white arrows), marked LS canal stenosis (doubleheaded black arrow), and minimal malalignment. An enlarged view to the right shows the canal stenosis more clearly (doubleheaded black arrow).

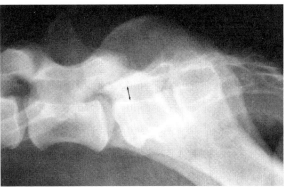

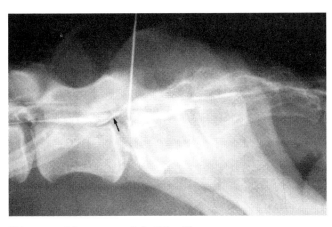

Disco-epidurographic Findings

Epidurography and discography show minimal LS instability and dorsal protrusion of the LS disc (arrow). The needle remains in position.

The diagnosis is a LS transitional segment with marked vertebral canal stenosis and a dorsally protruding LS disc resulting in a cauda equina syndrome.

Comments

Transitional LS vertebrae are thought to be inherited, at least in German Shepherd Dogs and Labrador retrievers because of the high frequency in those breeds and familial trends.

"Bootek's" hip joints appear normal ruling out arthrosis due to hip dysplasia as a cause of the clinical signs. Radiographs of the stifle joints were also normal, ruling out arthrosis due to cruciate ligament disease as a cause of the clinical signs. Hip and stifle arthrosis can cause hindquarter pain, reluctance to move, and muscle atrophy, clinical signs that also occur with cauda equina syndrome.

Case Description

"**Joshua**" is an 8-year-old male shepherd who has a 2-month history of sensitivity around the pelvic region. He shows pain when rising, lying down, or turning. Pain can be elicited by pressure over the LS region. He is depressed and unwilling to move

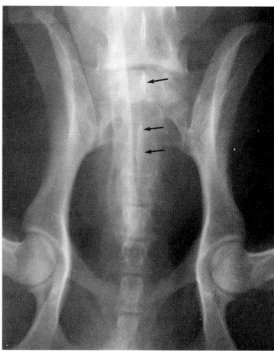

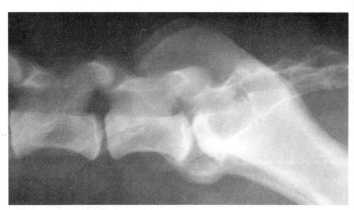

Radiographic Findings

The noncontrast radiographs show:

1. a transitional LS segment (note the separation of the spinous processes (arrows)
2. spondylosis deformans at the LS junction
3. minimal end plate sclerosis
4. no signs of vertebral canal stenosis

Stress LS radiographs showed minimal LS instability.

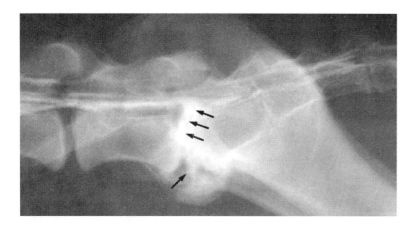

Disco-epidurography

The epidurogram and discogram (above) show contrast agent filling a severely degenerated, cavitary LS disc (arrows). Dorsal location of the contrast agent indicates dorsal displacement of the outer annulus to approximately one-half the height of the vertebral canal.

The diagnosis is an acquired lumbosacral stenosis resulting from a transitional LS vertebra plus the dorsal protrusion of a severely degenerated LS disc.

Comments

The degenerative changes surrounding the LS junction were not completely identified on the noncontrast radiographs and no indication of malalignment and only minimal instability were noted.

The compressive lesion at the LS junction was identified only following use of the discogram and epidurogram.

The hip joints are radiographically normal.

Case Description

"Harpo" is a 6-year-old male retriever with a 9-day history of an acute onset of pain and a history that he would not rise from the floor. Muscle atrophy is evident in the hindquarters on physical examination.

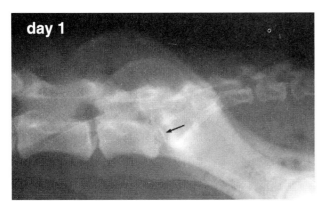

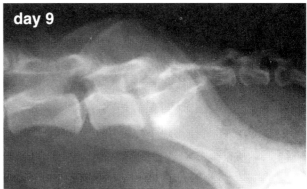

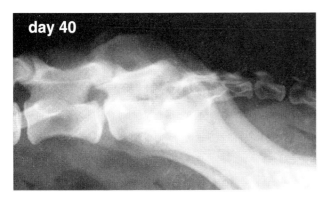

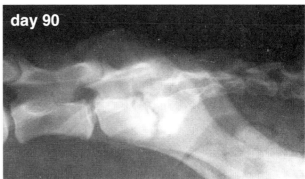

Radiographic Findings

The radiographs include stress studies and demonstrate a sequestrum (arrow) within an area of end plate destruction at the LS disc space. Disc space widening is present, however, no evidence of instability or malalignment is present. The diagnosis is an active LS discospondylitis.

Note the progression of change on the radiographs made 9 days later, 1 month later, and 7 weeks later. Despite antibiotic therapy, progression of end plate destruction is evident along with vertebral malalignment resulting in ventral displacement of the sacrum.

Comments

Paraparesis occurred suddenly 3 days after the original admission.

Staphylococcus aureus was cultured from the blood, urine, and from a biopsy specimen.

Contrary to what might be anticipated, "Harpo" improved clinically during the time that the radiographic changes around the LS junction were becoming more destructive. Four months after the original admission, "Harpo" was clinically normal. The possibility of LS instability should be considered during the healing phase and the dog should be caged to avoid excessive physical activity

Noncontrast Study Negative - Myelographic Study Positive

In many patients, the noncontrast radiographs of the spine do not demonstrate a lesion that could cause the neurologic signs. In these patients, if the owner is interested in pursuing a diagnosis and if surgery may be required to treat the lesion, myelography is the next most useful diagnostic tool.

Case Description

"**Sir Checkers**" is an 11-year-old male Basset hound with pelvic limb ataxia that quickly progressed to paralysis. A perianal adenocarcinoma had been surgically removed several months ago. The radiographic studies include the lateral views of a noncontrast study.

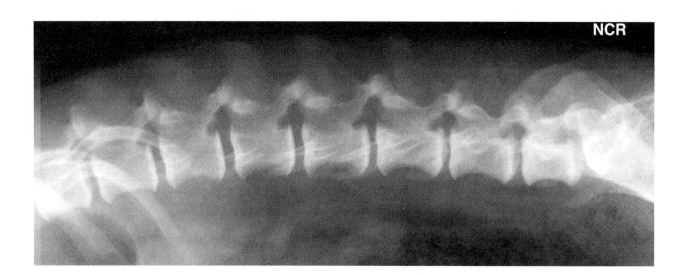

Radiographic Findings

No radiographic changes on the single noncontrast study (above) can be related to the clinical signs. It is important to note the absence of disc space narrowing, end plate sclerosis, or disc calcification any of which would suggest disc disease. Minimal prostatic hyperplasia was noted. The fecal-filled colon is in a normal position and does not suggest any sublumbar lymph node enlargement that could be secondary to the perianal tumor.

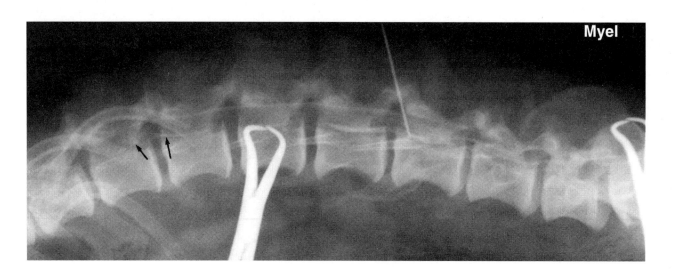

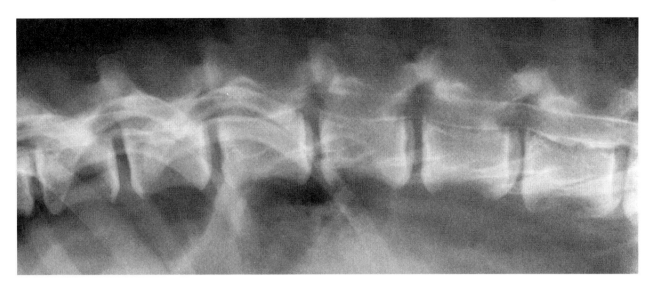

Myelographic Findings

The myelographic study includes a view (bottom opposite page) after the test injection with the spinal needle remaining in position and a second view (above) made after injection of the total amount of contrast medium. The elevation and narrowing of the spinal cord at L1-2 is seen best on an enlarged view (arrows, below). Both dorsal and ventral subarachnoid columns are narrowed.

The diagnosis is a Type II disc protrusion that was not suspected on the survey study.

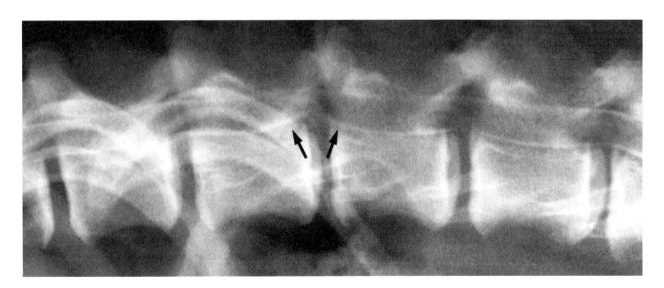

Case Description

"Princess" is a 10-year-old female Pekingese with a sudden onset of upper motor neuron paraplegia.

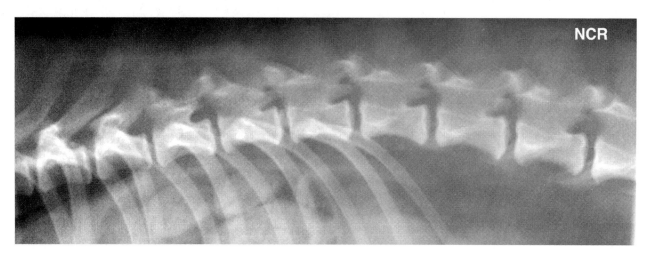

Radiographic Findings

The radiographic abnormality on the noncontrast study (above) is a calcified disc at T12-13 that seems to be contained within the disc space.

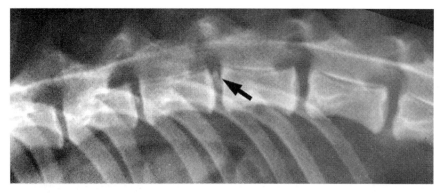

Myelographic Findings

The myelogram shows the calcified disc on the lateral view (arrow) and a right-sided extradural mass on the VD view (arrows), probably secondary to a disc herniation at T12-13. Cord swelling extends over 2 vertebrae. Note how the cord fills the vertebral canal in this chondrodystrophic dog, causing a break in the ventral subarachnoid column as it passes over each disc space.

The presence of calcified disc tissue within the disc space may be associated with: (1) a calcific nucleus with no herniation or protrusion and with all of the nuclear tissue within the disc, (2) a partially herniated or protruded nucleus with nuclear tissue in both the vertebral canal and remaining within the disc, or (3) a partially herniated or protruded nucleus with the nuclear tissue lateral or ventral to the disc with some nuclear tissue remaining within the disc.

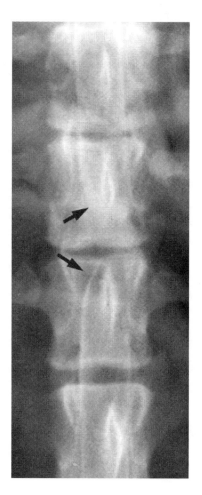

Case Description

"**Jody**" is a 4-year-old female dachshund with a 3-month history of back pain. Over the past 24 hours, she has become paraparetic, then paraplegic.

The noncontrast radiographs showed a series of calcified discs with narrowing of disc spaces at T11-12, T12-13, and possibly calcified tissue in the vertebral canal at L2-3.

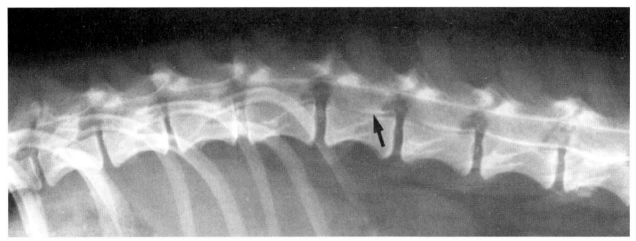

Myelographic Findings

The myelogram shows spinal cord swelling from T10 to L3. The ventral subarachnoid space is seen to terminate at L2 (arrow). Cord swelling following trauma or acute compression seems to spread approximately equal distances cranially and caudally from the point of impact. If this is the case, "Jody's" lesion is probably at T12-13 and, given her breed and the noncontrast radiographic findings, is probably a herniated disc. A lesion of this type in a chondrodystrophic breed with marked cord swelling is most often the result of a Type l, explosive, disc extrusion causing hemorrhage and edema within the spinal cord. The clinician should remember, however, that the myelographic appearance of cord trauma (i.e., cord swelling) is essentially that of an intramedullary mass, and that disorders other than trauma can produce intramedullary masses.

It is always helpful when the contrast agent is seen on both cranial and caudal aspects of a lesion since this provides specific information as to its character.

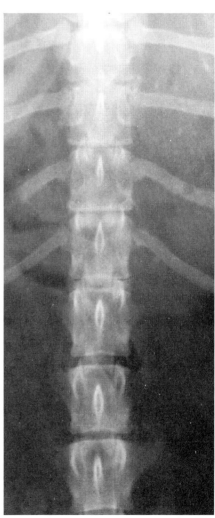

Question #1

Can you name three other causes for myelographic intramedullary mass patterns in addition to spinal cord swelling?

Case Description

"**Frau**" is a 10-year-old female Doberman Pinscher who was examined because of progressive pelvic limb weakness. A survey study was made of the spine.

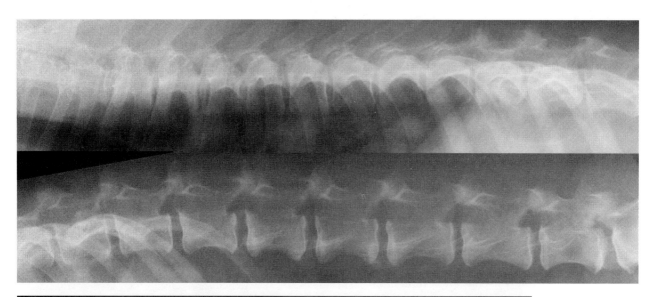

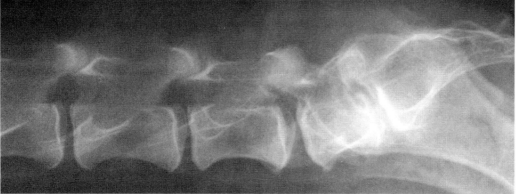

Radiographic Findings

The noncontrast radiographs have a number of features, some of which could be important clinically:

1. suspect calcification of the dorsal portion of the disc at L1-2
2. generalized osteopenia
3. multiple pulmonary nodules
4. transitional TL vertebra with a hypoplastic rib on the right and a well developed rib on the left
5. transitional lumbosacral vertebra

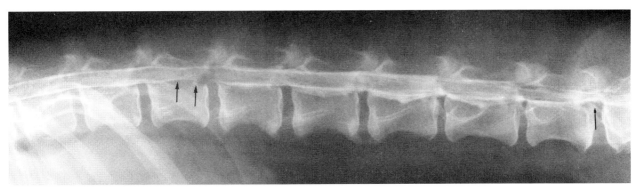

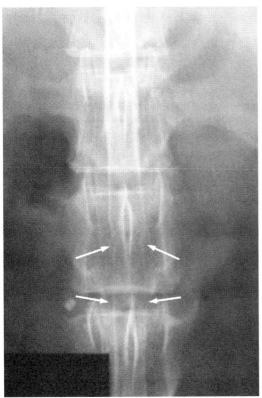

Myelographic Findings

The myelogram shows an extradural mass just caudal to the transitional TL segment on the lateral view (black arrows) causing elevation of the cord and on the VD view (white arrows) causing compression on both right and left sides. This creates the impression of a partial "ring" mass on three sides of the cord. The subarachnoid columns are abruptly narrowed which is atypical for a protruding disc. In addition, at the transitional LS segment, elevation of the ventral subarachnoid column and depression of the dorsal subarachnoid column on the lateral view indicate a spinal stenosis caused by a protruding disc and a hypertrophied interarcuate ligaments (arrow).

The tentative diagnosis was malignant disease with metastasis to the vertebral canal and/or meninges causing an extradural mass at L2, pulmonary metastatic disease, plus a clinically less-important LS stenosis. The diagnosis at necropsy was a metastatic malignant melanoma to the lungs and vertebral canal.

Question #2

Why might "Frau's" pelvic limb weakness be getting worse?

Comments

The presence of the pulmonary nodules suggests a malignant disease possibly related to the L2 extradural mass. The LS disc disease appears more chronic and associated with the transitional vertebral segment and would not cause the clinical signs seen in "Frau".

A thoracic radiographic study is indicated in every patient who is older and has chronic disease. The possibility of the detection of chronic pulmonary or cardiac disease is high. The detection of pulmonary metastatic disease is important in formulating a prognosis for treatment and recovery, information that is helpful to the owner.

Case Description

"Tasha" is an 8-year-old female Rottweiler with a sudden onset of paraparesis/ataxia that progressed to paraplegia within 4 days. The neurologic signs indicate an upper motor neuron myelopathy to the pelvic limbs.

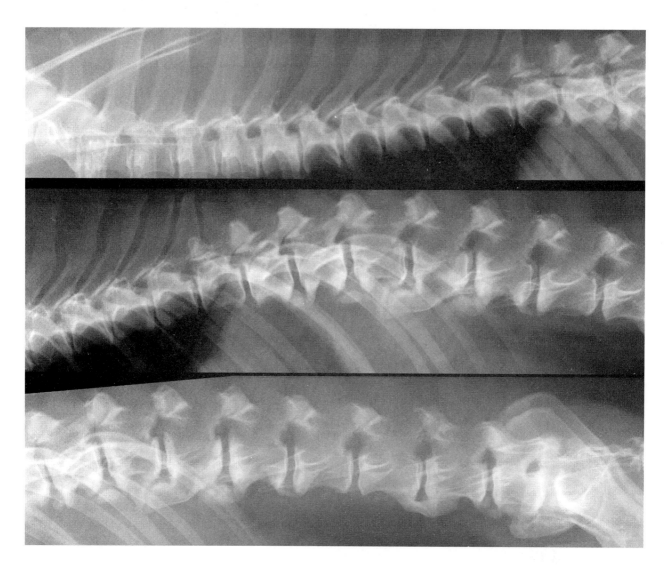

Radiographic Findings

The noncontrast radiographs show a widespread spondylosis deformans, LS disc space widening with ventral displacement of the sacrum suggestive of lumbosacral malalignment and canal stenosis, generalized osteopenia, and costovertebral arthrosis. None of these were thought to explain the acute onset of ataxia that was progressive.

Myelographic Findings

The myelogram (opposite page) shows an extradural compressive lesion primarily ventral and left-sided extending from the T8-9 disc space over the vertebral body of T9. The mass, as seen on the lateral views, causes abrupt cord narrowing and displacement somewhat different from that seen with a disc disease (black arrows). The VD and oblique views adds information as to the character of the extradural mass (white arrows).

The extradural mass is probably not disc tissue because of the location in the midthoracic spine, the location in the midportion of a thoracic vertebra, and the abrupt change in the width and location of the cord. For these reasons, a metastatic neoplastic lesion is more likely.

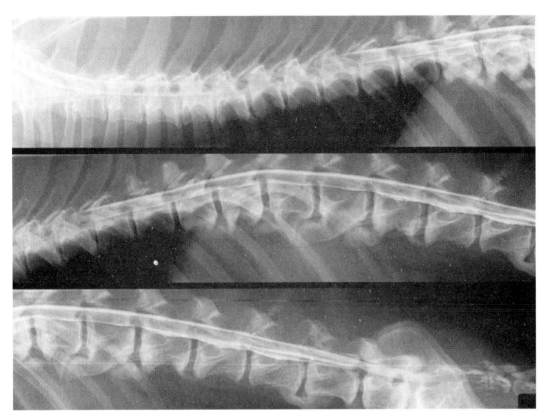

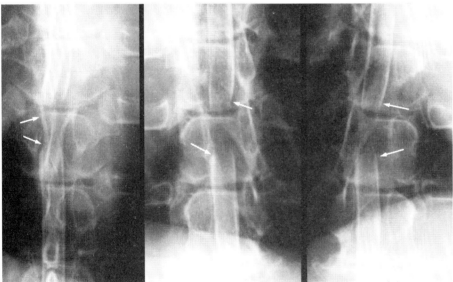

Comment

A left hemilaminectomy was performed and the mass removed, however, "Tasha" lost deep pain perception 6 days postsurgically and failed to respond to medication.

Tissue obtained at necropsy was examined and histopathology and immunohistochemistry confirmed the spinal mass to be a histiocytic sarcoma. Additional masses with the same pathologic characteristic were found in the spleen, kidney, lung and paravertebral muscle.

Thoracic radiographs were normal without evidence of metastatic disease.

Answer #1

1. Neoplasia
2. Infarction by fibrocartilagenous emboli
3. Inflammation/infection

Answer #2

The simplest explanation is that the tumor is enlarging and increasing the amount of pressure applied to the spinal cord, causing ischemia, demyelination, neuronal degeneration, and other pathologic changes. It is also possible for a mass that is not enlarging to cause progressive dysfunction through the same pathologic mechanisms.

A Postsurgical Patient

If the patient has had prior spinal surgery, radiographic images of the spine may be altered in a manner that is unexpected. Postsurgical infection can lead to radiographic changes typical of acute or chronic spondylitis or discospondylitis. Intervertebral disc fenestration often lead to disc space collapse. A healing fracture often heals with malunion of the fragments. The addition of metallic implants can also complicate visualization and interpretation of spinal radiographs.

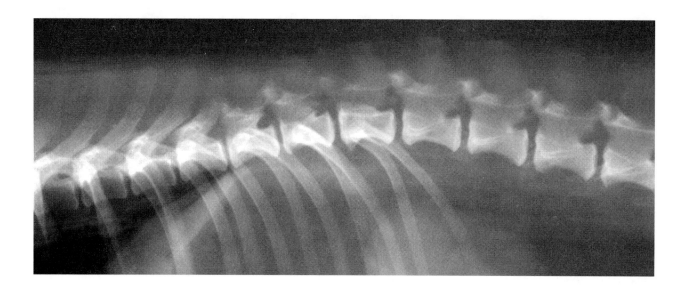

Case Description

"Princess" is a 10-year-old Pekingese with cervical pain for the past 3 weeks. She had a hemilaminectomy at T12-13 about 3 years ago for treatment of a herniated disc at that site. The radiographs of the thoracolumbar spine were a part of the total spinal study performed at this time.

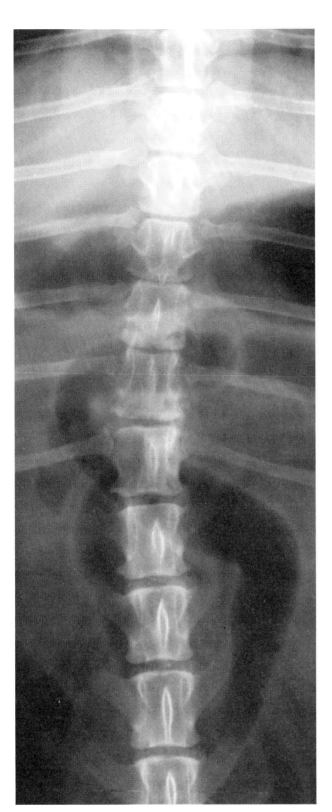

Radiographic Findings

The radiographs made today show the absence of the pedicle of T13 and the articular processes of T12-13 on the right side. The calcified disc material remaining on the floor of the vertebral canal at T13 is residual from the previous disc herniation. The scoliosis at T13-L1 is a post-operative condition.

Question # 1

Why is the pain localized in the cervical spine?

Comments

The vertebral malalignment is an uncommon sequel to hemilaminectomy and is probably related to the extent of the surgical trauma. An aggressive fenestration plus the hemilaminectomy appears to have resulted in extensive injury to the disc and paravertebral musculature leading to the instability.

Answer# 1

"Princess" acute spinal pain is not related to the old spinal surgery. An evaluation of her complete spinal series showed a C3-4 calcified herniated disc.

What Is Dural Ossification?

As the dog ages, the radiographic evaluation of the spine reveals more abnormalities, but unfortunately doesn't tell us which are the ones of clinical importance. Within the past year, "Romulus" has had hepatomegaly, a compensated mitral insufficiency, scrotal edema associated with a perianal swelling, weakness in walking, and pain in the pelvis. Radiographs of patients such as "Romulus" are necessary and still the clinician and owner need to understand that the lesions detected may not account for all of the problems presented by the dog.

Case Description

"Romulus" is a 13-year-old male shepherd dog whose major complaint today is pelvic limb ataxia and weakness. Degenerative myelopathy was suspected because of the breed and age, however, radiographs were made to rule out other lesions.

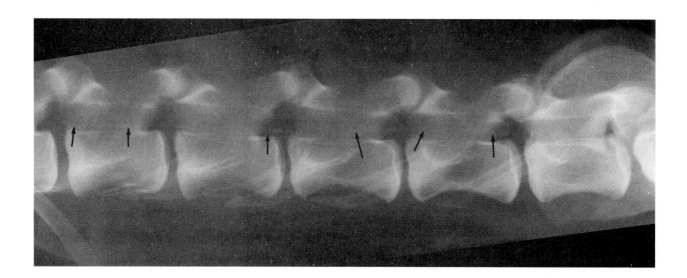

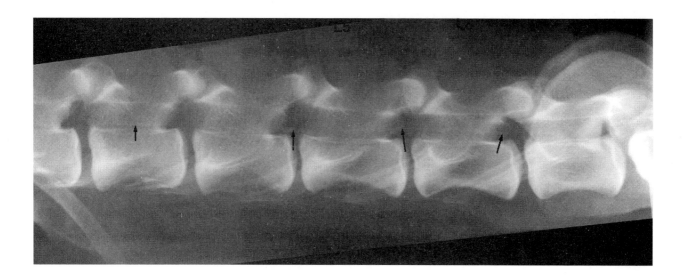

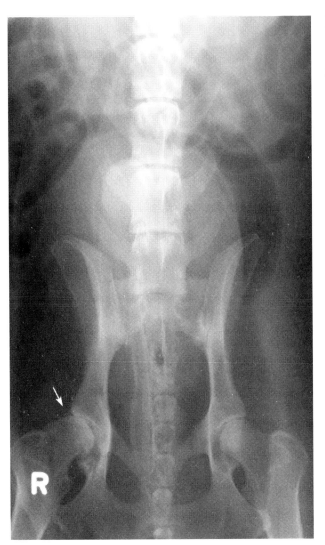

Radiographic Findings

Two lateral views from the spinal series are shown (opposite page). The radiographs have prominent, linear, radiopaque lines within the vertebral canal (arrows). One of these lines appears to elevate from the floor of the vertebral canal at L5-6 (arrow) suggesting a ventrally located mass. In addition, a severe unilateral arthrosis, probably secondary to hip dysplasia, is present in the right hip joint as seen on the VD view (arrow). The radiographic study is unique in that little evidence of disc degeneration is noted.

The radiographic diagnosis is dural ossification (osseous metaplasia of the dura). Interestingly, the dural ossification serves as a contrast marker within the dura and demonstrates an extradural mass at L5-6, possibly a chronic Type II disc herniation. In the past, dural ossification was incorrectly called pachymeningitis ossificans.

The hip joint arthrosis could certainly cause an abnormal gait, but would not cause neurologic deficits such as hyperreflexia.

Comments

Dural ossification is not considered a clinically important degenerative change. The extradural mass at L5-6 could have several causes. Disc tissue is suggested if the mass centers over a disc space and because of the frequency of disc disease in older shepherds. Because the mass is centered over the vertebral body in "Romulus", the lesion may have another cause and deserves a further diagnostic workup.

Osseous Metaplasia or Dural Ossification of the Spinal Dura Mater (Ossifying Pachymeningitis) in the Dog

Osseous metaplasia of the dura is characterized by the presence of bony plaques on the inner surface of the dura and occurs in over 60 % of both large and small breed dogs over two years of age. It is found most commonly in the cervical and lumbar areas, the most movable areas of the spine. The plaques are generally linear in shape with a longer craniocaudal dimension and have smooth surfaces. Radiographically, these plaques appear as thin radiopaque linear shadows seen dorsal and ventral to the spinal cord in which location they are seen "on end". They are most easily identified at the intervertebral foramina where they are not covered by the pedicles. Dural ossification can be confused with calcified disc tissue that has protruded. The ossified dura presents as a sharply delineated linear shadow, whereas the disc material causes a mound or mass of calcified tissue that is often amorphous in appearances.

Osseous metaplasia of the dura has incorrectly been implicated as the cause of progressive paresis of large and giant breed dogs and the term dural pachymeningitis used incorrectly, since the lesions are not inflammatory. Controversy remains regarding the clinical importance and some state that extensive dural ossification may cause pain, weakness and other neurologic deficits, which others feel that it never causes clinical disease. The authors feel that if one does include dural ossification in the differential diagnosis of pain and/or transverse myelopathy, the best approach is to eliminate all other possible causes before positively diagnosing dural ossification as the cause of clinical signs. Continued investigations have substantiated other causes for paresis, particularly German Shepherd Dog myelopathy and cervical spondylopathy.

Cervical Spondylopathy

Often the clinical signs plus the breed affected lead you to consider a particular diagnosis prior to your clinical investigation. Although this is reasonable, you should not narrow your list of differential diagnoses prematurely. The correct approach is to localize the neurologic lesion, then make a list of the possible disorders that could be producing a lesion at that site. Then, based on the animal's history, signalment, other problems, and any other pertinent information, this list is ordered from most to least probable and diagnostic procedures are selected and prioritized.

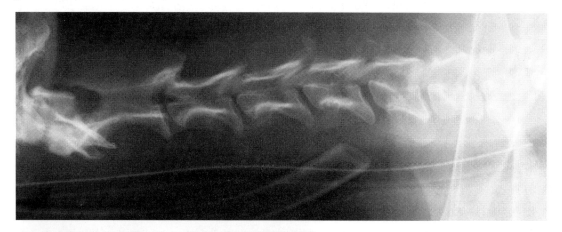

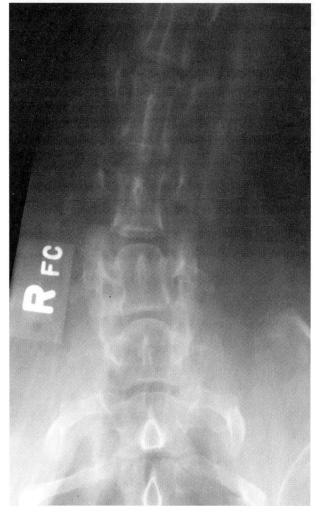

Case Description

"**Raina**" is a 7-year-old female Doberman Pinscher with recurring neck pain, a stiff thoracic limb gait, mild shoulder muscle atrophy, and mild pelvic limb paresis/ataxia. You localize her lesion to the caudal cervical spinal cord, and because of her breed, age and clinical signs, cervical spondylopathy is at the top of your list of differential diagnoses.

Radiographic Findings

The lateral and VD noncontrast radiographs on this page show a malalignment between C4-5 and C5-6 and narrowing of the C6-7 disc space.

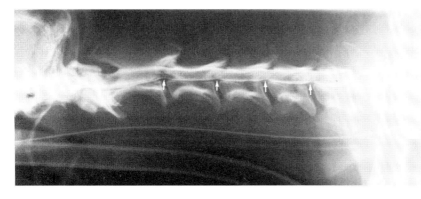

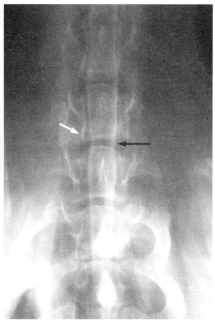

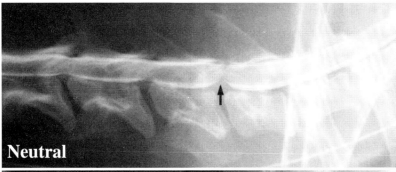

Neutral

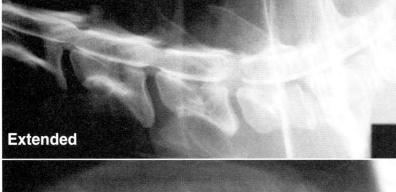

Extended

Myelographic Findings

The view of the cervical spine (above) shows small Type II disc protrusions affecting all discs (arrows). The enlarged lateral views of the myelogram show a large Type II disc at C6-7 where the spinal cord is narrowed (arrows) and displaced dorsally (arrow).

Enlarged lateral views were made in neutral, extended, and flexed positions of the head and show the variation in resulting spinal cord compression.

The laterally compressing masses seen on the VD view at C6-7 are caused by bony hypertrophy of the articular facets (arrow).

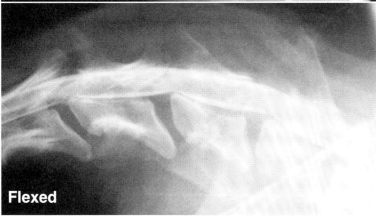

Flexed

Comment

Extension of the neck increases the degree of dorsal protrusion of the discal tissue and ventral protrusion of the hypertrophied ligamentum flavum between all of the cervical vertebrae. Thus a maneuver of this type in an anesthetized patient is done with some caution because of the possibility of causing an increase in compression of the spinal cord. Flexion causes separation of the cervical vertebrae and stretching of the protruding disc tissue and hypertrophied ligaments returning them to a more-normal position, relieving a part of the spinal cord compression. The features seen in "Raina's" cervical spine are classic for cervical spondylopathy of Doberman Pinschers.

Case Description

"**Domino**" is a 10-year-old female Dalmatian with recurring neck pain and proprioceptive placing deficits in all four limbs. The signs have been progressive over the past 10 months. The lesion was localized to C1-C5 spinal cord segments.

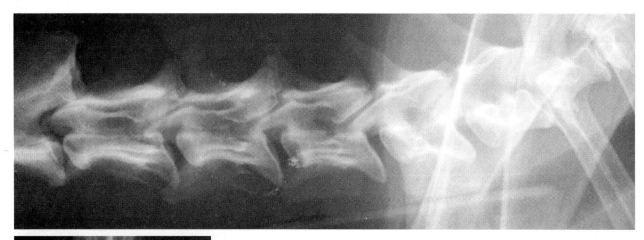

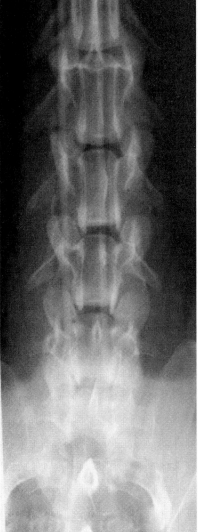

Radiographic Findings

The noncontrast cervical radiographs show no abnormalities.

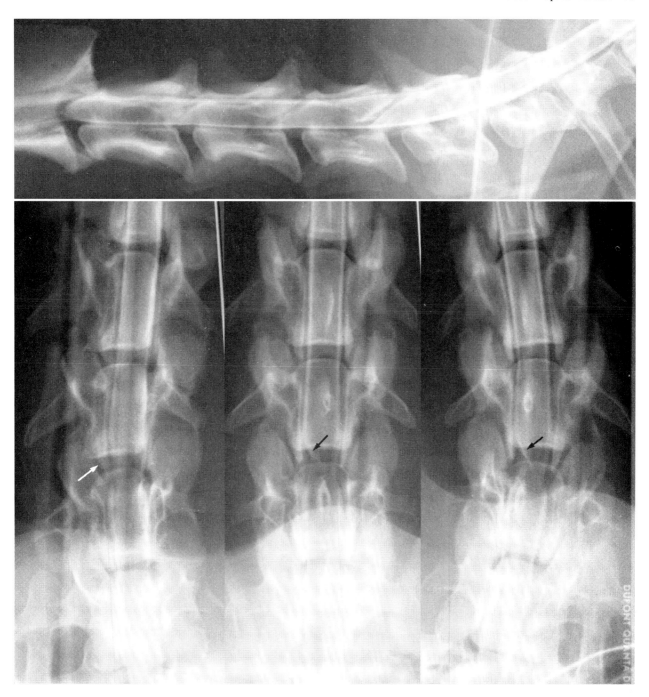

Myelographic Findings

The lateral view of the myelogram shows only a small dorsal disc protrusion at C2-3. However, the ventrodorsal views of the myelogram show a marked narrowing of the spinal cord and subarachnoid columns at C5-6 (arrow). The oblique views of the myelogram show the extradural mass to be particularly large on the right side causing minimal narrowing of the spinal cord and subarachnoid columns.

The cervical spondylopathy is characterized by a laterally compressive mass at C5-6 not evident on the lateral view.

Comments

At surgery, malformed articular facets were identified as causing cord compression, but more importantly was the presence of a large synovial cyst on the right side of the vertebral canal at the level of C5-6.

Without ventrodorsal views, the lesion would not have been identified. The increase in height of the spinal cord on the lateral view at C5-6 may represent the normal increase in cord size at that location or may represent displacement of the cord to the left with a resulting increase in the height of the cord.

Case Description

"Ridgeback Red" is a 10-year-old male Rhodesian Ridgeback with right hemiparesis. The lesion was localized to the C1-C5 spinal cord on the right side. Noncontrast radiographic studies were performed centering on the cervical spine.

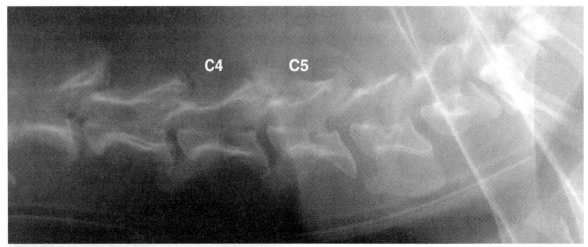

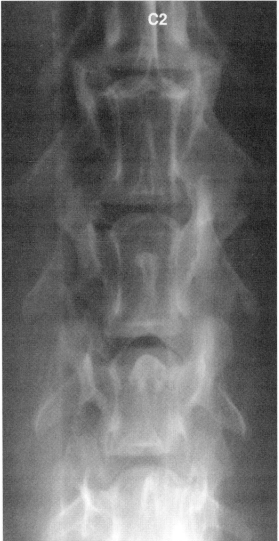

Radiographic Findings

The noncontrast studies show extensive deformity of the articular facets on the lateral view especially at C4-5. These deformities are also identified on the ventrodorsal views. The degree of vertebral canal stenosis is minimal, but the cranial diameter of the C5 vertebral foramen is smaller than the caudal diameter. No stenosis is seen on the ventrodorsal view.

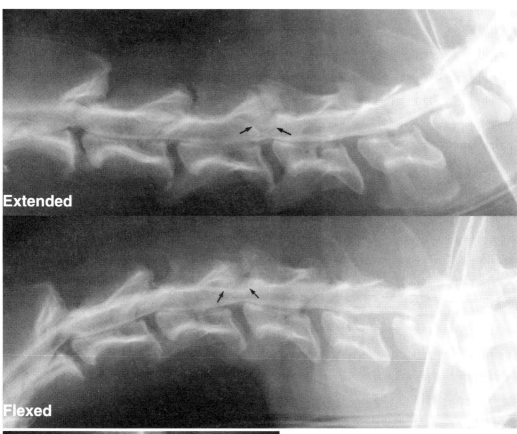

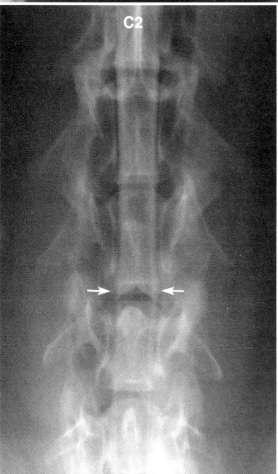

Myelographic Findings

The myelographic study includes extended and flexed lateral views and a VD view that show a massive soft tissue mass protruding ventrally into the vertebral canal at C4-5 (arrows), which probably represents hypertrophy of the interarcuate ligament and of the joint capsules around the vertebral joints. Flexing the neck separates the vertebral arches of C4-5 and stretches the interarcuate ligament and joint capsules, which reduces the canal stenosis and cord compression. The dorsal mass causes minimal widening of the cord as seen on the ventrodorsal view (arrows).

Comments

Clinically, "Ridgeback Red's" cervical spondylopathy resembles the disorder as seen in the Doberman Pinscher as opposed to the Great Dane in that his signs developed after middle age. However, his radiographic abnormalities are further cranial in the cervical spine than is usual, particularly in the Doberman. It is interesting that the increased stability at C4-5 has not resulted in disc degeneration with dorsal protrusion of the adjacent discs. Treatment of cervical spondylopathy, can be surgical or medical. Determination of the best surgical procedure is a subject of substantial controversy.

Cervical Spondylopathy (Cervical Vertebral Malformation — Malarticulation)

Since the early 1960's, an abnormality primarily of the caudal cervical vertebrae has been recognized in large and giant purebred dogs. The breeds involved have been generally large and have included the Great Dane, Doberman Pinscher, Saint Bernard, Weimeraner, Labrador Retriever, German Shepherd Dog, Boxer, Great Pyrenees, ChowChow, Basset Hound, Rhodesian Ridgeback, Dalmatian, Samoyed, Old English Sheepdog, Coonhound, and the Bull Mastiff. A higher frequency in males has been repeatedly suggested. The two breeds most frequently affected area the Great Dane and the Doberman Pinscher. In Great Danes, the clinical aspect of the syndrome seems to occur most commonly in young growing dogs, while it is a clinical problem of adults in Doberman Pinschers.

This syndrome has also been called the "wobbler" syndrome, cervical vertebral instability, progressive cervical spinal cord compression, cervical spondylosis, caudal cervical subluxation, Great Dane ataxia, cervical myelopathy, cervical spondylotic myelopathy, caudal cervical spondylomyelopathy, dynamic compression of the cervical spinal cord, and cervical spondylolisthesis. The term "wobbler" describes a non-specific clinical picture, and the terms instability and spondylolisthesis do not accurately reflect the complexity of the syndrome nor the fact that instability is often not demonstrable. The name cervical spondylopathy much more accurately reflects the complexity of the syndrome and therefore has become widely accepted. Instability of cervical vertebrae is seen in association with malformations of the vertebral bodies or articular facets and alteration of vertebral canal cross-sectional shape and area. This is seen most commonly in large dogs and especially in Doberman Pinschers and Great Danes. Cervical vertebrae 4 to 7 are generally involved. No one medical or surgical regimen is appropriate for all dogs affected with this syndrome. Effective management requires a basic understanding of the pathophysiology and the selection, modification, and individualization of medical and surgical techniques.

Pathogenesis

The basic lesions of cervical spondylopathy are most easily understood as developmental with degenerative changes superimposed. The syndrome worsens as a dynamic component influences the vertebral canal stenosis resulting in further cord or nerve root compression. The addition of a dynamic factor creates specific clinical signs, especially those resulting from hyperextension of the head and neck.

Deformation of the vertebral arches (including the articular processes and intervertebral joints) and hypertrophy of soft tissue structures (including the ligamentum flavum or interarcuate ligament, dorsal longitudinal ligament, dorsal annulus fibrosis, and the joint capsule of the vertebral joints)

all cause canal stenosis. Vertebral instability alone or in association with any of the bony or soft tissue lesions described above may be an initiating cause of clinical signs.

Neurologic Examination

The clinical signs in cervical spondylopathy reflect the intermittent, chronic compression of the cervical spinal cord, usually at the level of C6-7.

The affected dog shows deficits in both hopping and proprioceptive placing. Bilateral paresis and ataxia of the pelvic limbs cause an unsteady gait characterized by an abnormally long stride. The pelvic limbs are usually more severely involved than the thoracic limbs and show wearing of the toenails. The deficits in the thoracic limbs are less prominent, but consist of similar proprioceptive deficits, with knuckling and limb crossing as noted in the hind limbs. The dog may also be hypermetric because of damage to the spinocerebellar tracts.

The gait abnormalities are more noticeable if the dog is moved slowly or down an incline. Excluding the Doberman Pinscher, the signs usually present at 4 to 5 months of age. Other breeds have a later onset of signs.

The presence of cervical pain varies markedly. The absence of neck pain in some cases may be explained by the relatively slow progression of the disease as well as by the fact that the nerve roots, which are a source of cervical pain, are not directly involved. The classic flexed neck carriage in this syndrome can be explained by this position resulting in partial relief of pain from cord or nerve root compression.

The neurologic changes suggest lesions affecting the white matter of the cervical cord with involvement of the ascending proprioceptive tracts and descending motor tracts. Upper motor neuron signs usually predominate, but lower motor neuron lesions may cause muscle atrophy in the thoracic limbs. The more superficial and dorsolateral location of the proprioceptive tracts from the pelvic limbs may explain their vulnerability in this syndrome.

Radiographic Diagnosis

The diagnosis of cervical spondylopathy requires a noncontrast study that includes both lateral and VD views plus stress radiographs. Myelography is also required with both lateral and VD views plus stress views. The radiographic changes consist of: (1) malalignment of vertebral vertebrae, (2) change in the shape of the vertebral body with apparent loss of the cranioventral corner, (3) modeling with cranial stenosis of the vertebral foramina creating a funnel shape to the vertebral canal with asymmetry, (4) marked asymmetry of the articular facets with secondary periarticular new bone, (5) new bone formation (vertebral osteophytes) on the cranial ventral aspect of the vertebral body often appearing to be responding to a bony defect in this location, (6) end plate sclerosis resulting from the instability of the affected disc, and (7) Type II degeneration of the intervertebral disc including narrowing of the disc space and calcification of the nucleus pulposus. Vertebral instability places an important role in certain patients while it is of little importance in others.

Myelography, in conjunction with stress radiography demonstrates dorsally protruding intervertebral discs or ventrally protruding interarcuate ligaments or joint capsules. The use of stress positioning demonstrates the increase in vertebral canal stenosis and cord compression when the neck is extended. The use of hyperflexed lateral projections demonstrates the reduction in the degree of cord compression. The VD view during myelography shows the lateral compression associated with the articular facets and hypertrophy of the adjoining soft tissues. Traction radiographs also demonstrate the dynamic nature of the lesion, as the soft tissue compressive mass can be seen to be reduced by this type of positioning. This may be helpful to the surgeon in selection of a method of treatment, especially placement of a bone graft to maintain distraction of the vertebral bodies. The presence of compressive masses dorsally, ventrally, and laterally complicates the choice of a technique for surgical decompression.

Myelography identifies the nature of the extradural mass which may be due to: (1) Type II disc degeneration, (2) thickening of the ligamentum flavum and joint capsule, (3) thickening of the dorsal longitudinal ligament, (4) developmental bony abnormality, or (5) vertebral instability.

Pathologic Findings

The pathologic findings in the spinal cord are those expected with a compressive lesion. Wallerian type of degeneration of ascending and descending tracts is present due to the axon disruption at the site of the injury. The remainder of the axon and its myelin sheath distal to the cell body degenerates. In addition, a focal myelopathy results from the interference of the blood supply to the cord. The surgical decompression and stabilization appears to assist in the elimination of further neurologic injury and encourages remyelination of axons that are still intact. The necropsy findings suggest that increased mobility between vertebrae is not necessary for production of the lesions noted histologically, supporting radiographic findings that have suggested an absence of instability.

The absence of disc material within the vertebral canal has been noted, suggesting that this syndrome lacks features in common with an acute cervical disc herniation. Instead, the disc has a rounded appearance due to partial anular protrusion and possibly the presence of hypertrophy of the dorsal longitudinal ligament.

Causes of Vertebral Canal Stenosis Associated with Cervical Spondylopathy

Primary bone changes - Stenosis of the cranial vertebral foramina due to an excessive dietary intake

Vertebral body modeling - Change in the shape of the cranial ventral aspect of the vertebral body is due to an osteochondrosis-type lesion with failure to convert the cartilage model into a bony centrum that is normal in shape. The abnormal shape of the body causes a malalignment in the vertebral vertebrae and resulting spinal cord compression.

Secondary bony changes - Osteophytes and modeled articular facets are due to instability between the vertebral vertebrae. An increased ventral pressure from the caudal articular processes on the cranial articular process is important in creation of this new bony growth. Often, however, such bony growth does not cause spinal cord compression.

Hyperplasia of soft tissues - Without detection of osseous changes, hyperplasia of the soft tissues is due to laxity between the vertebral vertebrae, but not subluxation. The hypertrophy in the ligamentum flavum, seen most often in the Great Dane, is highly significant clinically and is best seen on the hyperextended projection made during the myelogram. Because the soft tissues are radiolucent, myelography is the only commonly-used diagnostic technique readily available for their detection.

Combination of changes - Compression from the: (1) anulus fibrosis ventrally, (2) ligamentum flavum dorsally, and (3) bony facets and fibrous joint capsule laterally create an hourglass compression. These are often noted in the Great Dane. Myelography is required to most completely visualize the exact nature of the compressive ring.

Summary - Cervical Spondylopathy in the Dog

1. Terminology
   a. cervical subluxation
   b. canine wobbler syndrome
   c. cervical spondylopathy
   d. cervical vertebral instability
   e. cervical spondylolisthesis
   f. stenosis of the cervical vertebral canal
   g. deformation of cervical vertebrae
   h. vertebral deformation
2. Incidence
   a. breed
      1. Great Danes
      2. Doberman Pinschers
      3. Saint Bernard
      4. Irish Setter
      5. Fox Terrier
      6. Basset Hounds
      7. Rhodesian Ridgeback
      8. Old English Sheepdog
   b. age
      1. from shortly after birth to 9 years
      2. Great Danes (under 1 year)
      3. Doberman Pinschers (3-9 years)
   c. sex
      1. male have a higher frequency
3. Clinical signs
   a. rate of appearance
      1. slowly progressive
      2. may develop more rapidly with disc protrusion
   b. proprioceptive loss
      1. rear limb incoordination (ataxia)
      2. wide base stance (abduction)
      3. hypermetric or prancing gait (often thoracic limbs)
      4. wearing toenails due to dragging toes
      5. difficulty on rising with ataxia during first few steps
      6. may be quadriplimbic with extensor rigidity
   c. pain (10%)
   d. with testing
      1. hopping and proprioceptive positioning show greatest deficit
      2. UMN signs predominate
      3. little pain noted

4. Gross lesions
   a. general
      1. usually last three cervical vertebrae
      2. malformation or malarticulation
      3. funnel-shaped vertebral canal with small cranial orifice
      4. malarticulation
         a. with stability
         b. with instability or slippage on hyperflexion
   b. vertebral joints
      1. osteoarthrosis with osteophytosis
      2. clinical ankylosis
      3. asymmetry or malformation of articular processes
      4. incomplete cartilage covering of articular processes (osteochondrosis)
      5. joint capsule hypertrophy or hyperplasia
   c. stenosis of vertebral canal due to hypertrophy of
      1. interarcuate ligament
      2. joint capsule
      3. dorsal longitudinal ligament (minimal involvement)
      4. dorsal anulus fibrosis
      5. laminae of vertebral arch
   d. vertebral body
      1. malformed cranial dorsal aspect of vertebral body especially C6
   e. intervertebral disc
      1. disc degeneration
      2. narrowing and calcification
      3. nuclear protrusion
      4. dorsal anulus fibrosus hypertrophy
      5. sclerotic end plates
      6. discs adjacent to clinically fused vertebrae degenerate
   f. vertebral malalignment
      1. usually C6-7 with the cranial aspect of the body of C7 displaced dorsally
      2. C4-5 or C5-6 affected to a lesser degree
      3. C3 has been described in the Basset and C 3-4 in the Great Dane
   g. cord lesions
      1. compression
      2. focal spinal cord injury

5. Etiology
   a. genetic
   b. nutrition
   c. long neck with heavy weight - "result of abnormal forces" -
   d. osteochondrosis
   e. trauma or minimal repeated traumatic event
6. Treatment
   a. medical
   b. surgical
      1. ventral decompression
      2. ventral decompression with fusion with or without distraction
      3. dorsal decompressive laminectomy
      4. dorsal decompressive laminectomy with arthrodesis of articular processes
      5. stabilization with screwing
      6. stabilization with dorsal spinous process plating
      7. stabilization with pins positioned by methylmethacrolate cement
      8. disc fenestration with hope of fusion

Cervicothoracic Lesions in Four Dogs

Radiographic diagnosis of lesions at the cervicothoracic junction is somewhat unique because of the difficulty in obtaining satisfactory positioning of the spine and because of the overlying shadows created by the shoulders. For these reasons, you are invited to look at four cases some of which had lower motor neuron lesions in the thoracic limbs and others in which the cervicothoracic lesion was something of a surprise.

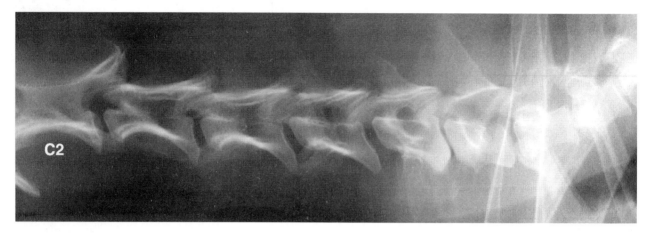

Case Description

"**Major**" is a 4-year-old male Doberman Pinscher who has incoordination in both pelvic limbs. Proprioception appears to be slow.

Radiographic Findings

The noncontrast lateral radiograph with the head in a neutral position shows narrowing of C6-7 disc space with end plate sclerosis and spondylosis deformans. Small amounts of calcified nucleus are dorsal to this disc. Note the malalignment at C5-6 with widening of the disc space. A flexed study (below) shows the full extent of the malalignment at C5-6 and indicates instability. The cranial vertebral foramina are small in both C5 and C6. The diagnosis on the noncontrast study is a suspect cervical spondylopathy with a Type II disc protrusion with canal stenosis especially marked at the cranial portion of C6 ("wobbler" syndrome).

Only a myelogram can demonstrate the specific nature of the cord compression and determine if it is due to a protruding disc at C6-7 or hypertrophy of the interarcuate ligament at C5-6. The disc causes a dorsal protrusion from the floor of the canal while the dorsal ligament plays a role in spinal stenosis by creating a dorsal mass that protrudes ventrally and both are exaggerated by dorsal extension of the head.

Comment

"Major" had a ventral fenestration and decompression at C6-7 and a spinal fusion using bone grafts. Unfortunately, he died from an acute bronchopneumonia 5 days after the surgery.

Note the apparent lucent cavities within the center of the bodies of C3-6. This is a normal radiographic pattern created by the short vertebral arches on these vertebrae.

"Major" is typical of a "wobbler" patient in that the neutral study suggests one location of the lesion while the stress studies indicates a second location.

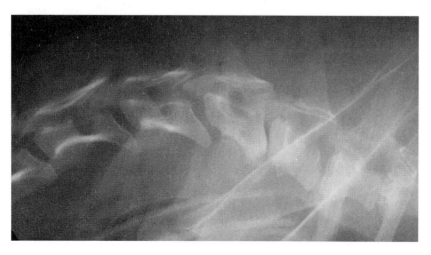

Case Description

"Tanya" is an 11-year-old female toy poodle that had a thoracic radiographic study made in a search for pulmonary metastatic disease secondary to the discovery of an adenocarcinoma located near the right temporomandibular joint. No clinical signs related to the spine were reported although she was debilitated and was receiving a general medical evaluation.

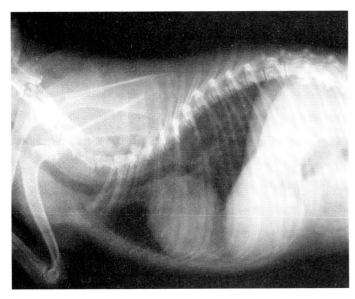

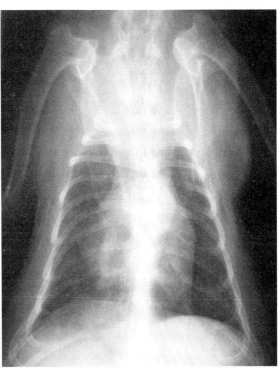

Radiographic Findings

As is typical for an older dog, "Tanya" has a lot of radiographic changes in the spine. The thoracic radiographs show a marked lordosis centering on the cervicothoracic region with a kyphosis centering on the T13. Collapse of the disc spaces at C5-6 and C6-7 are seen with a minimal spondylosis deformans at C6-7 (see enlarged view below). Note the vertebral canal is normal in height.

Hypoplasia of the spinous processes of T4 and T5 seems to be associated with incomplete formation of the arches including the articular facets. Collapse of the disc spaces at T12-13 and T13-L1 is complete with end plate sclerosis and spondylosis deformans. No radiographic evidence of pulmonary metastasis was seen.

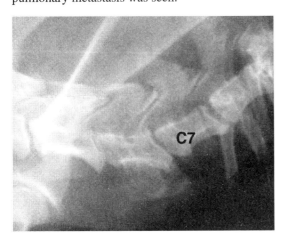

C7

Comment

"Tanya" is a classic patient in which you are searching for evidence of pulmonary metastatic disease and find instead a series of congenital and degenerative lesions that all may potentially be associated with prominent neurological signs or all can be clinically silent. The caudal cervical discs are completely destroyed with end plate contacting end plate but apparently without dorsal herniation of nuclear tissue. The TL discs have degenerated in a manner that is typical for small breeds of dogs with a resulting kyphosis, marked sclerosis of the end plates, vertebral osteophytes, but with no evidence of disc tissue within the vertebral canal. Congenital hypoplasia of the cervical and midthoracic spinous processes could be associated with pedicle hypoplasia and canal stenosis but that does not cause a problem in this dog. None of these patterns were thought to be threatening enough to suggest myelography. Still, it is interesting to think how "Tanya's" myelogram might appear.

The cranial mediastinum as seen on the dorsoventral view is widened. A change of this type in a smaller dog is often due to fat accumulation, however, "Tanya" is not particularly obese. Remember that she has an adenocarcinoma in the retropharyngeal region and the enlarged mediastinum may result from metastasis to lymph nodes.

Case Description

"**Baron**" is an 11-year-old male Doberman Pinscher with 6 to 7 months history of irregular gait in the hind limbs. The "toenails" are worn on all feet indicating proprioceptive deficits. He has a stiff gait in the front limbs and prefers to hold his head in a flexed position.

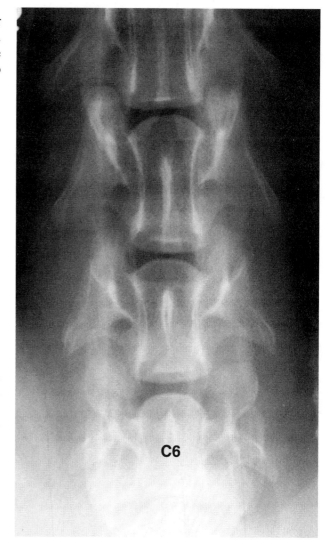

Radiographic Findings

The radiographic changes on the noncontrast studies (seen on this page) consist of collapse of C6-7 with secondary spondylosis deformans and sclerotic end plates. A myelogram was performed to further evaluate a possible disc protrusion at C6-7.

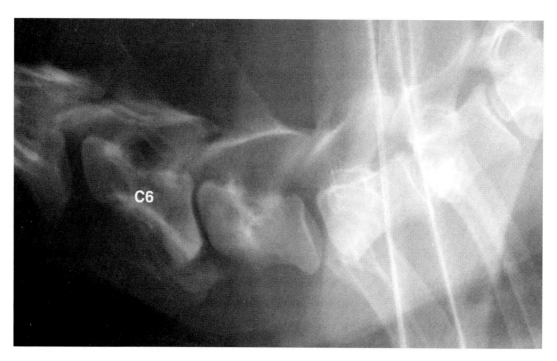

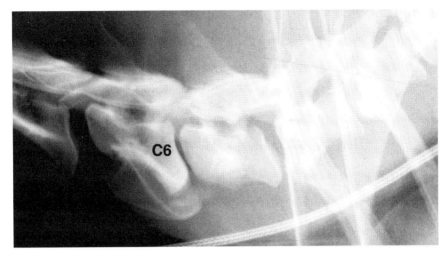

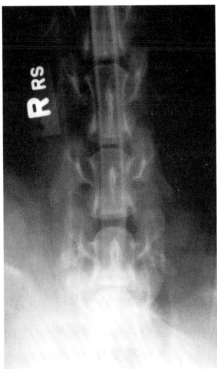

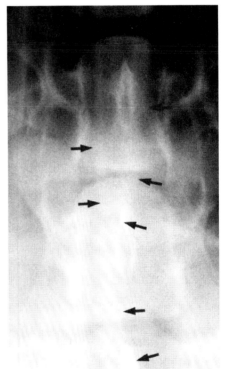

Myelographic Findings

The myelographic changes (seen on this page) include spinal cord elevation at C6-7 with compression and narrowing of both dorsal and ventral subarachnoid columns. The contrast columns are identified on the enlarged VD view (arrows) and show a large left sided extradural mass that appears to extend caudally to include the C7-T1 region (arrows).

The diagnosis is a cervical spondylopathy with a Type II dorsal protrusion of C6-7 disc and resulting cord compression. We are left with the idea that the extradural mass extends further caudally, but are not provided with good radiographic evidence. The failure to make additional ventrodorsal views centered at the cervicothoracic junction is a technical error in evaluation of this patient.

Comments

"Baron" was treated medically and was lost to "follow-up".

The myelographic injection was made at the cerebellomedullary cistern and 7cc was required to obtain a flow of the contrast agent caudal to the lesion. The possibility of postmyelographic seizures is greatly increased because of the increase in flow of the contrast agent into the subarachnoid space around the brain because of the resistance to flow caudally around the obstructive lesion.

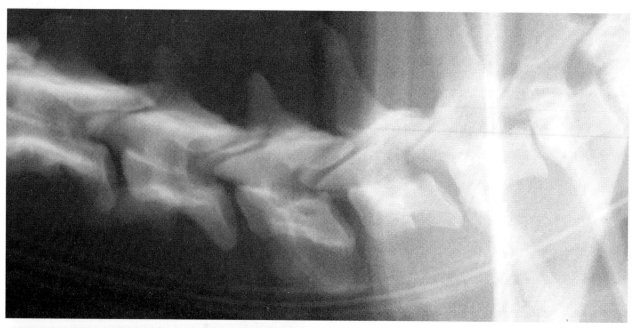

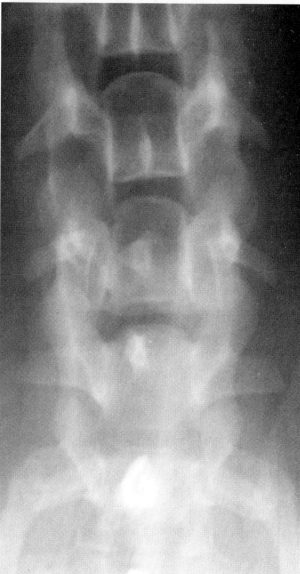

Case Description

"Bo" is a 1-year-old male spaniel who was playing and fell or was hit by another dog in a manner that appeared to cause a brachial plexus injury. The dog was immediately ataxic leading to quadraparesis with UMN signs in the hind limbs and LMN signs in the forelimbs. The left forelimb showed anesthesia. These signs lead to the study of the cervicothoracic region.

Radiographic Findings

The noncontrast radiographs seen on this page were thought to be radiographically normal and we proceeded to the contrast study.

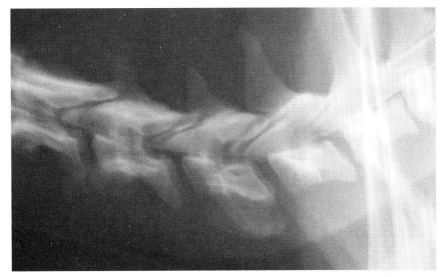

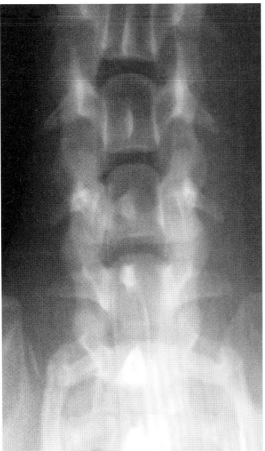

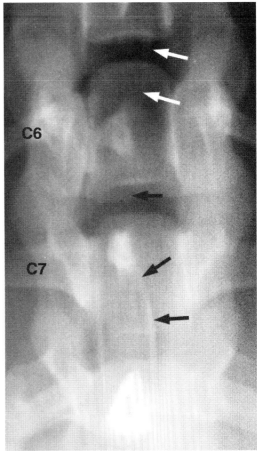

Myelographic Findings

The myelographic study shows a large left sided extradural mass at C6-7 best seen on the detail view (arrows). The centering of an additional view on the cervicothoracic junction is helpful in seeing the lesion more clearly.

Comments

Because of the clinical history, a traumatic disc protrusion, extradural hemorrhage, or nerve root injury were all considered. The clinical history in this case tended to make us incorrectly rule out infection, tumor, or degenerative disc disease. We were surprised to learn that "Bo" had a nerve sheath tumor, in addition to an extradural hemorrhage thought to be trauma-induced.

Unusual Features of Myelography

The introduction of a positive contrast medium into the subarachnoid space renders the space visible and is important in predicting the location and nature of a mass lesion. The myelogram is of value in the determination of whether a vertebral canal mass is located within the spinal cord (intramedullary) or outside the dura mater (extradural). Lesions are sometimes located outside the spinal cord but within the dura (intradural-extramedullary). Often, an extradural mass, such as a nerve sheath tumor, extends along a nerve root so that it occupies an intradural location as well.

Since the contrast agent is added to the fluid already within the subarachnoid space, it influences the fluid dynamics of the CSF. As with any fluid, it will flow to the location of least resistance and it will be influenced if a stricture alters or prevents its flow. Not enough thought is given to how the flow of the fluid influences its appearance on a myelogram. Unusual features are noted in this series of myelograms. Note that often these relate to the site of injection and the speed of the injection. The cause of the myelographic features is discussed at the end of the section.

Case Description

"Shadow" is an 8-year-old male shepherd examined by a myelogram because of incoordination in the pelvic limbs. The radiograph with the needle in position was made following the test injection. The other radiograph was made 5 minutes later following the completion of the injection and removal of the needle.

Question #1
What is incoordination and what causes it?

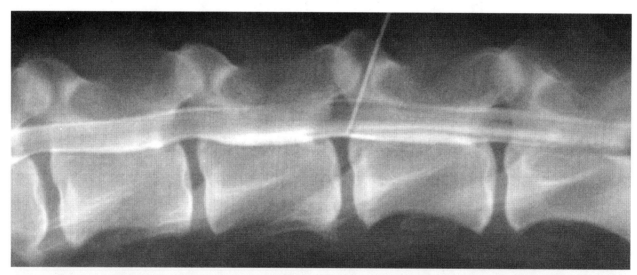

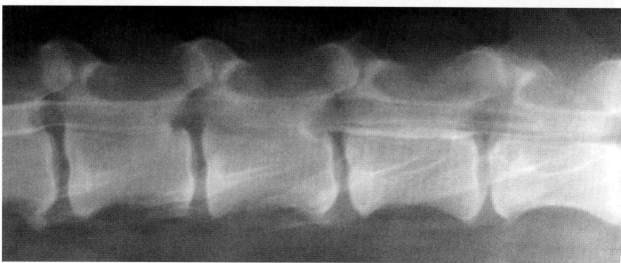

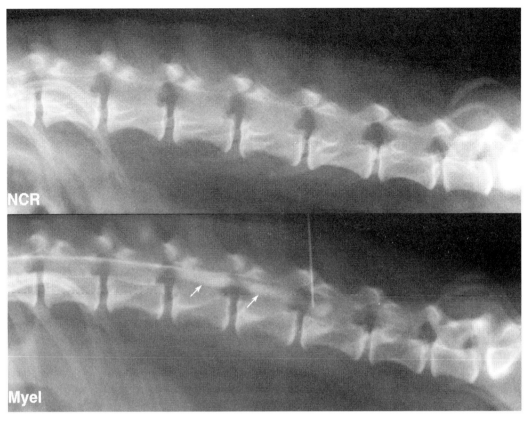

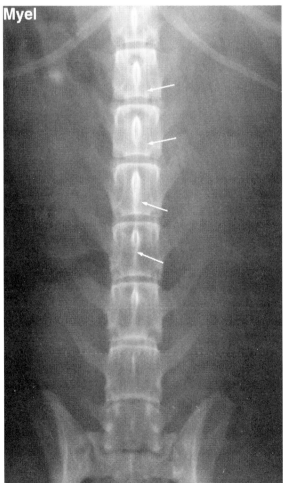

Case Description

"**Heidi**" is a 4-year-old female dachshund with paraparesis and a suspect TL disc. The noncontrast study (NCR) is followed by an attempt at myelography (Myel) in which the needle remains in position on the lateral view made after a partial injection. The needle was removed for the VD view. The distribution of the contrast agent is unusual (arrows).

Case Description

"**Buzzy**" is a 4-year-old male Lhasa Apso with paraparesis and a suspected TL disc. Noncontrast radiographs (NCR) were made and were followed by a myelogram (Myel). The needle was removed and the exposure was made immediately after a greater than expected back pressure was detected on the syringe.

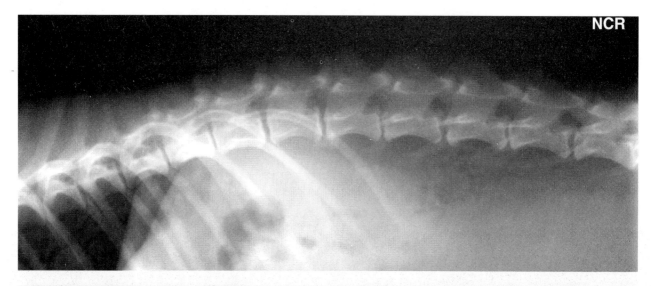

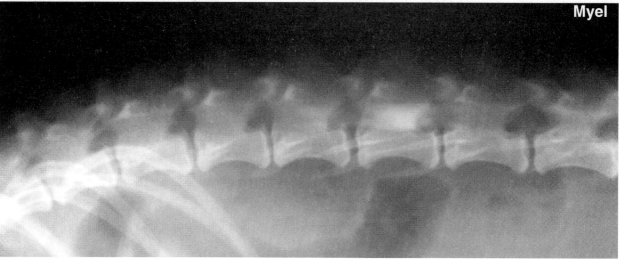

Case Description

"Sandy" is a 1-year-old female shepherd radiographed because of being in an automobile accident. She had a fracture of the maxilla and nasal bones. The arrows (detail view) point out shadows with a decreased density.

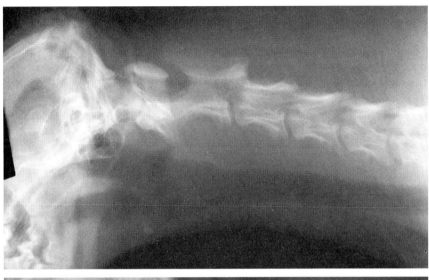

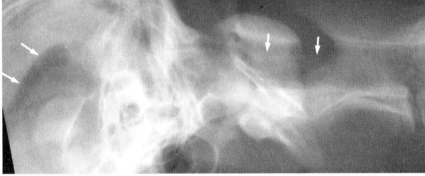

"Shadow" - Myelographic Findings

Pooling of the contrast agent was evident in "Shadow's" study made immediately after injection. The injection was made quickly and with some force which is questionable. Following completion of injection of contrast agent, the injured cord that was swollen because of edema and/or hemorrhage re-expands causing a thinning of the subarachnoid space. A pattern of this type with the expansion of subarachnoid space followed by collapse is indicative of severe cord injury and is not identified if you only have one immediate post-injection study to evaluate. "Shadow" did recover and had no further progression of the neurologic signs. Still, these studies suggest that myelography is a dynamic technique that has some risk and needs to be conducted carefully using a predetermined protocol.

"Heidi" - Myelographic Findings

"Heidi" had a myelogram performed with the needle tip in the center of the spinal cord and contrast agent was injected into the spinal cord. The contrast agent is identified in the subarachnoid space (arrows) as well as pooling within the spinal cord around the central canal (arrows). It is possible that the needle bevel permitted injection directly into the central canal. Despite the rather frightening appearance of the contrast agent accumulation within the cord, "Heidi" was discharged following medical treatment and lead a normal life until she was returned to the clinic 3 years later with recurrence of the back pain.

"Buzzy" - Myelographic Findings

"Buzzy" had a myelogram performed with the needle positioned at L4-5. A collapsed disc space had been noted at L2-3 and L4-5. A film made at 8 minutes after injection showed contrast pooling in a zone of myelomalacia while the remainder of the contrast agent had been resorbed. "Buzzy" did not respond to treatment and was euthanized.

"Sandy" - Myelographic Findings

"Sandy" has a unique myelogram as well as encephalogram. A pneumo-encephalogram and pneumomyelogram is seen on the detail view (arrows) followed the skull fractures. The last study was made (below) 10 days after the trauma and the air has resorbed. "Sandy" recovered and was released without further problem. How does the air gain entrance into the subarachnoid space?

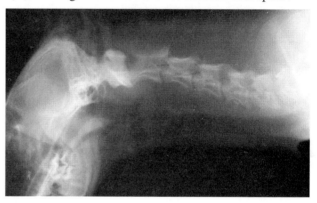

Answer #1

Incoordination is the inability to coordinate muscle activity during voluntary movement, so that smooth movements occur. Most often this clinical finding is due to disorders of the cerebellum or the spinal cord. The term ataxia is often used as a synonym for incoordination. In spinal cord diseases, incoordination is often accompanied by a decrease in muscle strength. In cerebellar disease, muscle strength is usually preserved.

Myelography with Disc Disease

Intervertebral disc disease is the most common indication for myelography in dogs because it is the most frequent spinal lesion. The specific indications for myelography in patients with a transverse myelopathy suggestive of disc disease are: (1) negative findings on noncontrast radiographs, (2) inconclusive findings on noncontrast studies, (3) multiple, widely separated herniated intervertebral discs diagnosed on noncontrast films with clinical signs that do not permit the determination of which disc is causing the neurological signs, and (3) the recurrence of clinical signs in dogs previously operated for herniated intervertebral discs in which a new herniation is suspected, or in which complications such as scar tissue formation may be present at the previous surgical site.

Another consideration in the determination of the use of myelography in diagnosis of disc disease is the age of the patient. In the younger patient you may be examining a dog with its first clinical problem with disc disease and a narrowed disc space or a small amount of calcified disc tissue within the vertebral canal may be indicative of the disc protrusion responsible for the clinical signs. However, the older dog has most likely had multiple discs that have undergone various stages of degeneration making it impossible to determine which one of the lesions seen on the noncontrast study is causing current clinical signs. Another consideration as the patient ages is that the frequency of transverse myelopathy due to other causes increases. The noncontrast study may correctly detect disc disease; however, that may not be the cause of the neurologic signs at this time and a cyst, abscess, or tumor may lie unobserved within the vertebral canal unless a myelogram is performed.

Recent review of a group of both old and young dogs has shown that when features identified on noncontrast radiographic studies are compared with those seen with myelography, the conclusions made from evaluation of the noncontrast study contain false positive or false negative findings in over 50% of the patients. The frequency of error increases in the nonchondrodystrophoid breeds and in the older dogs. Therefore, despite the possible exceptions listed above, it should be a rule that prior to surgery for suspected disc disease a myelogram should be performed.

Soft Tissue Tumors within the Vertebral Canal

Most soft tissue masses found within the vertebral canal are disc protrusions or extrusions which create an extradural mass. Extradural masses are external to the dura mater and displace the meninges and spinal cord by compressing these structures. Another group of soft tissue masses within the vertebral canal is that of tumors that originate from the meninges or neural tissue. These tumors may be extradural and appear similar radiographically to disc herniations. Tumors may also originate from tissue within the dura mater. Intradural tumors fall into two groups. Tumors internal to the dura mater but external to the pia mater are termed intradural-extramedullary tumors. Tumors internal to the pia mater are called intramedullary tumors. Most of the specific tumor types have a predilection for a particular location (e.g., spinal cord astrocytomas are intramedullary tumors). All of these tumors offer unique radiographic features on the myelogram. Few cause any pattern of change to the vertebrae and are therefore not identified on noncontrast studies.

Examine the noncontrast radiographs (NCR) and the myelograms (Myel) of these dogs to determine the nature of the tumor (arrows). With this knowledge, you have information regarding the feasibility of surgical removal of the mass and some indication as to tumor type.

Case Description

"**Torri**" is a 1-year-old female Doberman Pinscher with a 2 month history of progressive paraparesis.

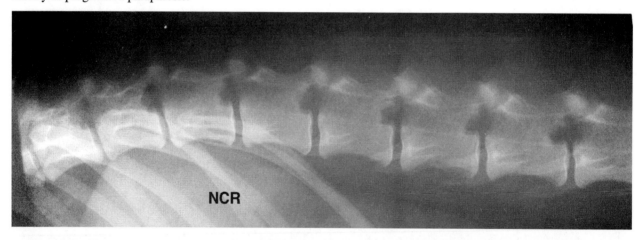

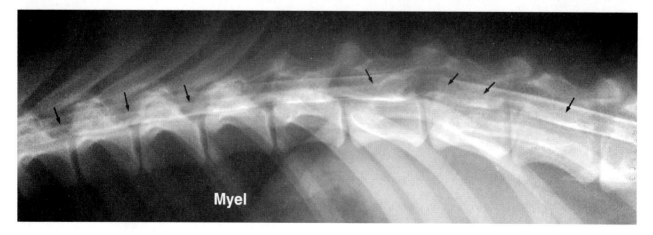

Case Description

"**Charlie**" is a 10-year-old male spaniel who became lame in the left thoracic limb five weeks ago. The lameness was followed by weakness that has progressed to a nonambulatory quadriparesis. The deficits are worse on the right side.

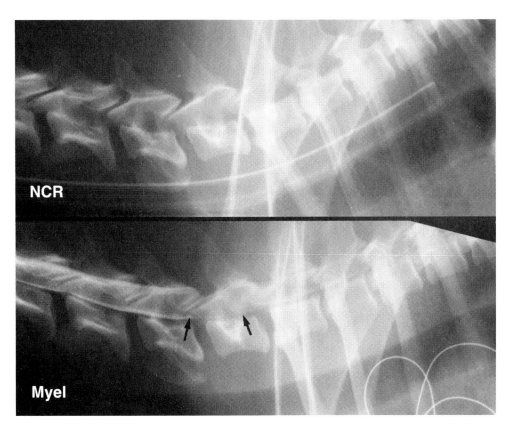

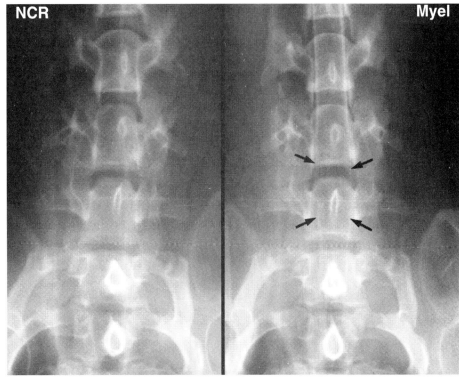

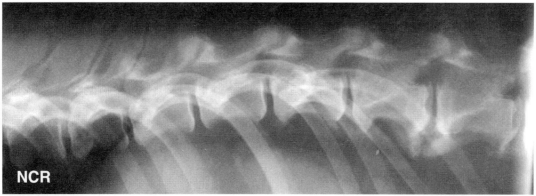

NCR

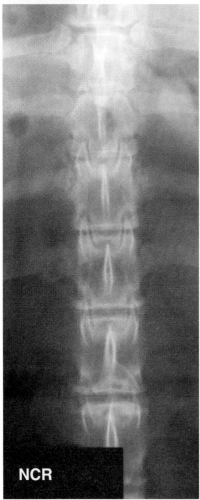

NCR

Case Description

"**Anastasia**" is a 9-year-old female Weimeraner who had a sudden onset of ambulatory paraparesis 2 weeks ago. Proprioceptive placing was absent in the pelvic limbs, the patellar reflexes were exaggerated, and pain perception appeared to be normal.

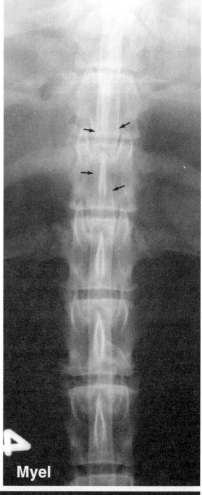

Myel

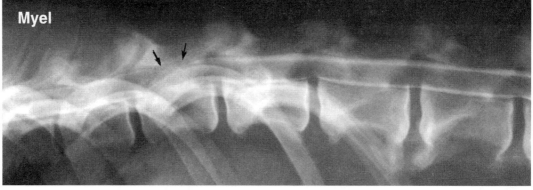

Myel

Case Description

"**Zeb**" is a 6-year-old male crossbreed dog with a history of quadriparesis/ataxia, shifting forelimb lameness, and a stiff-legged gait for nearly a year. Proprioceptive deficits were noted in all four limbs. He shows signs of pain on movement of the head. The lesion was localized to C1-C5. Because of the cervical location, the myelogram was performed via cerebellomedullary cistern injection.

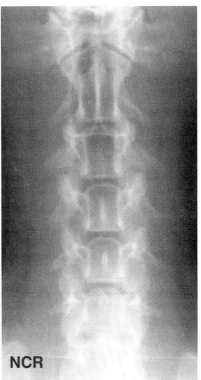

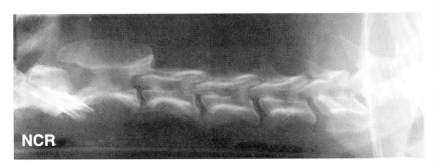

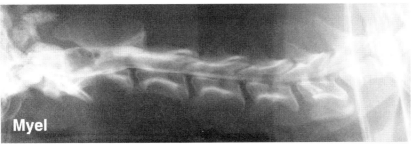

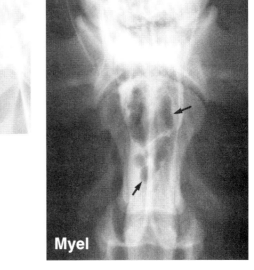

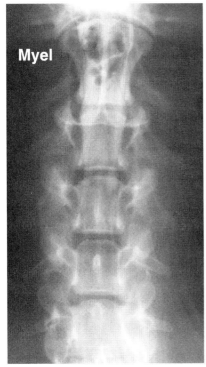

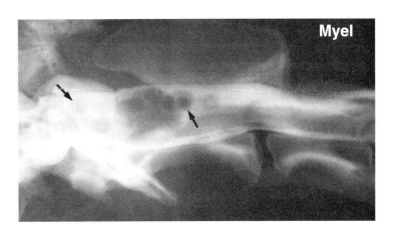

"Torri" - Radiographic Findings

"Torri" has a T12-13 lesion causing a small dorsal elevation of the ventral subarachnoid column and a narrowing of the dorsal subarachnoid column. This lesion could be a T12-13 disc protrusion. However, other radiographic features are helpful in making a diagnosis. The central canal has filled with contrast agent (arrows) and abruptly elevates over a midcord (medullary) mass. Also, the ventral subarachnoid column cranial to the mass is widened and suddenly narrows at the site of the lesion. Abrupt change in width of contrast columns is more suggestive of a tumor mass. The tumor was an ependymoma, 1 cm in length and 0.5 cm in diameter that replaced much of the cord and tapered to a point cranially and caudally. This was an intramedullary mass.

"Charlie" - Radiographic Findings

"Charlie" has a lesion at C6-7 that causes abrupt widening of the cord and thinning of the subarachnoid columns (arrows). The degree of widening of the cord is made more difficult to evaluate since it is at the site of the cervical enlargement. A diagnosis of intramedullary mass could be made except for the clinical history, site of the lesion, and one small radiographic feature. Starting with the radiographic feature, there is a tendency for the ventral subarachnoid column to widen slightly just as it comes in contact with the mass, thus appearing more as an intradural-extramedullary mass. Also the interface of the column with the mass is irregular, not smooth as would be expected if the cord were swollen. The clinical signs suggest a lesion that had laterality and finally, nerve sheath tumors are often found at the cervicothoracic junction. The tumor was a schwannoma that was associated with the nerve roots. Surgical removal was attempted but was incomplete.

Remember that an extradural mass must cause narrowing of the spinal cord. This cord narrowing may be seen on two views or may be seen on one view with widening of the spinal cord seen on the other view. In uncommon cases, the cord and subarachnoid spaces may appear of normal width on conventional lateral and VD views and cord or subarachnoid column narrowing may only be seen on oblique views.

"Anastasia" -Radiographic Findings

"Anastasia" has a mass lesion at T12 that causes focal displacement and thinning of the subarachnoid columns. The cord is compressed and shifted in position by a mass that is dorsal and left sided (arrows). These features are typical of an extradural mass, which would usually be considered to result from an expulsion of nuclear tissue from a disc. However, the signs of disc degeneration at that site are limited to a small vertebral osteophyte at T13 with no end plate sclerosis or disc space narrowing. Also, the dorsolateral location of the mass is a bit unusual for a disc herniation. Therefore, an extradural lesion has been identified but a specific diagnosis has not been reached.

At surgery a meningioma was removed. "Anastasia" developed pancreatitis and pelvic limb edema due to venous thrombosis and was necropsied 10 days postoperatively. No additional neoplastic tissue was found on sections of the spinal cord at that time.

On the lateral view, a rather unique bony shadow is seen at T13 that appears as a bone-dense mass within the vertebral canal. This mass is not seen within the vertebral canal on the ventrodorsal view. Careful examination of the right 13th costovertebral joint shows prominent hyperplasia of that articulation that creates a bony mass that is superimposed on the vertebral canal on the lateral view.

"Zeb" - Radiographic Findings

"Zeb" has a mass lesion at C1-2 that widens the dorsal subarachnoid column at the cranial and caudal edges of the mass. The altered contrast column resembles two golf tees laid broad-end to broad-end. This appearance is termed a "tee" sign. The contrast lines narrow but remain smooth ventrally while dorsally the narrowing is associated with a nodular pattern. The contrast columns as seen on the VD view are both narrow. The mass appears to have a nodular appearance resembling a bunch of grapes with several filling defects within the contrast column both cranial and caudal to the principal mass. The total mass causes displacement of the cord and subarachnoid column ventrally. These features are indicative of an intradural-extramedullary mass. The pathologic diagnosis was meningioma.

General Comment

A tumor produces its effect on the spinal cord or nerve roots by direct pressure on the neural elements and by interference with circulation. This usually causes a transverse myelopathy, although meningopathy or radiculopathy is also possible, producing predominately pain and lameness such as "Charlie" had. As with transverse myelopathies in general, the signs are usually bilateral and may be asymmetric. Unilateral signs may appear early in the course of the disorder. The rate of progression is usually slow, but occasionally clinical signs appear suddenly, as with "Anastasia", and progress so rapidly that they resemble severe infectious myelopathies or even traumatic myelopathies. Rarely, a tumor such as feline lymphosarcoma invades and ascends or descends the vertebral canal, producing clinical signs suggestive of a disseminated myelopathy.

When to Use Compression Technique?

Techniques are available that you can utilize to improve radiographic quality. In addition to a compression study, oblique views and "cone-down" views are used.

Case Description

"**Cindy**" is a 7-year-old female beagle being radiographed for diagnosis of lumbar pain.

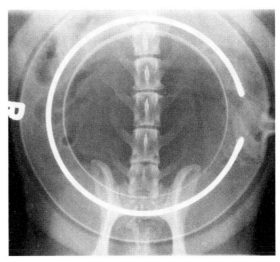

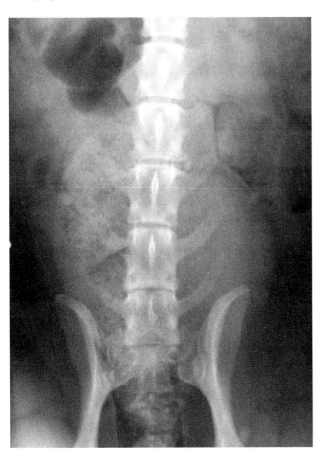

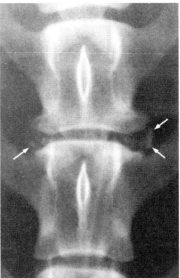

Radiographic Findings

The noncontrast VD radiograph on the right shows a suspect calcified disc at L4-5 but does not clearly identify a protrusion.

Compression Study

A compression study (above) using a circular compression paddle permits identification of lateral herniation of calcified disc material seen best on the detail view (arrows).

Comments

The lateral herniation is unlikely to be clinically important but it clearly demonstrates the degeneration of the disc and explains the density adjacent to the disc. This pair of radiographs shows how the use of a compression paddle can move fecal material and gas-filled bowel loops aside and permit better visualization of the spine on a VD view. The compression paddle has a metal ring and an inflatable bladder that protrudes permitting movement of abdominal organs. Note the additional effect of collimating the primary x-ray beam through the use of a smaller field of exposure.

Question #1

What is the next step in diagnosis of "Cindy's" problem?

Answer on next page.

Answer #1

Analysis of lumbar CSF fluid. The CSF of animals with disc protrusion is variable and depends on the rate at which the cord compression occurred, the severity of the cord compression, and the time since the compression occurred. The pattern of abnormality is essentially that of trauma with acute protrusions (generally Type I) or trauma with chronic compression (generally Type II). The CSF associated with chronic compression may be normal or have a mild to moderate elevation of total protein content. If the CSF changes are inflammatory in nature, other causes of inflammation must be included on the list of differential diagnoses (e.g., microbial myelitis, parasitic myelitis, granulomatous meningoencephalomyelitis, immune-mediated myelitis, or neoplasia). The pattern of CSF changes associated with chronic disc protrusion may also be produced by degenerative myelopathies and neoplasia.

Patterns of Myelographic Changes

The introduction of a positive contrast medium into the subarachnoid space renders the space visible and allows evaluation of lesions that may be divided into three groups: (1) intramedullary, (2) intradural-extramedullary, or (3) extradural disease. The pattern of change is of value in the prediction of the etiology of the mass lesion and specifies the location of a vertebral canal mass relative to the spinal cord (intramedullary) or outside the dura mater (extradural). Lesions are sometimes located outside the spinal cord but within the dura (intradural-extramedullary). Often, an extradural mass extends along a nerve root so that it occupies an intradural location as well. This unique pattern is most frequently identified with a nerve sheath tumor.

Extradural masses are usually noncontained nucleus pulposus from degenerating intervertebral discs (Type I disc disease) or a contained nucleus pulposus within a protruding anulus fibrosus (Type II disc disease). Chronic Type I disc disease eventually forms a fibrotic mass referred to as a Type III disease. Extradural masses can be recognized radiographically because they: (1) displace the spinal cord on at least one view, (2) narrow one or more of the subarachnoid columns, and (3) narrow the spinal cord on at least one view. A unique feature of an extradural mass occurs if it causes marked displacement of the spinal cord to the degree that the cord is compressed and actually appears widened on the opposite view. The features just described may be limited to only a single vertebral segment or may extend for a longer distance of the spinal cord, depending on the nature of the extradural mass. Minimally protruding discal tissue may cause a narrowing of the subarachnoid columns and slight displacement of the spinal cord, but do not cause narrowing of the spinal cord. This type of finding is common in the older patient and may indicate a lesion of less clinical importance.

In addition to commonly found ruptured nucleus pulposus or protruding discal tissue, other types of extradural masses include: (1) benign osteochondromas, (2) primary bone tumors, (3) metastatic bone tumors, (4) primary or metastatic tumors originating within the soft tissues around the spinal cord, (5) bony or fibrous callus secondary to trauma or surgery, (6) hemorrhage/hematoma, (7) exudate/abscess, (8) developmental spinal stenosis plus those forms of stenosis caused by a congenital vertebral vertebrae such as block or cleft vertebrae, hemivertebrae, or transitional vertebrae, (9) hypertrophied ligamentum flavum, (10) synovial cysts, and (11) hypertrophied joint capsule from the true vertebral joints.

Intradural-extramedullary masses occur within the subarachnoid space and are recognized radiographically by the typical sharply defined golf "tee" sign or "cup" sign, as the contrast in the subarachnoid space widens as it comes in contact with the mass. The contrast column tapers as it moves away from the mass, producing the "tail" of the golfer's "tee". These lesions tend to be eccentric and are usually seen best on one projection. They commonly are malignant and are often meningiomas or nerve sheath tumors.

Intramedullary masses lie within the spinal cord and thus produce a widening of the cord as seen on all projections. The subarachnoid column is uniformly narrowed due to the expanding tumor mass. The most common intramedullary masses are malignant tumors such as meningiomas, ependymomas, astrocytomas, or metastatic tumors as well as syringomyelia cysts. A swollen cord following trauma may present with narrow subarachnoid columns and appear as an intramedullary mass.

Patterns of bony changes are seen with vertebral canal masses that are due to an enlarging tumor mass that result in an increase in the height or width of the vertebral canal. Another pattern of change is seen with slowly protruding disc tissue that is projected dorsolaterally and often causes an increase in the size of the intervertebral foramen as seen on the lateral view.

Radiographic Changes in Disc Diseases

A certain group of features can be examined on the noncontrast radiograph in an effort to diagnose disc disease.

Width of the intervertebral disc is an important parameter to be evaluated on survey radiographs. Narrowing of the width of the disc space can be confirmed by noting a normal width in the surrounding discs. In an older dog, decreased width of the disc spaces is often present as the discs slowly degenerate and is not a reliable radiographic sign of disc herniation with or without the presence of vertebral osteophytes on adjacent vertebral end plates or sclerosis of the end plates. Thus, a narrowed disc space with or without calcification in a young dog is more suggestive of an acute disc protrusion than is narrowing in an older patient. A narrow disc space can also be associated with a traumatic disc herniation or can be an early sign of discitis.

Shape of the disc space can be a diagnostic aid. Usually the adjacent vertebral end plates are parallel to each other, indicating that the disc has the same width dorsally as ventrally. A recently herniated or ruptured thoracolumbar disc often appears to have a decrease in the width of the disc dorsally and the disc appears wedge-shaped. In a young patient without the presence of secondary changes associated with chronic disc degeneration, this wedging can be an important diagnostic finding on the radiograph.

Calcification within the nucleus pulposus follows chondroid metaplasia and is much more extensive in some breeds than in others. The appearance of calcification of the nucleus pulposus may be seen most easily on the lateral projection and appears as a: (1) haziness, (2) well defined density in the midportion of the disc, (3) focal density in the dorsal or ventral portion of the nucleus, (4) ring shadow around the noncalcified center of the nucleus, or (5) amorphous pattern of calcification. Associated with these features, sharp spikes of calcified tissue within the disc may extend dorsally toward the spinal canal and suggest early nuclear herniation. Calcification of the disc can take many appearances and still be clinically insignificant because rupture or significant herniation has not occurred.

Following further degeneration of the disc, the calcified nucleus may be seen dorsally in which location it may have clinical importance. A calcified nucleus located laterally or ventrally only indicates disc degeneration without any protrusion or herniation into the spinal canal.

Types of disc degeneration

The types of disc disease in chondrodystrophoid breeds are usually chondroid with fibroid degeneration uncommon in the older dogs. The type of disc disease is usually Type l with Type II uncommon. In nonchondrodystrophoid breeds, the disc disease is usually fibroid with chondroid degeneration being uncommon. The type of disc disease is usually Type ll with Type l disease rare. Breed types influence the: (1) type of nuclear degeneration, (2) type of bony maturation, (3) relationship in size between spinal cord and vertebra, and (4) different location of spinal cord termination.

The various types of disc degeneration are:
1. Chondroid metaplasia (early)
    a. calcified nucleus pulposus
    b. intact anulus fibrosis
    c. preserved disc space
    d. normal end plates
2. Chondroid metaplasia (late)
    a. calcified nucleus pulposus
    b. partially ruptured anulus fibrosis
    c. possible nuclear herniation
    d. normal to narrowed disc space
    e. normal to sclerotic end plates
    f. no spondylosis deformans
3. Chondroid metaplasia with nuclear herniation (Type I disc disease)
    a. nucleus pulposus is sequestered within the vertebral canal
    b. disc space normal to narrow
    c. end plate normal
    d. no spondylosis deformans
4. Fibroid metaplasia (early)
    a. normal radiographic appearance
5. Fibroid metaplasia (late)
    a. degenerated nucleus pulposus
    b. degenerated anulus fibrosis
    c. disc space narrow
    d. end plates with sclerosis
    e. spondylosis deformans
6. Fibroid metaplasia with nuclear protrusion (early Type II disc disease)
    a. nucleus pulposus remains within the distorted, protruding anulus
    b. disc space normal to narrow
    c. end plates normal to sclerotic
    d. spondylosis deformans absent to minimal
7. Fibroid metaplasia with nuclear protrusion (late Type II disc disease)
    a. nucleus pulposus remains within the distorted, protruding anulus
    b. narrowed to collapsed disc spaces
    c. end plates minimal to moderate sclerosis
    d. spondylosis deformans minimal to moderate
8. Chronic disc protrusion (Type III disc disease)
    a. calcified nuclear tissue in vertebral canal
    b. narrow disc space
    c. end plates sclerotic
    d. spondylosis deformans prominent

Which Lesion Is Important?

These cases address the problem of an animal with a myelopathy having a congenital lesion of the spine that may or may not be the cause of the myelopathy. Many spinal malformations do not involve or affect the spinal cord. Therefore, these lesions must be assessed carefully, while considering that another lesion may be the real culprit. The first step in assessing the role of a congenital lesion in the cause of a myelopathy is accurate neuroanatomic localization of the lesion via a complete neurologic examination. If the location of the congenital lesion identified radiographically does not agree with the neuroanatomical location of the lesion, than the search for the cause of the neuroanatomic lesion must continue.

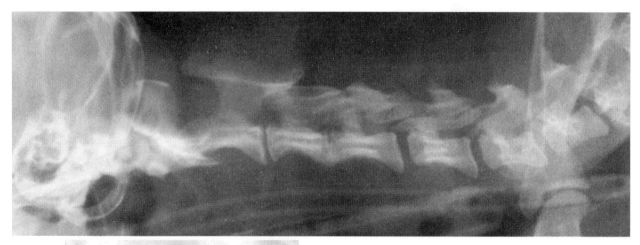

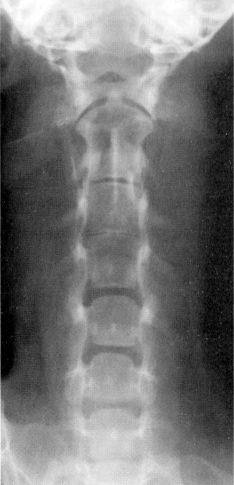

Case Description

"**Trinket**" is a 2-year-old female toy poodle that was radiographed because of weakness in the pelvic limbs that prevented her from going up stairs. Lately the owner has noted "Trinket" seemed painful when handled.

Radiographic Findings

The radiographs show a block vertebra malformation, i.e. failure of embryonic segmentation of C3-4. The malformation involves the vertebral bodies and the vertebral arches.

Comments

The majority of block vertebrae do not cause any clinical problem. In "Trinket", the block vertebra was not associated with vertebral instability, malalignment or stenosis of the vertebral canal, any of which could cause spinal cord compression and pain. "Trinket" did have herniated discs at L1-2 and L2-3, which were believed to be the cause of her neurologic problem.

Case Description

"**Melissa**" is a 6-year-old cocker spaniel cross with a 4-months history of intermittent back pain.

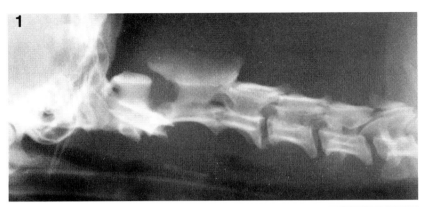

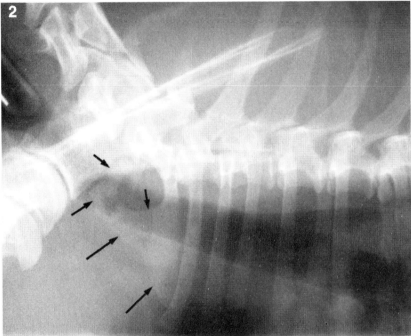

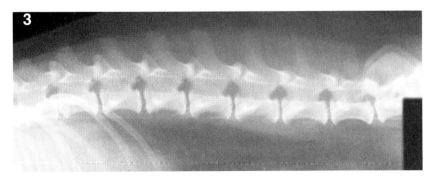

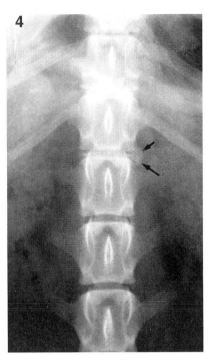

Radiographic Findings

The radiographs show; (1) block vertebra at C2-3 (figure 1), (2) congenitally malformed first rib on the right that articulates with a cervical rib from C7 (arrows) (figure 2), (3) 8 lumbar type vertebrae (figure 3), and (4) a calcified disc at T12-L1 that is seen on the VD view to have herniated laterally (arrows) (figure 4).

"Melissa" has several congenital spinal anomalies, none of which are of clinical importance. The disc disease of the T12-L1 disc is severe but appears to have herniated laterally to the right. The owners left us without a diagnosis and decided to take "Melissa" home without further work-up.

Question #1

Name a vertebral malformation that is much more likely to cause a myelopathy than is a block vertebra.

Answer #1

Hemivertebrae, because the malaligned vertebrae may compress the spinal cord, or the spinal column may be unstable in the area of the hemivertebrae allowing vertebral luxation with resultant cord compression.

Four Dogs with Spondylosis Deformans

Heavy new bone formation is often noted on radiographs of the spine where the vertebral spurs attempt to bridge intervertebral disc spaces. Often the pattern of new bone surrounds a disc that has undergone degeneration characterized by disc space narrowing and end plate sclerosis. Thus, the spurs often appear to be stabilizing a weakened disc. Only the bony portion of the reactive lesion is radiographically opaque, while the fibrocartilaginous portion remains radiolucent.

The pattern is most easily identified on lateral views of the lumbar spine because of its superimposition over the soft tissues of the abdomen. The spurs also project laterally but are difficult to identify on the VD view because of the overlying bowel shadows. Spondylosis deformans is also easily identified in the cervical spine. Spondylosis deformans in the thoracic spine is less well developed and may not be seen because of the use of a less-powerful x-ray beam in making thoracic studies.

Of minimal clinical importance, the reactive bone is found in all dogs and cats becoming more prominent with increasing age. The bony spurs are an important radiographic pattern since they can superimpose either destructive or productive patterns of more clinically important disease.

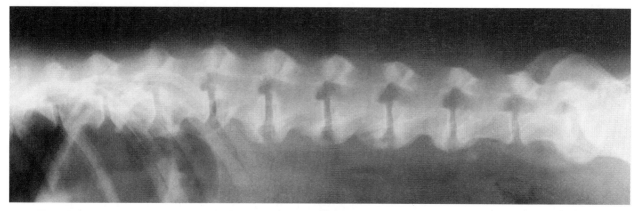

"Tara" is a 12-year-old female retriever with a history of depression. The abdominal radiographs show the typical appearance of spondylosis deformans. The disc spaces are not as collapsed in this patient as usually seen with spondylosis deformans.

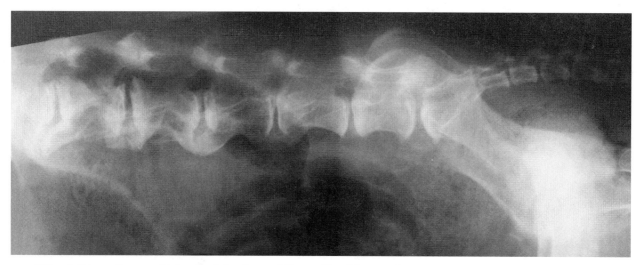

"Shorty" is an 8-year-old female Saint Bernard Dog with a history of surgical removal of a mammary gland tumor. Note that if the spurs mature and bridge the disc spaces, the ventral cortex of the vertebral bodies is modeled and the cortex of the spondylosis deformans forms a neocortex for the vertebrae.

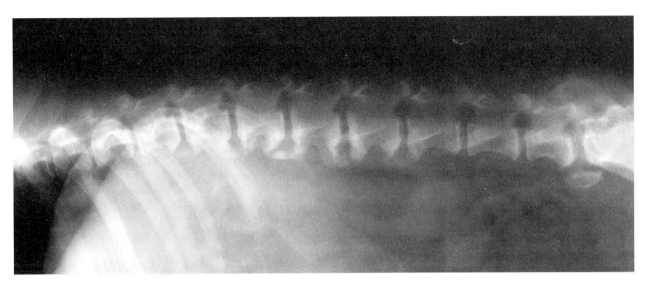

"**Ferdinand**" is a 13-year-old male spaniel with a history of vomiting ultimately proven to be the result of an intestinal adenocarcinoma. The spondylosis deformans at the LS junction is somewhat unique in that the new bone does not appear to be attached. This pattern is commonly seen at this location.

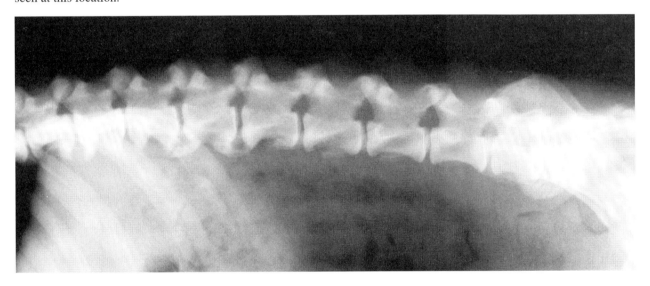

"**George**" is a 9-year-old male spaniel with a history of surgical removal of a leiomyosarcoma. The spondylosis deformans has formed more strongly at the TL and LS junctions. This is a typical pattern of presentation. Note that there is often periarticular new bone around the articular facets dorsally.

Comment

Spondylosis deformans occurs very commonly in middle-aged and older dogs, and commonly does not produce any clinical problem. Therefore, in animals with spinal pain or myelopathies and spondylosis deformans, every diagnostic effort is made to identify a cause for the clinical problem other than the spondylosis. Spondylosis deformans could cause radicular pain or radiculopathy if the osteophytes compress a spinal nerve as it emerges from its intervertebral foramen, but this is either uncommon or rarely diagnosed as such. Spinal cord compression by osteophytes protruding into the vertebral canal is extremely rare.

Spinal Problems in Cats

Here are a group of feline spinal cases. Given minimal history, examine these radiographs and try to make your diagnosis. Only noncontrast studies were performed. You may decide that a myelogram is necessary in order to make your diagnosis.

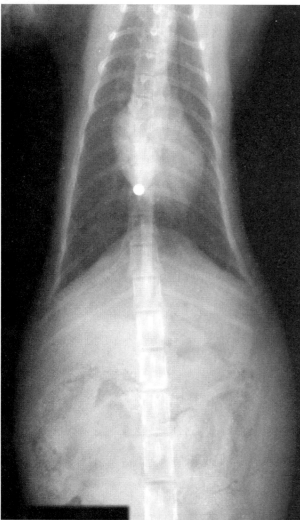

Case Description

"**Deleon**" is a domestic, short-haired cat with UMN paraplegia. A small wound is evident near the left scapula. "Whole body" radiographs were made at the referring clinic.

Question #1

Name 4 causes of sudden paraplegia or quadriplegia that would not be apparent on noncontrast spinal radiographs.

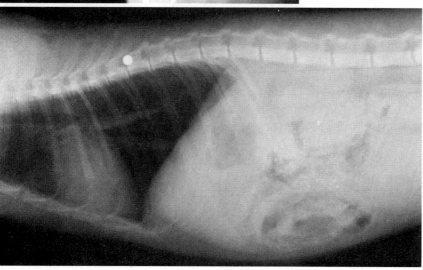

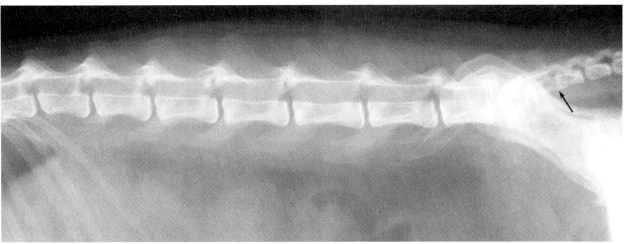

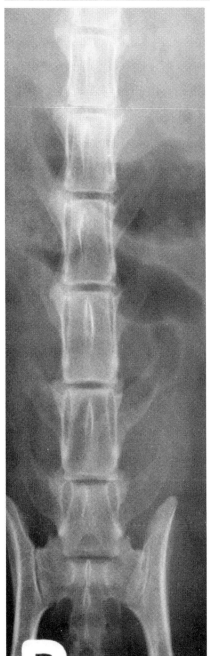

Case Description
"**Trisha**" is an 11-year-old female domestic, long-haired cat with a history of back pain. A detail VD view of L3-6 is included.

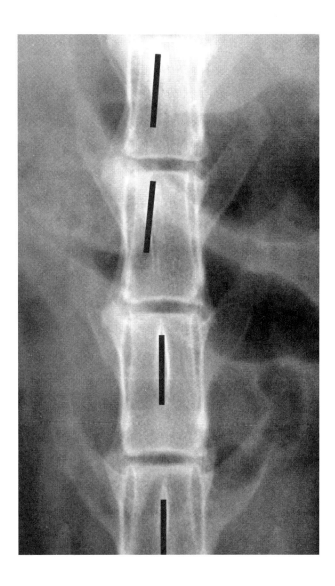

Case Description

"**Blatz**" is an 11-month-old female domestic, long-haired cat with a 10-day history of frequent attempts at urination. The tentative diagnosis is cystic calculi and cystitis. Detail lateral and VD views of the last lumbar vertebrae and pelvic are included.

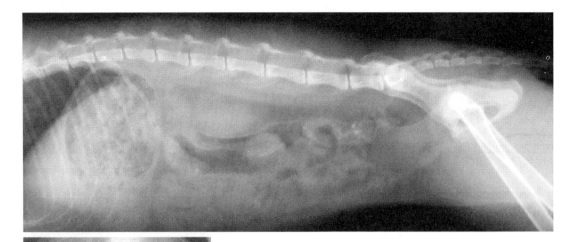

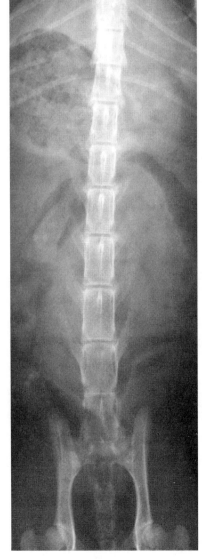

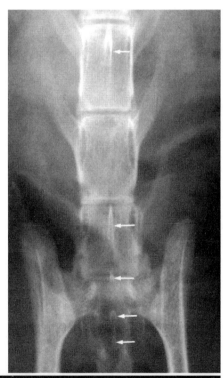

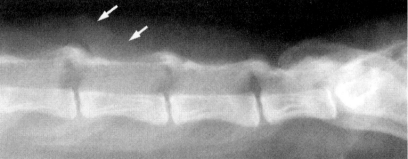

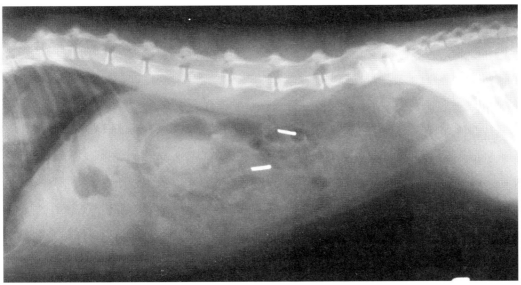

Case Description

"**Amber**" is a 2-year-old female domestic, long-haired cat with an acute history of being unable to walk normally. A detail view of the LS region is included below.

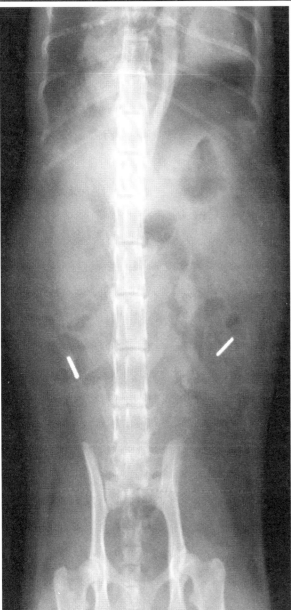

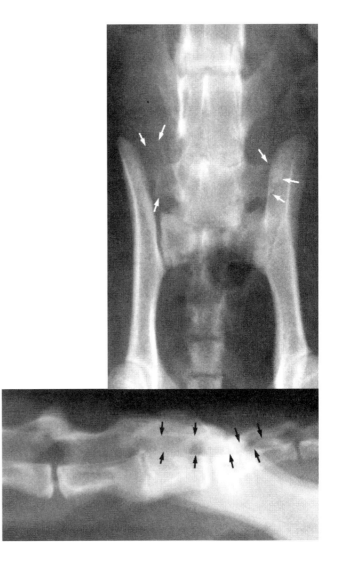

"Deleon" - Radiographic Findings

Most of the thorax and abdomen are seen on the radiographs. The small round metallic object is located within the vertebral canal at T9 and is the result of being shot by a pellet from an air gun. It seems difficult to explain how the small shot gained entrance into the canal. Localization of the foreign body requires the use of two orthogonal views. It is always risky to use "whole-body" radiographic studies of a cat, in which the cranial and caudal parts of the body are not included on the radiograph.

"Trisha" - Radiographic Findings

The radiographic findings are minimal but diagnostic. Note the malalignment of the spinous processes at L4-5 on the ventrodorsal view (lines). The disc space at L4-5 remains intact. This pattern is diagnostic of vertebral fracture-luxation. It may be appropriate to perform a myelogram in "Trisha" to determine the extent of cord injury following the apparent trauma.

"Blatz" - Radiographic Findings

The radiographs show a normal appearing spinous process at L5 (arrow) with an absence of a spinous process at L6 and widening of the pedicles indicating the possibility of a spina bifida. While the spinous process at L7 appears normal in size and shape (arrow), the pedicles are widened in that location as well. The spinous process on the first sacral vertebra appears hypoplastic (arrow) while the spinous processes on the second and third sacral vertebrae appear normal (arrows).

"Blatz" may have a spinal cord malformation associated with her vertebral malformation. However, urinary problems of recent onset in a mature animal are unlikely to be caused by a congenital malformation. She should first be worked up thoroughly for a genitourinary tract source of her problem, particularly if she does not have any neurologic deficits. If a diagnosis is not forthcoming, the spinal column, spinal cord, and cauda equina should be then be examined further.

"Amber" - Radiographic Findings

The radiographic findings may appear to you to be contradictory. The last two lumbar-type vertebrae are fused dorsally and ventrally with incompletely developed end plates with only a remnant of the disc space. The vertebral canal is stenotic as seen on the lateral view (black arrows). Paravertebral reactive bone has blended the two vertebrae together. Post-traumatic, post-infectious, and congenital causes should be considered.

Examination of the last thoracic vertebra shows a malpositioned hypoplastic rib on the left suggesting a congenital anomaly. On re-examination of the last lumbar vertebra on the ventrodorsal view, the transverse processes are short and stubby with wing-like processes that attempt to articulate with the sacrum (white arrows). All of these features suggest transitional vertebrae at the TL and LS junctions.

Careful examination of the margins of the radiographs show a pneumothorax with left caudal lung lobe congestion and mediastinal shift to the left. This is probably a traumatic pneumothorax with pulmonary hemorrhage and edema from the trauma. No post-traumatic changes are noted in the spine. Cerebrospinal fluid analysis and a myelogram are indicated to further examine the vertebral canal and spinal cord for the cause of "Amber's" problem in what may be a post-traumatic patient.

Note the prominent "white" lines in both VD and lateral views of the abdomen due to hemoclips.

The owner's decided against further diagnostic procedures. "Amber" was therefore treated medically and she eventually recovered. The owner was advised of the possibility of development of a clinically important vertebral canal stenosis that could cause a cauda equina syndrome later in her life.

Answer #1

1. Ischemic myelopathy (e.g., fibrocartilagenous embolism)

2. Neoplasia

3. Some disc protrusions: (1) Type I protrusion of calcified disc tissue that spreads out within the vertebral canal and therefore does not form a radiodense mass, (2) Type II protrusion (anular bulging) in which the protruding material is not radiodense, (3) or Type I protrusion of fibrous disc material in which the protruding material is not radiodense.

4. Concussive or hyperflexion/extension injury to the spinal cord

Cranial Cervical Mass

The cranial portion of the cervical spine is the most difficult area to evaluate on a myelogram if the injection has been made in the lumbar region. An insufficient amount of contrast agent may be injected resulting in a lack of radiopaque dye in the cervical region. Even if an appropriate volume is injected, the contrast agent may leak through the needle tract into the epidural space, or pool in the caudal subarachnoid space, also resulting in a lack of fluid in the cervical region. Examine these radiographs with these problems in mind.

Case Description

"Cubie" is a 10-year-old male Kuvasz with a 3 months history of progressive quadriparesis. He became completely recumbent 1 week ago. Clinical signs improved with prednisone therapy. "Cubie's" owner thought that he had cervical pain and had become increasingly lethargic over the past 2 years. The owner also reports that "Cubie" has lost 15 kg of body weight within the past months. A C1-C6 myelopathy was diagnosed on the basis of the neurologic examination.

The noncontrast radiographs showed a bony irregularity involving the left caudal articular facet of C1, but this lesion appeared to be a congenital anomaly or a post-traumatic lesion. No evidence of active bone destruction was present.

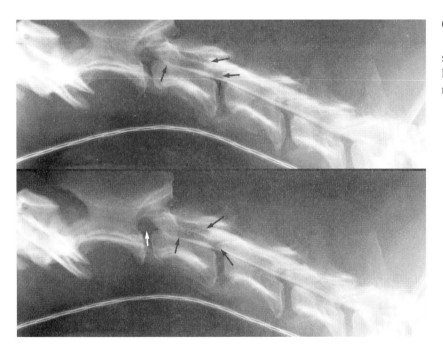

Question #1

What type of neurologic signs should "Cubie" have in his thoracic limb, upper motor neuron or lower motor neuron? In his pelvic limbs?

Myelographic Findings

Two injections in the lumbar region were required to achieve filling of the cervical region. Irregular thickness of the dorsal contrast column at C3 (black arrows) and narrowing of the ventral contrast column at C2 (white arrow) are present and indicate an intramedullary mass within the cranial cervical spinal cord. The mass appears to be restricting the flow of contrast medium.

On a ventrodorsal view (not shown), the contrast column on the left was attenuated from C3 cranially, supporting the diagnosis of an intramedullary mass.

The diagnosis is an intramedullary mass from C3 cranially toward the brain stem, with the cranial limit of the mass not identified.

Comments

"Cubie" was scheduled for removal of the mass, however, he developed pneumonia. The combination of lesions convinced the owner to not proceed with surgery and "Cubie" was discharged without a definitive diagnosis.

Re-examination of the VD radiograph showed an asymmetry of C1 strongly suggestive of a healed fracture. The myelographic lesion was therefore thought to be most likely a hematoma secondary to the trauma.

Answer #1

Upper motor neuron signs in all four limbs.

Discospondylitis with Instability

If discospondylitis becomes extensive enough, and especially if it affects the true vertebral joints, vertebral malalignment and instability results. Examine this case with this possibility in mind.

Case Description

"Yellow dog" is an 8-year-old female Labrador retriever with a 1-month history of not acting as active as usual. Today she became paraplegic. Neurological examination revealed a T3-L3 myelopathy. Noncontrast radiographs were made.

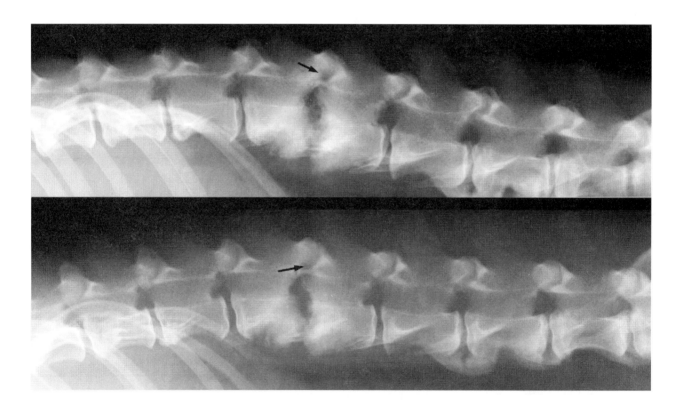

Radiographic Findings

Two lateral views of the caudal thoracic and lumbar region are included for your review. The noncontrast radiographs are diagnostic of malalignment at L2-3 with shortening of the vertebral bodies, end plate destruction, disc space collapse with destructive changes at the vertebral joints (arrows). The degree of instability or cord compression are not indicated. Stress studies were not performed because of fear of injury to the spinal cord. Instead, a myelogram was performed with the dog protected from movement of the spine during the study (see next page).

Question #1

Why did "Yellow Dog" become acutely paraplegic?

Question #2

In addition to spinal decompression and stabilization, what other therapy is essential for "Yellow Dog" to recover?

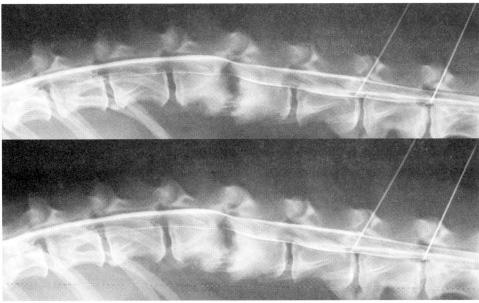

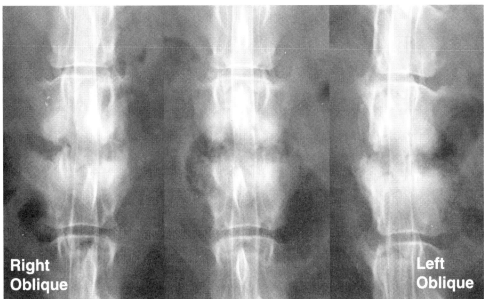

Right
Oblique

Left
Oblique

Myelographic Findings

The vertebral malalignment suggests instability and spinal cord compression on all views resulting from the discospondylitis that affects both the disc and the vertebral joints. Note spinal cord compression on both views with only slight narrowing of the subarachnoid columns. Two spinal needles were positioned in an effort to obtain a satisfactory myelogram.

Comments

A hemilaminectomy was done at L2-3 with stabilization achieved by placement of a bridge of methylmethacrylate on the lateral aspect of the spine with lag screws placed through the implant into the bodies of L1 and L4. Within 4 months, the disc space completely filled with bone tissue, creating a bony ankylosis.

Answer #1

The most likely cause of "Yellow Dog's" acute neurologic dysfunction is vertebral subluxation at the site of the discospondylitis. Usually discospondylitis does not cause neurologic deficits because it does not affect the spinal cord, only the disc and adjacent bone and soft tissue. The dorsal longitudinal ligament and meninges seem to protect the spinal cord from the infection. If the infection destroys enough spinal column tissue, instability and subluxation can occur, traumatizing and compressing the spinal cord.

Answer #2

Appropriate antibiotic therapy.

"Lucy"

Case Description

"Lucy" is an 8-year-old female Maltese that ran directly into a larger dog 12 hours ago and has been unable to walk since that time. She is in sternal recumbency. Her neck is not painful on palpation or on manipulation. The thoracic limbs have increased extensor tone, reduced placing reactions, and reduced voluntary motion. The left biceps reflex is absent, the right is present. The triceps reflexes are difficult to elicit but thought to be present. Withdrawal reflexes are present. The pelvic limbs have reduced placing reactions and reduced voluntary movement with normal spinal reflexes. The lesion was localized to the C6-7 area with possible involvement of C1-C5.

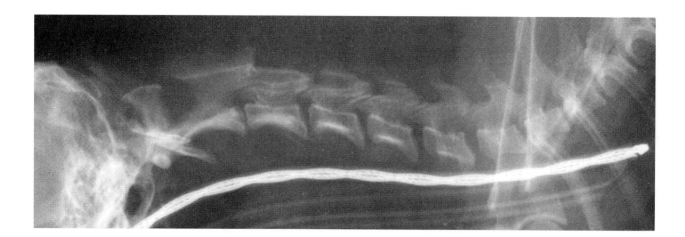

Radiographic Findings

Dorsal tipping of the cranial aspect of C4 and C5 causes minimal vertebral malalignment with wedging of the C3-4 and C4-5 disc spaces. The VD view was normal.

Note the short craniocaudal length of the C1 vertebral arch and the thinness of the occipital bone. These findings are typical for occipito-atlanto-axial dysplasia found frequently in some toy breeds. The odontoid process was normal as seen on the VD view.

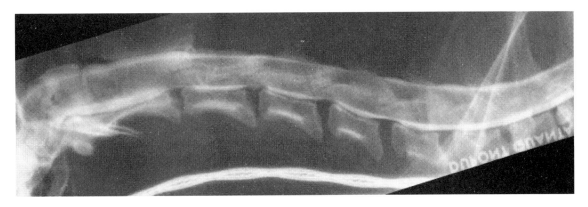

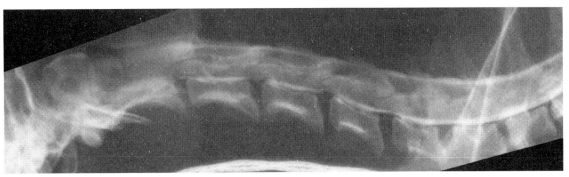

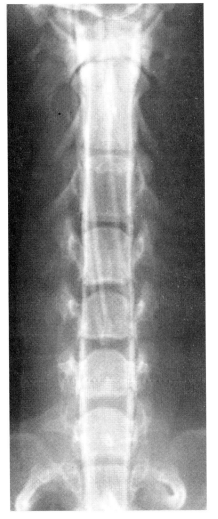

Myelographic Findings

The spinal cord appears swollen on both views suggesting a large intramedullary mass that extends from C3 to C6. The cord enlargement causes the contrast columns to be thin and displaced abaxially. Slight dorsal displacement of the ventral contrast column is seen as the cord drapes over each of the cervical discs.

Comment

The myelographic findings are consistent with cord swelling following the traumatic event. "Lucy" was discharged as a non-ambulatory quadriparetic with instruction for home care and a follow-up examination requested in 4 weeks. The owner did not return but advised the clinician that "Lucy" was clinically "ok" at that time.

The intramedullary mass pattern could be caused by a malignant process. However, the association of the clinical signs with trauma and a normal CSF made that possibility less likely and supported the diagnosis of spinal cord hemorrhage.

Spondylitis and Discospondylitis

Radiographs are helpful in determining if lesions of spondylitis and discospondylitis are becoming more destructive or are in a healing phase. While the bony changes caused by the disease process are delayed and do not provide an accurate indication of the actual stage of the lesion, sequential radiographic studies permit you to determine the general progress of the disease. Use of sequential studies is especially important in the diagnosis of certain inflammatory lesions, as you will learn from this series of patients.

Case Description

"Yasu" is a 3-month-old male Saluki with a history of Parvovirus infection at 6 weeks of age. During recovery he developed multiple abscesses and a high fever, and became painful over the back. He can walk, but he is depressed and has decreased proprioceptive placing in the pelvic limbs.

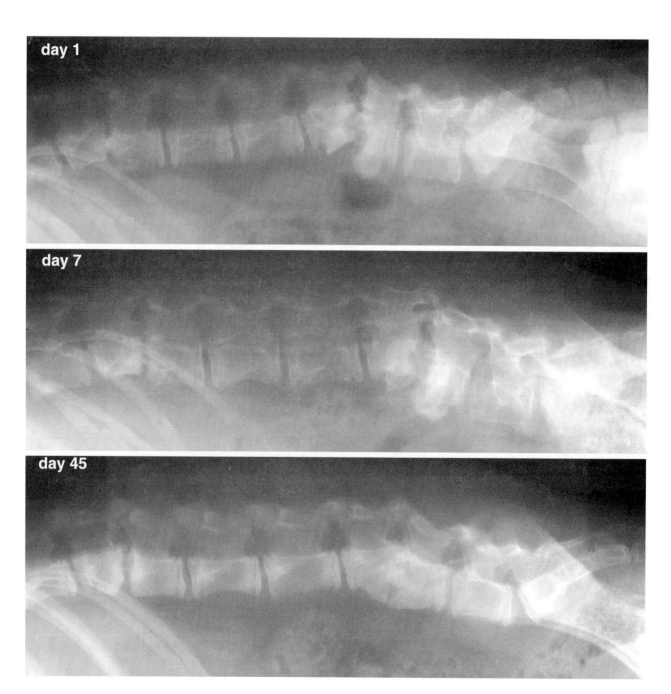

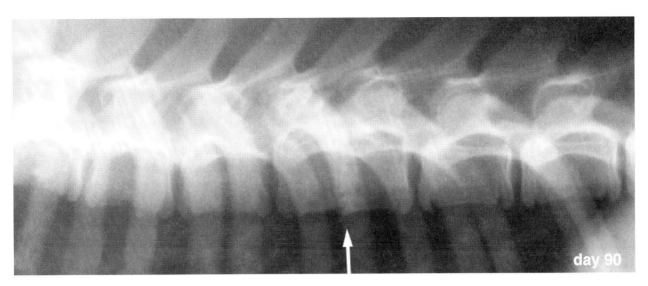

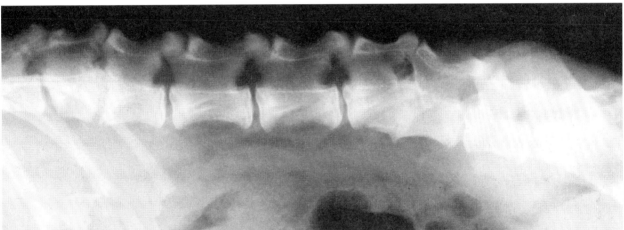

Radiographic Findings

The radiographs are made on day 1, day 7, day 45, and day 90. The series shows the progressive destruction at L1-2 and L5-6 with collapse of the disc spaces, end plate destruction, shortening of the vertebral bodies, and vertebral malalignment. A prominent kyphosis has developed at L5-6. New lesions were identified at T7-8 (arrow) and T13-L1 on day 45.

The diagnosis is a hematogenous discospondylitis with lesions in a stage of repair as well as in a stage of development.

Comments

The addition of new lesions in a hematogenous discospondylitis suggests the continued presence of an active infectious lesion elsewhere in the body that continues to spread to the new locations. It is possible, however, that the current sites of discospondylitis are acting as the active lesion(s), that is, "seeding" the new location.

Vertebral destruction and malalignment can be extensive and without great neurological importance if the lesion results in an "open" vertebral canal. "Yasu", however, had signs of cord compression resulting from vertebral instability as indicated by the neurological examination.

Case Description

"Baboose" is a 1-year-old male Bull Mastiff who was presented to the clinic with a 2 to 3 day history of lethargy, anorexia and nonspecific pain, a leukocytosis of 17,500, a neutrophilia of 13,475, and a fever. The dog was discharged following symptomatic treatment but was returned 5 days later with back pain, difficulty rising, and proprioceptive placing deficits in the pelvic limbs. Radiographs were made at that time and at 1, 2, 4 and 6 months later.

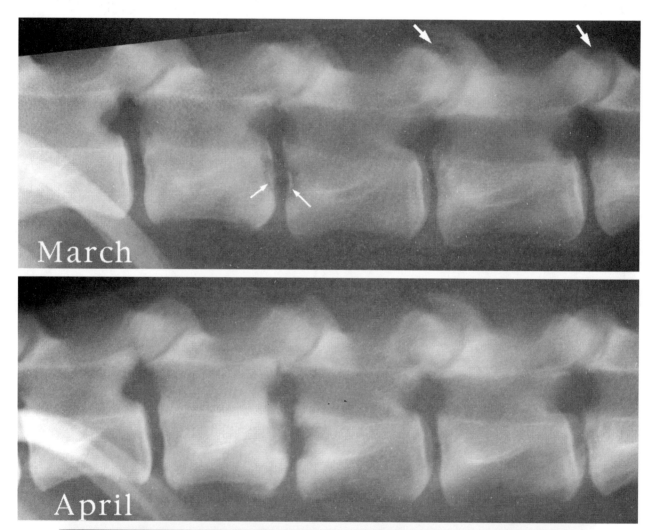

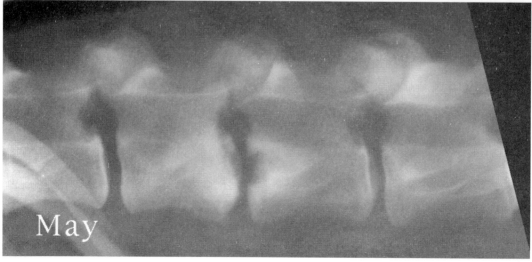

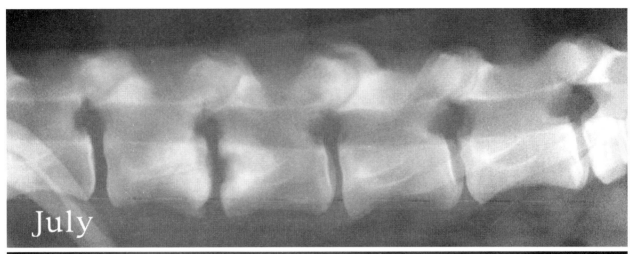

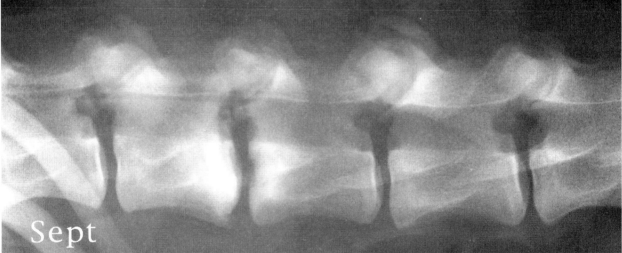

Radiographic Findings

The first radiographs show areas of focal end plate lucency at L2-3, L3-4, and L4-5 with destruction within the articular facets (large arrows). Sequestra are noted in the end plates (small arrows).

The subsequent radiographs show the progression of change at the sites of the major lesions with sclerotic zones surrounding the destructive lesions. The development of vertebral osteophytes and narrowing of the disc space suggests a stabilization of an injured L2-3 disc space. The destructive lesions in the end plates tend to fill with new bone. Periarticular osteophytes are seen to form around the vertebral joints.

The diagnosis is a hematogenous discospondylitis with healing.

Comments

These radiographs show the typical features of active and healing discospondylitis. The first radiographic study you make of a patient may show any of these stages, especially if the lesions are of different ages.

"Baboose's" blood cultures were positive for a coagulase positive Staphylococcus sp. A Brucella canis titer was negative. The geographic location and the travel history of the animal influence the probability of a positive Brucella canis titer.

Compare how "Baboose" as a 1-year-old was able to limit the spread of his lesions with rather minimal injury to the end plates and true vertebral joints while "Yasu" was younger and perhaps had a compromised immune system.

Case Description

"**Beau**" is a 5-year-old male hound with a clinical history of a swelling in the right lumbar area and a painful abdomen. He is febrile at the time of admission and abdominal radiographs were ordered.

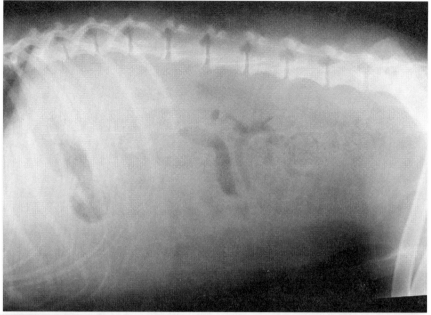

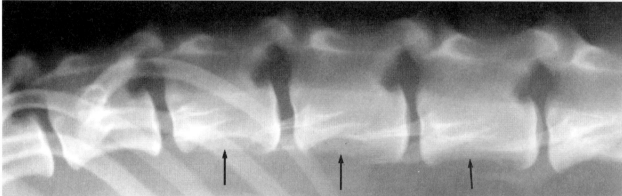

Radiographic Findings

The abdominal radiographs show new bone production ventrally on the vertebral bodies of L1-3. This is better seen on the enlarged view (arrows). Note the disc spaces at L2-3 and L3-4 are slightly narrowed.

This radiographic pattern is diagnostic of spondylitis secondary to a migrating grass awn (seed head). In a geographical climate in which a grass awn migration is an unusual lesion, the next most common causes would be hematogenous discospondylitis, spread of an inflammatory lesion from a paravertebral soft tissue abscess, or, much less likely, reactive new bone from a paravertebral tumor.

Comments

The minimal narrowing of the disc spaces at L2-3 and L3-4 may be associated with early non-inflammatory disc degeneration or may be an early part of a discitis syndrome.

Did you note the loss of abdominal detail that could suggest acute peritonitis or inflammation associated with the foreign body migration?

While the spondylitis could be hematogenous or secondary to a puncture wound, this location and pattern of new bone production is typical for aspiration of a foreign body and its subsequent migration to the vertebral site of attachment of the crura of the diaphragm.

Discospondylitis and spondylitis rarely include penetration of the meninges as a part of the syndrome. Therefore, the typical clinical picture for these 2 diseases is that of osteomyelitis, not meningitis or myelitis. Neurologic deficits are rare in these patients, but obviously spinal disease must be considered in all animals with back or abdominal pain.

Case Description

"Teal" is a 1-year-old female retriever with pain and lameness in all limbs. Thoracic and abdominal radiographs were made.

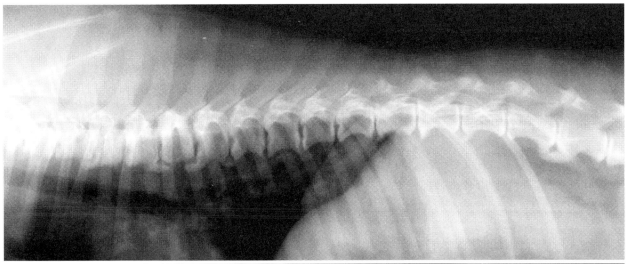

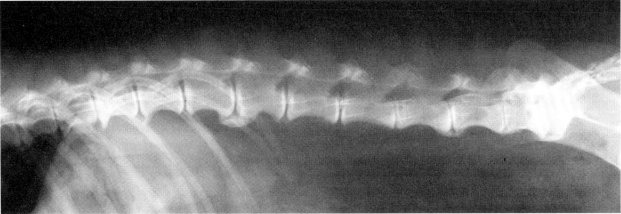

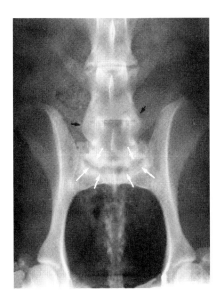

Radiographic Findings

The radiographs show:
1. marked narrowing of all disc spaces
2. extensive end plate destruction in the lumbosacral disc space (white arrows)
3. end plate destruction in all thoracic vertebrae
4. spondylosis deformans or reactive post-inflammatory vertebral osteophytes
5. bony bridges around the injured disc spaces (black arrows)

Because of the generalized nature of the disease, the diagnosis is a chronic hematogenous discospondylitis with reactive vertebral osteophytes secondary to the instability caused by the disc destruction.

Comments

The collapse of the lumbar disc spaces could represent a type of developmental disease; however, the end plate destruction in the thoracic and lumbosacral regions confirms an active inflammatory lesion and suggests that all discs are affected by the inflammatory disease, but are at different stages.

Spondylitis, Discitis, and Discospondylitis

The diagnosis of spondylitis/discospondylitis or discitis is suggested by the history and clinical signs and confirmed by radiography. Since the infection can reach the vertebrae or intervertebral discs by several different avenues, the presenting signs and the radiographic appearance of the lesions varies widely. Affected animals usually present with a several-week to several-month history of loss of condition and stamina, reluctance to run or jump, and hindquarter weakness. Pain can be elicited on palpation of the infected vertebrae and, occasionally, a draining tract is present in the paraspinal musculature or the flank. Body temperature is often elevated and the hemogram may show a regenerative left shift. Neurologic signs are uncommon but when present are those of meningeal irritation or transverse myelopathy. The myelopathy may be due to myelitis or to compression by reactive bone and inflammatory tissue. CSF analysis may support the diagnosis of concurrent meningitis or myelitis.

The signalment may vary from that of a young dog with canine distemper to an older dog with cystitis to a patient following disc fenestration. Subtleties such as depression, loss of appetite, and weight loss may be confusing early in the course of the disease and diagnosis of a spinal infection may not be considered. Something as simple as reluctance to walk in a patient with no pre-existing or documentable musculoskeletal or neurological problems is often the first clinical signs. Since many of these lesions are self-limiting, it is possible that the majority of lesions are never diagnosed. In many cases, the diagnosis of infection is made clinically before the diagnosis is confirmed radiographically. Other typical patients present with only abdominal or back pain and the radiographic diagnosis is surprising to the clinician. The majority of these cases are referred for radiographs from the medicine clinic rather than from orthopedics or neurology.

Infection following plant material as a foreign body

Spondylitis or discospondylitis caused by a migrating plant awn usually affects the cranial lumbar vertebrae. The route by which the awn reaches this site appears to be inhalation of the grass awn followed by passage through the lungs, into the pleural space, along the dorsal crura of the diaphragm, with a permanent lodging being adjacent to the second to fourth lumbar vertebrae.

The radiographic appearance of spondylitis that is associated with a paravertebral abscess (plant material) is rather specific. First, a fine periosteal new bone forms along the ventral aspect of the midportion of the affected vertebral bodies. The periosteal new bone covers the lateral aspects of the vertebral bodies as well, but the new bone is more difficult to identify on the ventrodorsal projections because of overlying bowel shadows. New bone continues to form, often reaching a thickness of one-half of the height of the vertebral body. At this time, the inflammatory process may have penetrated the vertebral body and it may be possible to identify the underlying destructive changes within the vertebral body. If untreated, the combination of destructive and productive bone changes can involve the dorsal laminae and spinal processes.

The disc is usually not affected by the inflammatory process. In some chronic lesions, discal involvement may cause radiographic changes such as narrowing of the disc space followed by the appearance of small punctate lucent foci within the normally dense vertebral end plates. Further advancement of the lesion within the disc space occurs uncommonly and collapse of the disc space, eventual end plate destruction, and shortening of the vertebral bodies is uncommon.

Healing can take place at any time during the course of the disease. Most lesions heal without involvement of the disc with the healing phase only showing smooth periosteal new bone on the vertebral body. Others heal after disc destruction, and the final appearance is that of shortened vertebral bodies collapsing around a destroyed disc with a large exuberant callus forming around the lesion. During healing, the productive bone is often without form or pattern and resembles the callus that forms around a poorly stabilized fracture within a long bone.

It is not possible to determine the stage of activity of the lesion by evaluation of the radiographic features.

Hematogenous spondylitis or discospondylitis

Bacteremia is an important cause of spondylitis/discospondylitis where venous drainage of the pelvic region may shower the vertebral column with bacteria via the vertebral veins. Brucella canis has been found to cause discospondylitis, probably due to bacteremia secondary to genital infection.

If the infectious process is hematogenous, noncontiguous vertebral vertebrae are frequently involved. The most common pattern is narrowing of the disc space and end plate destruction that occurs as the primary feature. Since the disc is assumed to be a nearly avascular structure, this is difficult to understand unless you accept the possibility that prior disease or injury of the disc has resulted in a neovascular response in the damaged disc. It is known that in the reparative process, new fibrous tissue fills the disc space bringing with it a neovascular pattern that may have a sluggish flow of blood with conditions favoring the settling out of infectious emboli. The pathogenesis of hematogenous discospondylitis is probably heavily dependent on this repair activity within the disc.

It is possible for the inflammatory lesion to begin first within the vertebral body just adjacent to the vertebral end plate where it presents as a focal destructive lesion. Expansion of the lesion results in involvement of the end plate and disc.

Regardless of the site of origin of the lesion, advancement of the lesion usually leads to destruction of the vertebral end plates and adjacent trabecular bone within the vertebral body and collapse of the disc space. Sequestration is often seen in the subchondral bone adjacent to the disc. Periosteal new bone is not obvious early, and the lesions remain centered around the intervertebral disc until the later stages of the disease when involvement of the adjacent vertebrae with new bone has occurred. Healing may occur at any stage in this form of vertebral infection and results in bony reaction typically appearing as stabilizing vertebral osteophytes. Healing often occurs with bony ankylosis across the disc space. The activity of the disease is difficult to ascertain from the radiographic features.

Post-fracture

If the infectious process is secondary to a fracture, the pattern of radiograpic changes are principally those of fracture healing and the changes due to the inflammatory infectious process are difficult to see. Sequestra are uncommon because the trabecular bone has a good vascular supply. Reactive new bone is mixed with callus formation and not clearly identified. Features of bone lysis due to the inflammatory process are mixed with those associated with the fracture repair.

This is a difficult radiographic diagnosis and the clinical diagnosis is better made on the basis of failure of a healing vertebral fracture to follow an expected course temporally. Clinical signs might include unexpected pain with fever and a draining tract. The use of consecutive radiographic studies may assist in the detection of spondylitis during fracture healing.

Post-disc fenestration

If the infection occurs following disc fenestration it usually begins as a primary discitis and the pattern of change begins with an early subtle collapse of the disc space with the appearance of small punctate lucencies within the vertebral end plate that indicate the inflammatory process has spread to bone and is now a spondylitis. Complete destruction of the disc, end plate destruction, shortening of the vertebral bodies, and loss of bone from the adjacent vertebrae may follow. The appearance of the healed lesions depends on the stage of destruction when healing begins with the possibility of only a narrowed disc space, vertebral osteophyte formation, or complete intervertebral bony fusion resulting. Other postsurgical infection may occur following hemilaminectomy, plating, pin placement, or bridging techniques. The features of the infection are unique to the type of surgery.

Post-trauma

Inflammation of the vertebrae may occur following trauma such as puncture wounds. The location and progression of the lesions is dependent on the nature of the injury. Bite wounds in small dogs and cats are the most frequent history of these injuries. The lesions may begin in either the disc, bone, or soft tissue and may come to involve all of these tissues before healing of the lesion occurs.

Radiographic changes of spondylitis or discospondylitis due to adjacent soft tissue foreign body infection (grass awn)

    1. Radiographic characteristics

      a. typically L2-4 vertebrae

      b. adjacent vertebrae involved

      c. reactive new bone midbody (ventrally and laterally)

      d. soft tissue paravertebral abscess

      e. normal vertebral alignment

      f. destructive lesion in the body (late)

      g. narrowed disc space (late)

      h. end plate destruction (late)

      i. vertebral osteophyte formation (late reactive change)

    2. Differential diagnosis

      a. primary vertebral tumor

      b. secondary vertebral tumor

      c. hematogenous spondylitis

Radiographic changes of primary discitis (hematogenous, post-traumatic, or postsurgical)

    1. Radiographic characteristics

      a. disc affected is dependent on etiology

      b. end plate destruction

      c. narrowed disc space

      d. destructive change in body (late)

      e. shortened vertebral body (late)

      f. reactive new bone (late)

      g. vertebral osteophyte formation (late)

    2. Differential diagnosis

      a. post-traumatic callus

      b. chronic disc disease

Radiographic changes of spondylitis/discospondylitis due to hematogenous spread

    1. Radiographic characteristics

      a. "skip" lesions (non-contiguous pattern)

      b. destructive lesions (body and end plate)

      c. reactive new bone

      d. spread of lesion to arch

      e. narrowed disc space (late)

      f. shortened vertebral body (late)

      g. vertebral osteophyte formation (late)

      h. malalignment (late)

      i. widened disc space if healing is delayed (late)

    2. Differential diagnosis

      a. primary vertebral tumor

      b. secondary vertebral tumor

"Percy"

Case Description

"Percy" is a 9-year-old male domestic, short-haired cat with thoracic limb paralysis and pelvic limb paresis. He has a 3-week history of lethargy and progression of the clinical signs. The neuroanatomical diagnosis is a C1-5 myelopathy.

Radiographic Findings

The cortices and end plates are thin and an abnormally strong trabecular pattern is seen in the bones of the spine. These patterns suggest a generalized skeletal disease and may be result of dietary deficiency or may be an osteoporosis due to disuse. No focal destructive or productive lesions are evident. The height of the cervical vertebral canal appears to be increased especially at the level of C2-3. A slight kyphosis is evident at T2-4.

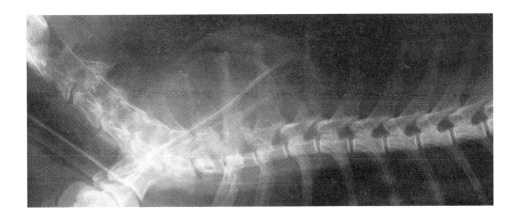

Myelographic Findings

Filling of the cervical subarachnoid space was accomplished from a lumbar injection. An increase in size of the spinal cord and thinning of the contrast columns are evident from caudal C1 to C5. The duplication of the pattern on both lateral and VD views is diagnostic of an intramedullary mass.

A tumor mass either primary or metastatic was considered the most likely diagnosis with lymphoma felt to be most likely. However, an intramedullary mass of this length, is uncommon in either the dog or cat.

Comments

The diagnosis was an astrocytoma.

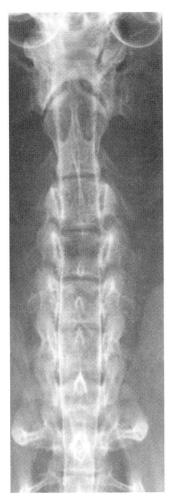

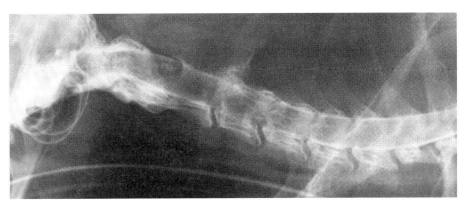

Spinal Problems in Puppies

Spinal pain and/or paresis in the puppy suggest a different group of diseases than these same signs in adult dogs. While neoplastic and degenerative lesions all but drop from the list of differential diagnoses, congenital and traumatic lesions rise to the top.

Case Description

"Pooh" is a 5-month-old female Labrador retriever with paraparesis since the owner acquired her at 8 weeks of age. Her pelvic limbs are hyper-reflexic, but sensation is apparently normal. The signs are not progressive. The lesion is localized to the T3-L3 spinal cord.

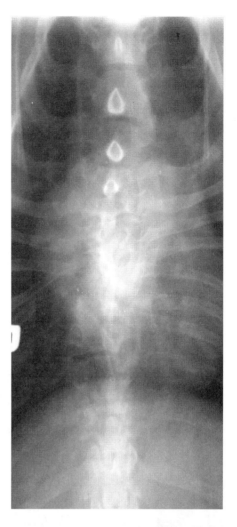

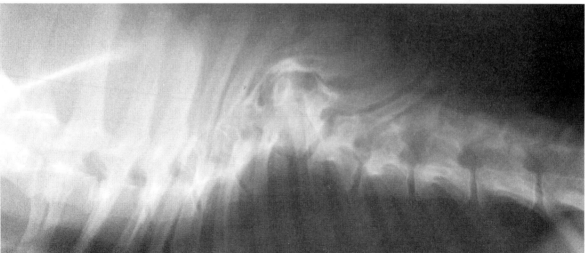

Radiographic Findings

The lateral and VD noncontrast radiographs of the thoracic spine show a congenital anomaly at T4-9 with a large, combination block and hemivertebrae at T6-8 causing a marked kyphosis. The three hemivertebrae seem to blend together creating a body with a ventrally projecting bony apex as seen on the lateral view. The malformed 7th rib is misplaced dorsally and cranially on the right side. The diagnosis is a congenital anomaly with a marked vertebral canal stenosis that may be primary or may be secondary to the displacement of the unstable hemivertebra. Myelography is necessary to determine the degree of canal stenosis and the possibility of surgical correction.

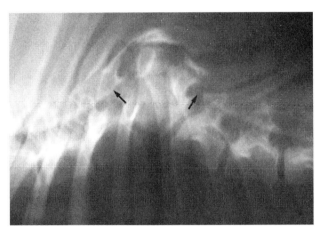 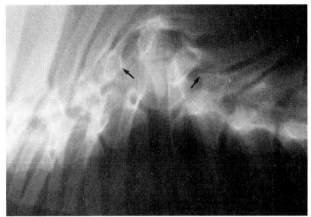

Myelographic Findings

Two lateral views from the myelographic studies are enlarged and show elevation of the narrowed subarachnoid columns (arrows) and spinal cord narrowing due to the vertebral canal stenosis.

Comment

The ventrodorsal view in either noncontrast or contrast studies of a case like this is of little value in determining cord compression because of the marked kyphosis and the resulting superimposition of the shadow from the heart and midthoracic vertebral vertebrae. A CT study is of little value because of the difficulty in positioning the spine due to the vertebral malalignment.

Case Description

"Amy" is an 8-month-old female Basset hound who was found by the owner 4 days ago unable to walk. The owner thought she had a fractured neck. "Amy" had a previous episode of being found "dazed", unable to walk, and crying but she had recovered satisfactorily in 24 hours according to the owner. On examination, she is a non-ambulatory quadriparetic with no proprioceptive placing reactions in any of her limbs. Her spinal reflexes are intact. The lesion was localized to the C1-C5 spinal cord. Noncontrast radiographs were made of the area, including the "open-mouth" view showing the occipito-atlanto-axial region.

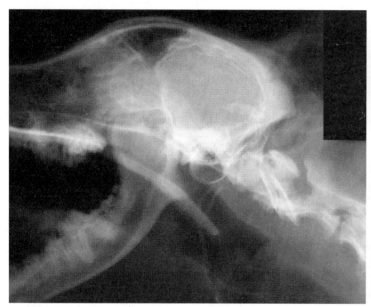
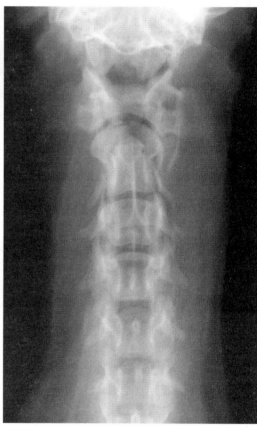

Radiographic Findings

The noncontrast radiographs demonstrate the absence of the odontoid process. The normal site of its attachment on the axis is indicated on the detail view (arrows, next page). The open-mouth view is helpful in viewing the lesion.

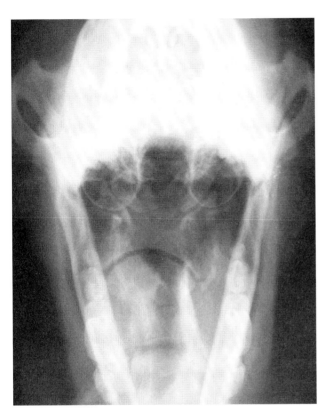 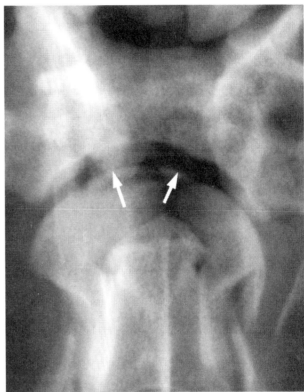

Comments

Stress studies would demonstrate the degree of abnormal vertebral movement allowed by this anomaly, but are not required for a diagnosis and the positioning could be damaging to the spinal cord.

It is possible that the odontoid process is present but cartilaginous in which situation it would not be seen on the radiograph. While theoretically possible, this has not been proven clinically to occur.

Commonly, occipito-atlanto-axial congenital lesions are not noted when the puppy is very young because of the protection provided by the mother and owner. When the puppy is older and begins to "roam more freely", it may then suffer some trauma, often relatively minor in degree, with resulting severe injury to the spinal cord.

Case Description

"Ju Lin" is a 6-week-old female Pekingese puppy who has been ataxic in the pelvic limbs since birth. She is unique for her breed since she does not have a tail. Because of her size, the entire body is easily included on the radiographs.

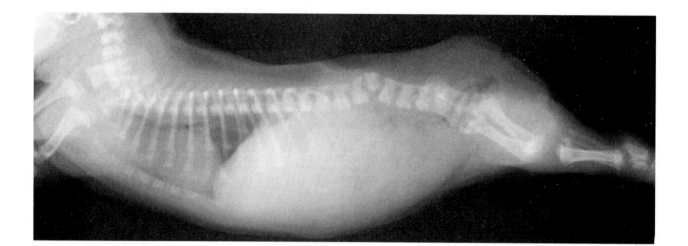

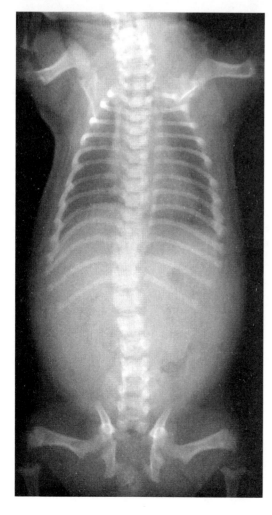

Radiographic Findings

The radiographs show a series of congenital anomalies:
1. a congenital hemivertebra at L4 with a marked kyphosis and probable stenosis of the vertebral canal
2. spina bifida at L4-7
3. sacral and coccygeal agenesis

The congenital hemivertebra at L4 is seen better on the enlarged views on the next page and is probably associated with vertebral canal stenosis. The spina bifida is detected by the wider than normal pedicles and the absence of spinous processes and may be associated with a cord lesion. The sacral and coccygeal agenesis may also be associated with a congenital cord lesion.

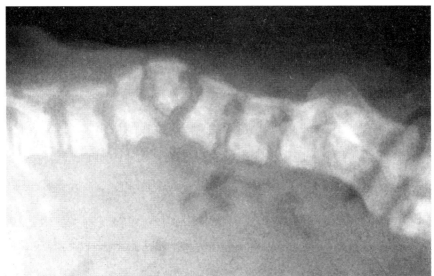

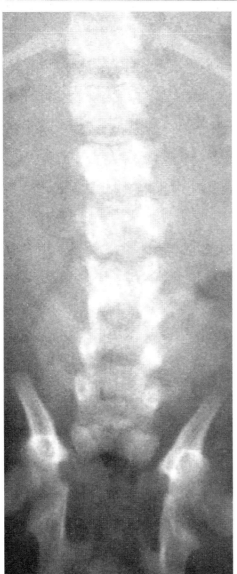

Comments

It is not possible to know which of the bony lesions is the most important or if there are associated lesions of the spinal cord not identified on these radiographs.

In patients with such extensive malformations, particularly if the spinal cord is malformed, the prognosis for neural improvement or recovery is very poor.

Case Description

"No-Name" is a 5-month-old English Mastiff who has marked lumbar scoliosis. No neurological signs are evident and the puppy was presented only because of the "strange-looking" back and way of walking .

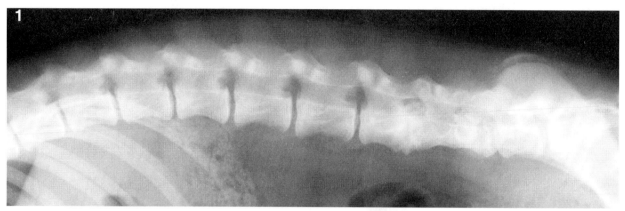

Radiographic Findings

The radiographs show a series of congenital anomalies:

1. eight lumbar-type vertebrae (1)
2. a single rib on the last thoracic vertebra (2).
3. a wedge shaped body of L5 is only partly separated from L6 (1,2)
4. wedge shaped L6 and L7 that failed to separate, with a single spinous process (1,2)
5. an L8 transitional vertebra that is wedge-shaped with the right transverse process blunted and the left transverse process more normal in shape (2,3)
6. articulation of the left transverse processes of L7 and L8 with the ilium (3)
7. a stenotic lumbosacral vertebral canal (4)
8. oblique attachment of the pelvis to the sacrum (3)

The VD enlarged view shows the single spinous process of the block vertebrae (black arrow) and the abnormal articulation of the transverse processes to the ilium (white arrows). The enlarged lateral view shows the stenotic vertebral canal (black arrows).

The diagnosis is a complex congenital anomaly in the lumbar spine without apparent clinical importance at this time.

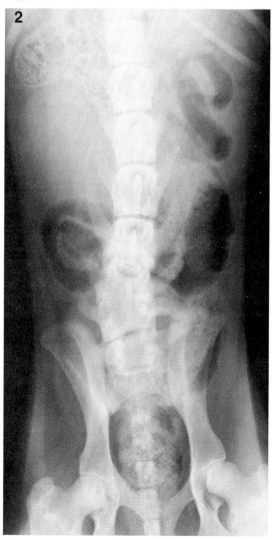

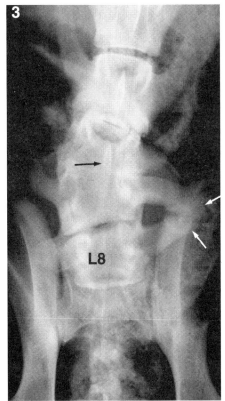

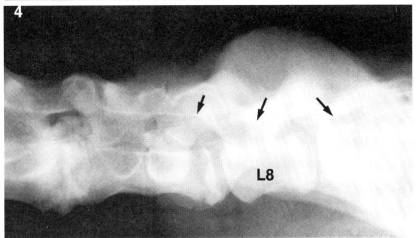

Comment

Despite their weird morphology, if the vertebrae enclose a normally developed spinal cord, have a vertebral canal of sufficient size, and the vertebrae remain stable in position, the patient probably will develop no neurological signs relative to the bony lesions. However, in "No-Name" there is potential concern for the development of a cauda equina syndrome at the lumbosacral junction as the dog ages because of the congenitally abnormal LS disc and altered SI joints. This potential problem should be explained to the owner.

The positioning of the pelvis is at an angle to the spine which may permit one femoral head (left) to subluxate. This is of importance in a larger breed dog with a greater potential for hip dysplasia.

Hemivertebra

Hemivertebra is a congenital anomaly seen most often in the screw-tailed breeds, particularly in the thoracolumbar spine. The vertebral body is incompletely formed and has a wedged shape when seen from either lateral or ventrodorsal view. Radiographically, the hemivertebrae and adjacent vertebrae appear to be formed of normal bone tissue. The disc spaces are usually well preserved or widened. Adjacent vertebrae frequently have an altered shape that conforms to the defect found in the congenitally affected vertebral body. The vertebral end plates are smooth and have an increased density.

Differential diagnosis includes pathologic or traumatic fracture that causes collapse of the vertebral body. However, those lesions have disruption of the ventral or lateral cortical shadows, disruption of the trabecular pattern, and the possibility of disruption of end plates.

Hemivertebrae are often incidental findings; however, they may be associated with moderate-to-severe angulation of the spine (scoliosis, kyphosis, or lordosis) and occasionally with vertebral canal stenosis and instability of the involved vertebrae, producing spinal cord compression or intermittent trauma. Affected animals usually have a progressive or intermittent transverse myelopathy. Myelography is useful in determining the presence of spinal cord compression produced by the hemivertebra.

Vertebral osteophytes may form in an effort to stabilize an unstable hemivertebra. Osteophytes may be also found in patients with vertebral instability secondary to a malformed vertebra associated with a healed fracture, malformed vertebra secondary to a severe discospondylitis, or a malformed vertebra secondary to a chronic disc degeneration. The absence of any reactive osteophytes suggests either an acute situation or one that is stable.

1. Radiographic characteristics of hemivertebra
   a. wedge-shaped vertebral body (on lateral or VD view)
   b. end plates are normal
   c. disc spaces may be narrow or not uniform in width
   d. reactive osteophytes often form
   e. may be severe kyphosis or scoliosis or lordosis
   f. trabecular pattern undisturbed
   g. adjacent vertebrae have compensatory changes
2. Differential diagnosis
   a. traumatic compression fracture
   b. pathologic fracture
      1. tumor
      2. infection

Spina bifida

The two ossification centers that represent the lamina may fail to fuse causing a midline cleft of varying prominence. Anomalies of the vertebral arch and the spinal cord are profoundly influenced by the development of the neural tube. The vertebral arch or spinal cord may be affected individually or together. If there is no soft tissue malformation present, the term "spina bifida occulta" describes the lesion while associated cord or meningeal lesions, such as a meningocele or myelomeningocele, result in use of the term "spine bifida manifesta."

Failure of fusion of the arch is most common in the LS region where the defect may be small, producing only a cleft dorsal spinous process, or a vertebra in which most of the vertebral arch is absent. The defect may involve a single vertebra, often L7, or may affect that vertebra plus part or all of the sacral vertebrae. An extensive defect is best recognized on a ventrodorsal view where it is characterized by the absence of the shadow created by the spinous process. In a severe lesion, two smaller bony densities that represent the ununited lamina are present lateral to the midline. A third pattern is seen when the spinous process is larger than usual but divided with a radiolucent line between the two closely fitting ununited processes. Either one vertebra or several adjacent vertebrae may be affected. Complete absence of the lamina and spinous process can be detected on the lateral view as well.

In small animals, spina bifida is usually an incidental finding. However, if neurologic signs referable to the spinal cord or cauda equina are present and spina bifida is discovered, the possibility of concomitant spinal cord malformation should be considered. The condition of the spinal cord and meninges can be determined radiographically with the use of subarachnoid myelography and epidurography.

1. Radiographic characteristics of spina bifida
   a. normal vertebral body
   b. affected arch
      1. spinous processes are formed but do not fuse
      2. spinous processes do not form completely
         a. pedicles are positioned laterally
   c. end plates are normal
   d. disc spaces are normal
   e. absence of reactive osteophytes
   f. without vertebral angulation
   h. without change in adjacent vertebrae
2. differential diagnosis
   a. none

Failure of Separation of Vertebrae (Block Vertebra)

Complete or partial failure of embryonic separation of two or more vertebral bodies may occur as a congenital anomaly throughout the vertebral column. Block vertebra results if segmentation of the somites is disturbed usually leaving the trabecular pattern uninterrupted throughout the length of the block vertebrae. In some cases, the trabeculae may be interrupted by a radiolucent line representing partial development of the disc and thin dense shadows representing incompletely formed vertebral end plates. The combined length of the vertebral bodies may just equal the length of two normal vertebral bodies minus the intervertebral disc, but usually the length is markedly shorter.

An important pattern is that the bone tissue is normal in appearance with no evidence of change in thickness of the cortex, bony destruction, periosteal proliferation, or a repair or modeling pattern. In most dogs, the vertebral canal is preserved without any stenosis. Thus, a block vertebra is generally stable, rarely of clinical significance, and usually only an incidental finding. An exception is the detection of a midthoracic lesion with marked kyphosis, instability, and canal stenosis. If instability or canal stenosis is suspected, myelography is indicated to evaluate either of these clinically important features.

The failure of vertebral separation may involve only the vertebral bodies or may also involve the vertebral arches. If only the bodies are affected, the dorsal arches form in a near normal manner with production of articular facets and angulation occurs between the affected vertebral bodies with a focal kyphosis. In this pattern, a degree of hemivertebrae may be associated with the anomaly causing further shortening of the body and more prominent kyphosis. If in addition to the changes in the bodies, the spinous processes fail to separate normally the arches usually appear hypoplastic. The shortening of length of the vertebral arches results in a malalignment of the vertebral bodies causing a lordosis and wedging of the discs. Lateral angulation or scoliosis may also result.

Differential diagnosis includes fusion of vertebrae following: (1) surgical intervention such as extensive fenestration, (2) malunion healing of a fracture, or (3) healing of a discospondylitis. In such cases, the fusion would be characterized by callus formation or reactive new bone and osteoclastic changes in the end plate. However, in patients following disc fenestration or discospondylitis, the resulting fusion is difficult to distinguish from a congenital block vertebrae.

1. Radiographic characteristics of block vertebrae
   a. disc space is absent or narrowed
   b. end plates are absent, less dense, or of diminished thickness.
   c. periosteal or reactive new bone is absent
   d. trabecular pattern is usually continuous
   e. resulting angulation may cause a focal scoliosis, kyphosis, or scoliosis
   f. arch may be equally or unequally involved in the anomaly
2. Differential diagnosis
   a. malunion healed fracture
   b. healed discospondylitis
   c. healing of postsurgical
      1. fenestration
      2. postsurgical fusion

Spinal Lesions Identified on Abdominal Radiographs of Cats

While disease of the abdominal organs is the most common cause of abdominal pain and abdominal organ dysfunction, spinal disease can cause clinical signs suggestive of abdominal disease. The lumbar vertebrae and the sacrum are rather easy to evaluate on an abdominal radiograph, and in these cats in particular, the clinical importance of any apparent spinal lesion must be carefully assessed. Look at these abdominal studies and decide about the clinical relevance of any spinal lesion that you see. Enlarged views are included in 3 cases to assist in your radiographic evaluation.

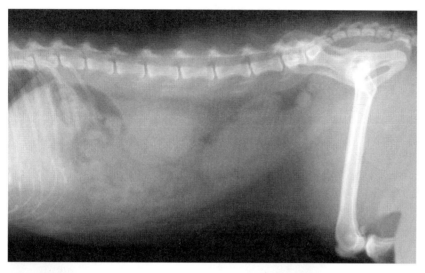

Case Description

"Friskie" is a 12-year-old male domestic, long-haired cat with histiocytic lymphoma that is being treated with chemotherapy and radiation therapy. The abdominal radiographs are made in a search of a suspected abdominal mass.

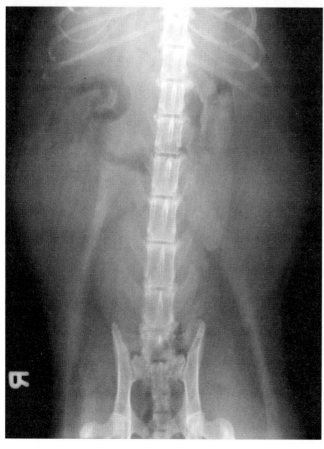

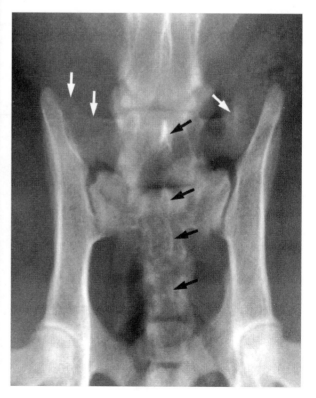

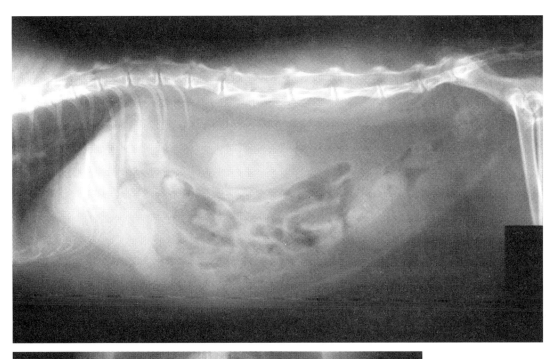

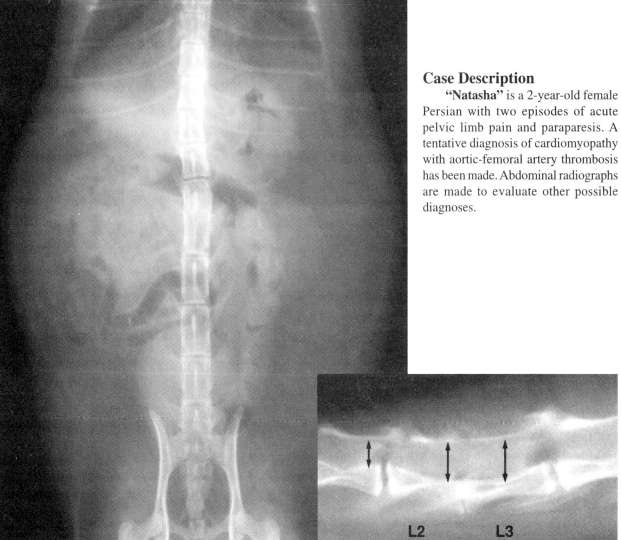

Case Description

"**Natasha**" is a 2-year-old female Persian with two episodes of acute pelvic limb pain and paraparesis. A tentative diagnosis of cardiomyopathy with aortic-femoral artery thrombosis has been made. Abdominal radiographs are made to evaluate other possible diagnoses.

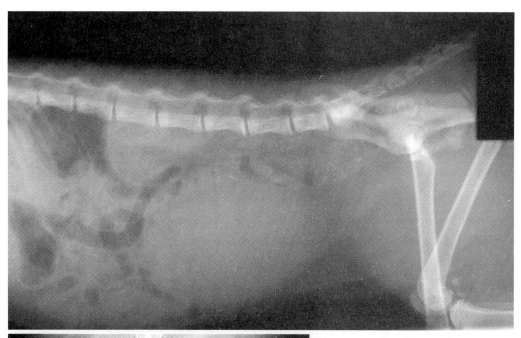

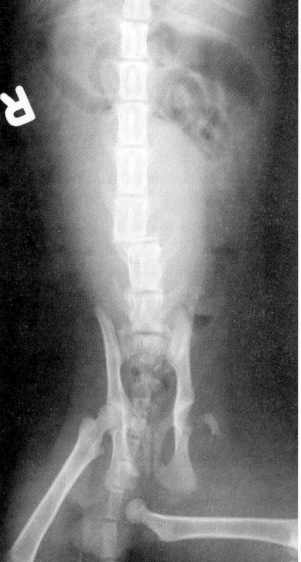

Case Description

"Bandit" is a 7-month-old male domestic, short-haired cat who is unwilling to walk on his pelvic limbs. His owner's think a car may have hit him.

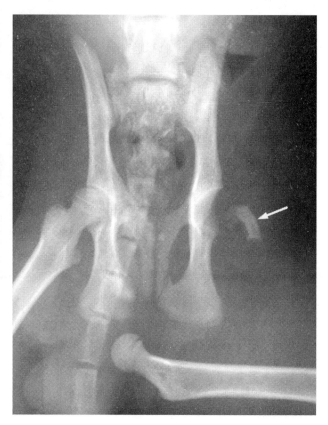

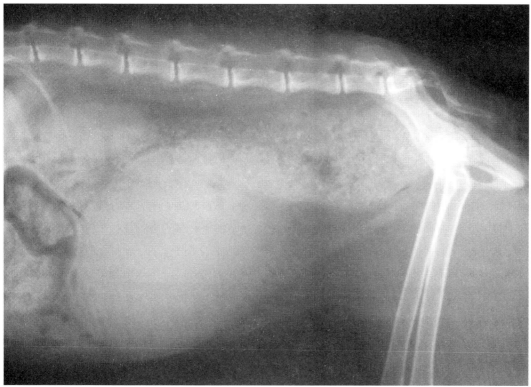

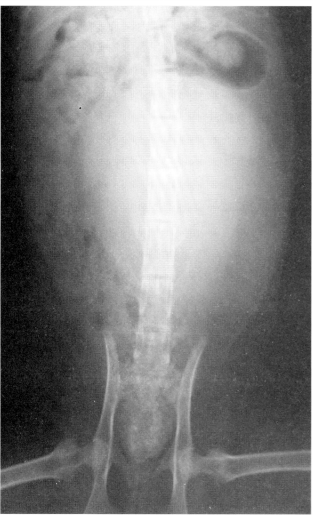

Case Description

"**Pipper**" is a 14-month-old male Manx with a 5-month history of persistent cystitis and bowel and urinary incontinence. He appears paretic in the pelvic limbs.

"Friskie" - Radiographic Findings

"Friskie" has a midabdominal mass causing caudolateral displacement of both kidneys and caudal displacement of the transverse colon. The mass was later proven to be associated with a primary lymphoma. It is interesting that "Friskie" has a transitional vertebra at the thoracolumbar junction with a single rib on the first lumbar vertebra, and another transitional segment at the lumbosacral junction with large wing-like processes bilaterally (white arrows). An additional anomaly is a sacrum that has only 2 vertebrae. The spinous processes of the transitional vertebrae, sacrum, and first coccygeal vertebra are identified (black arrows). Note the degree of vertebral canal stenosis at the site of the transitional lumbosacral segment. While these lesions are potentially important in the dog because they may play a role in the development of a cauda equina syndrome, this is a much less likely problem in the cat. Congenital spinal anomalies often occur in multiple sites often assisting in the determination of the etiology of the lesions.

"Natasha" - Radiographic Findings

"Natasha" has focal lordosis and scoliosis at L2-3. The spinous processes have failed to separate and the interposed disc space is narrow with incompletely formed end plates. The vertebral canal is enlarged at this site (double-headed arrows), but no evidence of instability is seen. Thus, this lesion is a congenital block vertebra that is thought to be clinically unimportant. Note the last thoracic vertebra is a transitional one with a rib only on the left.

The small bowel in the cat tends to "clump" together when it is empty, being forced ventrally by the sublumbar fat accumulation.

"Natasha" was treated for the cardiomyopathy and aortic thrombosis.

Question #1

The L2-3 lesion in "Natasha" is felt to be stable. What radiographic features would suggest instability?

"Bandit" - Radiographic Findings

"Bandit's" radiographs show a physeal fracture from the caudal aspect of the L5 vertebral body, with lateral displacement of the caudal fragment to the left. The distended urinary bladder may be due to spinal cord injury, or reluctance to urinate because of pain and difficulty posturing. A complete neurologic examination should be done.

Note the difficulty of diagnosing "Bandit's" spinal fracture if you had only the lateral view. The luxation of the left femoral head is atypical with the femur displaced caudally.

Question #2

What is the bony fragment adjacent to the left acetabulum (arrow)?

"Pipper" - Radiographic Findings

"Pipper" has congenital anomalies of the sacrum and the caudal vertebrae. The urinary bladder distention and megacolon are evident on the radiograph suggesting that the sacral spinal cord/cauda equina is also malformed, producing lower motor neuron deficits of the bladder and terminal intestinal tract. "Piper" has a typical clinical picture for Manx cats with sacral dysgenesis/agenesis, although most of these cats have clinical problems from the time they are neonates. The ability to see the sacral spina bifida on the ventrodorsal view is made difficult because of superimposition by the contents of the rectum.

Answer #1

Spondylosis deformans (reactive bony spurs), sclerotic end plates, change in the width of the disc space on stress views, or change in position of the vertebral bodies on stress views.

Answer #2

"Bandit" is young and without skeletal maturation. The bony fragment (arrow) is avulsion of the previously ununited greater trochanter from the femur.

Changes in the Vertebral Arch

The vertebral arch is formed of the pedicles that attach to the vertebral body and the lamina that complete the arch by joining dorsally at the site of origin of the spinous process. Changes in size or shape of the vertebral arch are much less common than those of the body and are much more difficult to identify on the radiograph. The lesions are divided into groups in which there is: (1) a shorter arch and resulting canal stenosis, (2) an incompletely formed arch in which the lamina have not joined (spina bifida), (3) union of the lamina but a hypoplastic or aplastic spinous process, (4) fusion between the arches of adjacent vertebrae, (5) new bone production secondary to inflammatory or neoplastic lesion, (6) new bone production resulting in a limitation of motion between adjacent vertebrae, and (7) destruction associated with inflammatory or neoplastic lesion.

Congenital anomalies are of two types: (1) block vertebrae with union of adjacent spinous processes, and (2) spina bifida in which the two lamina from a single vertebra fail to join and an incomplete dorsal arch results. Cervical spondylopathy causes an arch with a shorter height cranially and a smaller vertebral foramen. The chondrodystrophoid dog has a vertebral arch size in which the height of the vertebral canal throughout the spine is smaller. Other breeds show this lack of height only at specific locations. The resulting focal lesions may or may not have clinical importance.

Massive overgrowth of new bone around the articular facets alters the size and shape of the vertebral arches and these dogs may fit into the category of disseminated idiopathic skeletal hyperostosis (DISH). These "bone formers" generate new bone involving the dorsal arch of all vertebrae. Basstrup's disease is the eponym used to describe the formation of a pseudoarticulation between the spinous processes. These bony pseudofacets form on adjacent processes where they appear to articulate. Large breeds of dogs are most commonly affected and it appears to be a disease of older age dogs. The clinical importance remains unknown. The radiographic importance lies with the fact that the pseudofacets often form at the base of adjacent spinous processes in the lumbar region where they create a dense mass between the true vertebral joints. On the lateral radiograph they may falsely be interpreted as being a disease in the true synovial joints.

Fractures of the vertebrae alter the shape of the arch with eventual patterns of bone healing. Postsurgical patients may show the effect of a hemilaminectomy or complete dorsal laminectomy.

Tumors or infection of bone may cause destructive lesions in the pedicles, lamina, and spinous processes that are difficult to identify. Healed discospondylitis lesions may result in fusion of adjacent arches.

Reactive new bone may be secondary to a primary bone tumor or invasion of soft tissue tumor into the bone. Soft tissue tumors originating within the vertebral canal rarely cause any reactive new bone. The most common cause of reactive bone follows the spread of intrapelvic tumors as they metastasize locally to lumbar vertebrae. The other common cause of reactive new bone is from inflammatory lesions that spread from the soft tissues. In all of these, the reactive bone on the vertebral body is more prominent than is the new bone on the arch.

While tumors of bone cause patterns of destruction or production, tumors that originate from the soft tissues within the vertebral canal may cause a craniocaudal shortening of the pedicles on the affected side causing an enlarged intervertebral foramen the result of a spinal nerve sheath tumor. Cord or meningeal tumors can assume a large enough size that they cause an expanding type of change in the arch to accommodate the mass lesion. In these cases, the roof of the vertebral canal arches dorsally and /or the floor arches ventrally to accommodate growth of the tumor.

Vertebral arch - patterns of change

1. Incomplete development - pedicles and lamina
   a. chondrodystrophoid skeletal maturation
   b. congenital hypoplastic arch
   c. spina bifida
2. Incomplete development -spinous processes
   a. spina bifida
3. Incomplete development - vertebral foramina
   a. cervical spondylopathy
4. United arches and spinous processes
   a. block vertebrae with failure of arches to separate
   b. fusion secondary to
      l. healed spondylitis
      2. healed fracture
5. New bone production
   a. spondylitis
   b. reactive bone
      1. associated with primary bone tumors
      2. associated with invasion of soft tissue tumor
6. Bone destruction
   a. focal destruction
      1. associated with primary bone tumors
      2. associated with invasion of soft tissue tumor
   b. increase in size of intervertebral foramina
      1. due to nerve sheath tumor
      2. due to dorsolateral herniation of disc tissue
   c. increase the diameter of the vertebral canal
      1. due to neural tumor
      2. due to vertebral canal tumor
7. Unique lesions
   a. DISH
   b. Basstrup's syndrome

Spinal Changes Seen on Thoracic Radiographs in Four Cats

The thoracic spine is at least partially visible in studies of the thorax in cats. Often the study is made in patients to evaluate pulmonary or cardiac disease, or may be made as a part of the establishment of a database. The changes identified can be congenital, degenerative, post-inflammatory, or post-traumatic. Uncommonly, features of neoplastic disease are seen. Some lesions cause vertebral canal stenosis while others lead to instability causing cord compression and neurologic signs. Examine these cats and decide if the changes in the thoracic vertebrae are clinically important and require additional study. Detailed views are included in 3 cases.

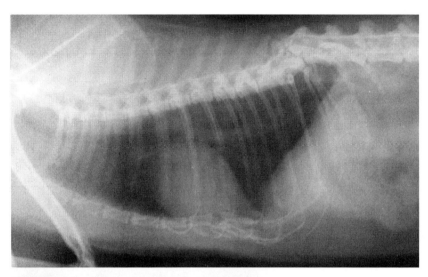

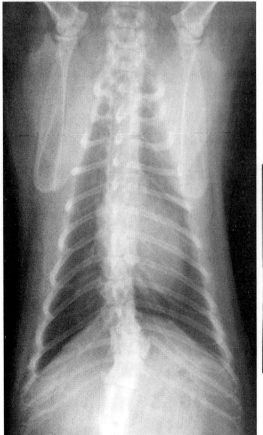

Case Description

"**Midnight**" is a 5-year-old female domestic, short-haired cat with progressive paraparesis. This referral study was intended to be a spinal survey.

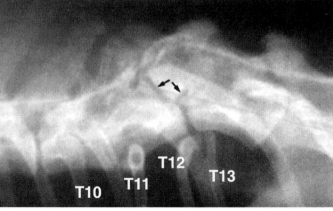

Case Description

"S Hui" is a 1-year-old male domestic, long-haired cat in whom a thoracic study was made to establish a database.

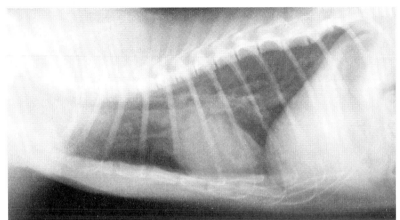

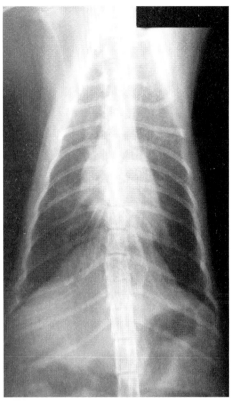

Case Description

"Butterball" is a 2-year-old male domestic, short-haired cat who was anorectic causing emaciation. The thoracic study was to establish a database.

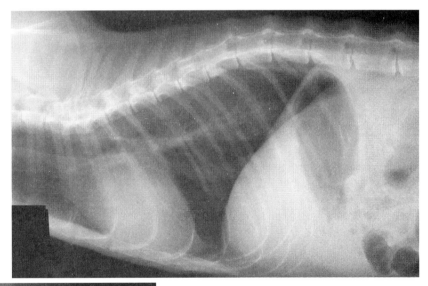

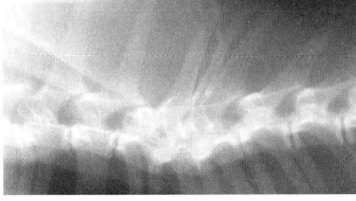

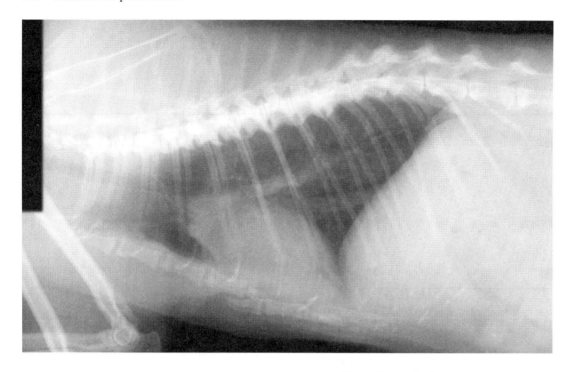

Case Description

"**Oatmeal**" is a 15-year-old female domestic, short-haired cat with progressive pelvic limb weakness and lethargy for the past week. She is hypersensitive to touch of the skin over the LS region. Proprioceptive placing deficits are present in the right pelvic limb.

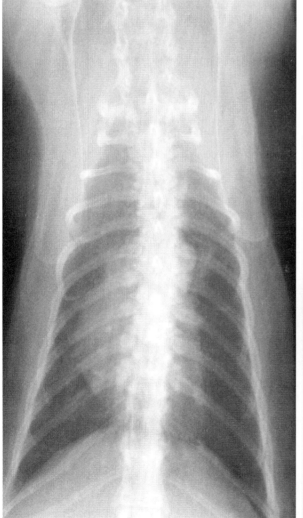

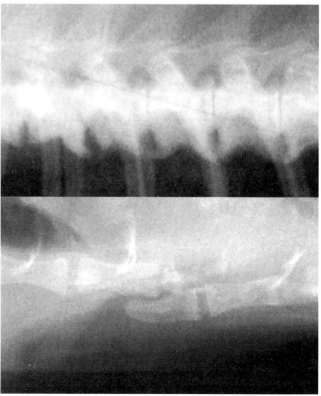

"Midnight" - Radiographic Findings

"Midnight" has a congenital lesion causing kyphosis and scoliosis of the spine. The bodies of T10 and T11 are elongated. The body of T12 is hypoplastic with dorsal angulation and the apex of the body directed ventrally (arrows). The body of T13 is elongated and angled ventrally. The wedge-shaped hypoplastic body of T12 is a potentially weakened locus because both cranial and caudal forces tend to displace the vertebral body dorsally causing increasing vertebral canal stenosis.

Note the position of the ribs on the ventrodorsal view. Counting them suggests that the hemivertebra is wedged laterally as well as dorsoventrally, with the apex on the right. Note the anomalous sternum with only 7 sternebrae. Congenital sternal lesions can be associated with congenital diaphragmatic lesions. Congenital anomalies in the axial skeleton are often multiple.

Hemivertebrae are often incidental findings, but occasionally they cause vertebral canal stenosis and compress the spinal cord. Also occasionally, the involved vertebral column may be unstable and the hemivertebrae may become suddenly or progressively displaced, compressing the enclosed spinal cord. "Midnight" has progressive paresis, which may be caused by a progressive, dorsal luxation of her hemivertebra to its current position. The hemivertebra appears to be causing vertebral canal stenosis, but myelography would be necessary to confirm this impression.

"S Hui" - Radiographic Findings

"S Hui" has a pattern of patchy infiltrates in both lung fields that probably represent an active pneumonia. The spinal changes are the result of a hypoplastic vertebral arch at T11 and fused arches between T11 and T12 resulting in a focal lordosis. As a result, the disc spaces at T10-11 and T11-12 collapsed. The vertebral canal remains open; in fact it appears to be wider than the canal cranially and caudally. The spinal changes are congenital and should not be clinically important in this cat during his life. If the spinal lesion was secondary to trauma or an inflammatory lesion, reactive bone should be present.

"Butterball" - Radiographic Finding

"Butterball" was emaciated and had chronic bowel disease causing the clinical signs. The block vertebrae at T4-6 have hypoplastic arches causing a focal lordosis. While the floor of the vertebral canal dips ventrally, the roof of the vertebral canal remains a straight line. Thus, the vertebral canal is actually enlarged at the site of the congenital lesion. The detection of the hypoplastic spinous processes and the absence of any reactive new bone confirms a congenital lesion.

"Oatmeal" - Radiographic Findings

"Oatmeal" has a cardiac shadow and pulmonary structures that are unremarkable for a cat this age. The aortic arch has a "knob-like" appearance because the heart has assumed a more horizontal position with progressive aging. The collapse of the disc spaces, development of vertebral osteophytes, and end plate sclerosis is extensive (see detail view), but not remarkable for a cat of this age. The malformed sixth sternebra is the result of an old fracture-luxation with persistent dislocation (see detail view). The degeneration of costal arches is typical for an aged cat. The radiographs do not demonstrate the cause of the clinical signs.

The owner did not know of any trauma that might have caused the sternal fracture-luxation.

Myelography in Cats

Myelography is performed in the cat in a manner similar to that used in the dog. Either the cerebellomedullary cistern or the lumbar subarachnoid space can be used as sites for injection. The cord is large when compared with the size of the vertebral canal making subarachnoid filling likely (as opposed to epidural filling), although it is possible to have a partial epidural injection and a non-diagnostic study. Disc disease is common in the cat and follows a pattern similar to that seen in nonchondrodystrophic dogs, however, most protrusions or extrusions are ventral or lateral to the disc and do not result in injury to the spinal cord. Most myelographic studies in the cat are done when spinal injury or malignant disease is suspected. Both noncontrast and myelographic studies were made in these cases. Evaluate the spinal studies in these cats and try to arrive at a diagnosis.

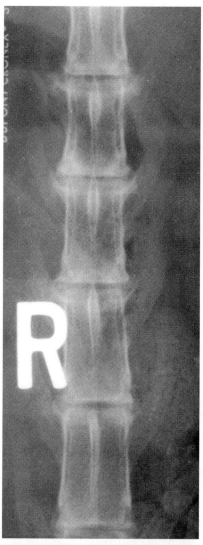

Case Description

"**Tennile**" is a 14-year-old female domestic, short-haired cat with progressive paraparesis over the last 10 days. Proprioceptive placing is absent in the pelvic limbs. Crossed extensor reflexes are present in both pelvic limbs. The noncontrast studies are seen on this page and the myelogram on the next page.

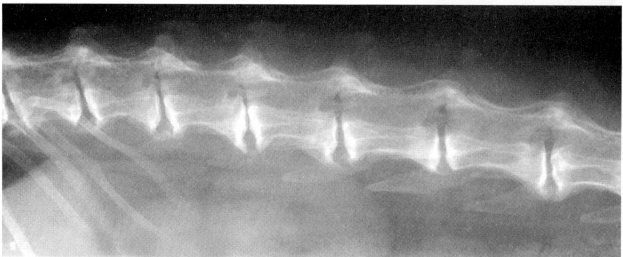

Question #1

Does "Tennile" have an upper motor neuron lesion or lower motor neuron lesion of the pelvic limbs?

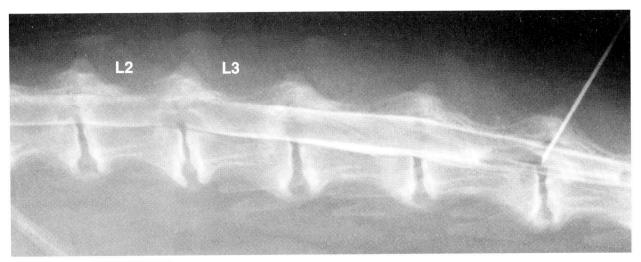

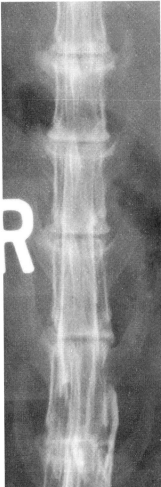

"**Tennile**" - lateral, VD, and detail views from the myelogram are shown.

Left Oblique   **Right Oblique**

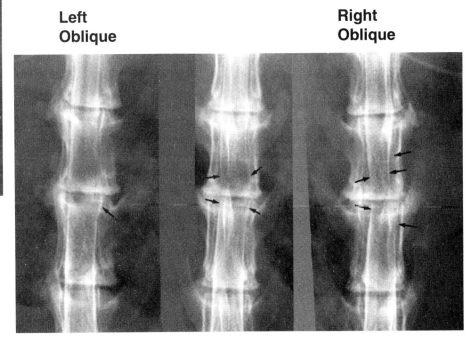

Case Description

"M-1" is a 1-year-old female domestic, short-haired cat who suffered a spinal injury 2 weeks ago after falling from a height of 4 meters. She was dazed after the accident. Following the accident, she had slight ataxia that has developed into a paraparesis of the pelvic limbs. Both noncontrast radiographs (NCR) and a myelogram (Myel) were made.

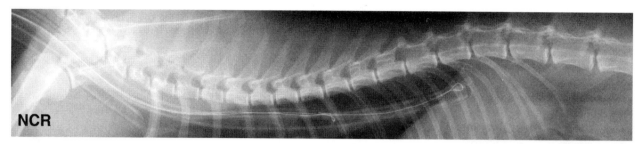

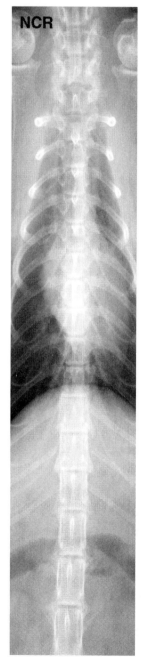

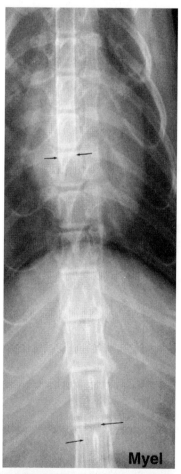

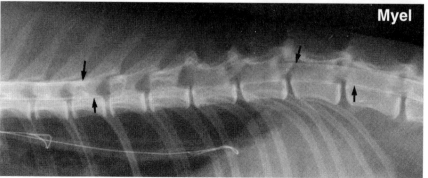

Case Description

"Sam" is a 5-year-old male domestic, short-haired cat who has a history of spinal trauma 4 years ago. Since that time he has not walked normally. In the past month, however, "Sam" has become progressively more paraparetic with hyperesthesia over the back. He has upper motor neuron signs in the pelvic limbs. Both noncontrast studies (NCR) and a myelogram (Myel) were performed.

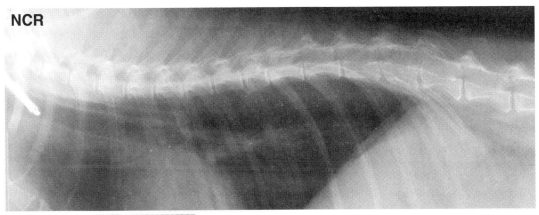

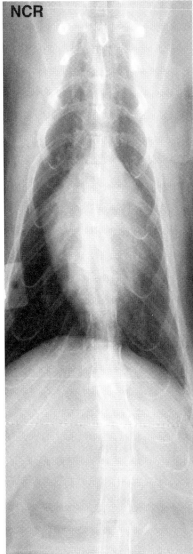

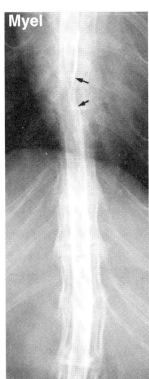

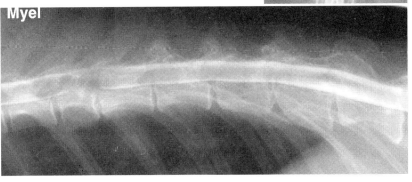

Case Description

"**Annie**" is a 7-year-old female Persian with a 5-month history of a progressive right forelimb lameness. Proprioceptive placing of the limb is decreased and pain perception in the limb may be decreased. The noncontrast study (NCR) is above and the myelogram (Myel) below.

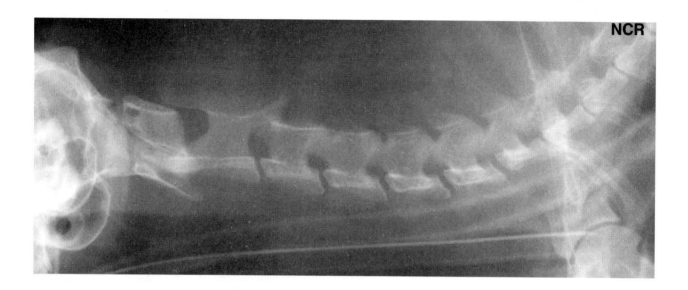

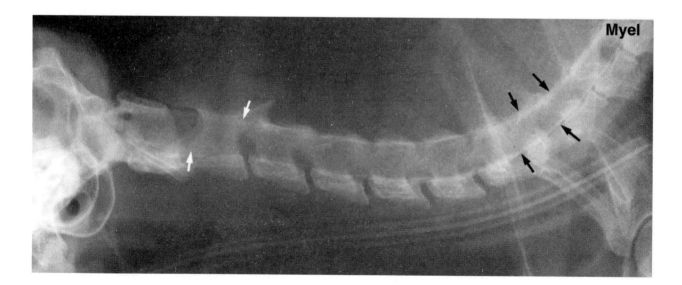

"Tennile" - Radiographic Findings

"Tennile" has spinal changes typical of a geriatric cat, with disc space narrowing, end plate sclerosis, and spondylosis deformans. Disc space collapse at L2-3 is somewhat more prominent than the others. If you think of the position that cats assume when sitting, it is rather easy to understand the modeling of the bodies of T11-L1 that led to development of the wedge shaped vertebrae with the ventral apex. The disc spaces become wedged in the opposite direction with the apex dorsally if the spine is extended. The bones are osteopenic, which is again typical for age.

Since a cause for her myelopathy was not apparent on the noncontrast radiographs, a myelogram was done. The extradural mass seen on the myelogram at L2-3 is ventral and right-sided with a small dorsal, left-sided component. The mass is most likely a disc protrusion (arrows).

Note the small air bubble located at L6 and the larger air bubble at the tip of the needle at L5. While the appearance of the small air bubble is typical, the larger bubble at L5 is more suggestive of an intradural-extramedullary mass. Fortunately later studies showed movement of both filling defects confirming them to be air bubbles. Injection of air during myelography is a preventable technical error.

The owner refused treatment and "Tennile" was released from the clinic.

"M-1" - Radiographic Findings

"M-1" has normal noncontrast studies but has an intramedullary type lesion seen on the myelogram that extends from T9 to T12 (arrows) and causes widening of the spinal cord and narrowing of the subarachnoid columns (arrows). The amount of subarachnoid compression caused by the lesion made it necessary to inject contrast agent from both the cerebellomedullary cistern and the lumbar subarachnoid space in order to identify the cranial and caudal limits of the lesion. While a tumor could have this appearance, intramedullary hemorrhage was thought to be a more likely diagnosis because of the clinical history. "M-1" was treated medically and discharged partially improved.

"Sam" - Radiographic Findings

"Sam" has two spinal lesions. The body of T9 is collapsed with some reactive periosteal bone surrounding a vertebral body that contains a permeative pattern of destruction. The other lesion is at the thoracolumbar junction with dorsal fusion and partial collapse of those vertebrae resulting in a slight scoliosis with the concavity to the right. The modeling of the body of T13 is typical for age. The T9 lesion was believed to be malignant, while the thoracolumbar lesion was thought to be post-traumatic.

The myelogram shows marked vertebral canal invasion at T9 by a mass lesion, with subsequent displacement and compression of the spinal cord by a left sided mass (arrows). The bony changes in addition to the extradural mass suggest a primary bone tumor expanding into the vertebral canal.

The myelogram at the thoracolumbar lesion is normal without any evidence of canal stenosis or cord compression.

On the noncontrast radiographs, there is a question of which lesion is clinically important, T9 is most suggestive since it looks like a compression fracture that could be either traumatic or pathologic. Trauma, infection, or more likely tumor should all be considered in the differential diagnosis. The fusion of the dorsal arch at T13-L1 is of little help in reaching a determination of the etiology of that lesion and those changes could be post-traumatic, postinfectious, or developmental.

The myelogram clearly demonstrates the clinical importance of the lesion at T9. The biopsy diagnosis was a Schwannoma. The bone destruction seen in this cat is somewhat unusual with a tumor of this cell type.

Question #2

If both of "Sam's" lesions, the T9 lesion and the T13-L1 lesion, were causing spinal cord compression, would he have upper motor signs or lower motor signs in the pelvic limbs?

"Annie" - Radiographic Findings

"Annie" has a normal noncontrast cervical radiographic study; however, the myelogram shows extensive cord swelling from C1 to T1 with subarachnoid column thinning (white arrows). A huge intramedullary mass is probably the cause of the myelographic abnormalities. The more normal subarachnoid columns are seen caudal to T1 (black arrows). At necropsy, a neoplasm was found that consisted of highly pleomorphic cells and infiltrated the surrounding spinal cord parenchyma. The tumor was considered to be an undifferentiated sarcoma.

Comment

All of these cats seem to have clinical signs that are minimal when considering the size of the lesion within the spinal canal.

Answer #1

The crossed extension reflex is an abnormal reflex that appears subsequent to moderate or severe and/or chronic lesions to upper motor neurons.

Answer #2

Upper motor neuron signs. Both lesions are in the pelvic limb upper motor neuron area, T3-L3.

Spinal Neoplasia in the Cat

Spinal neoplasia is relatively uncommon in cats but may affect either bone or soft tissues. Lymphosarcoma is an exception and frequently affects the spinal cord or nerve roots and may occur at any point along the vertebral axis. Bone tumors may occur as either primary or secondary. The frequency of either type of vertebral tumors is less than that in the appendicular skeletal system and while uncommon, malignant bone tumors are seen more often than benign bone tumors. Primary bone tumors may be of the expected cell types: osteosarcoma, fibrosarcoma, or chondrosarcoma. The secondary, or metastatic, tumors to bone may be hematogenous or the tumor may extend from soft tissues to a surrounding vertebrae.

Spinal neoplasia may also originate within the meninges or spinal cord or nerve roots where they may be primary or metastatic. Many cats with spinal lymphosarcoma may have additional organ system involvement, suggesting that the spinal lesions may be metastatic in nature. In others, the spinal tumor may be the single lesion suggesting a primary cord involvement.

Certain of the tumors cause marked bony changes while others are seen only with myelography. With the use of this special procedure, the tumor may be identified and described as an extradural, intradural-extramedullary, or intramedullary tumor. While tumors need to be included within a differential diagnosis of causes of a transverse myelopathy, they remain an uncommon cause of clinically detected myelopathy in the cat.

Multiple Osteochondromatosis in the Cat

Multiple cartilaginous exostoses in cats are a unique form of neoplasia and differ markedly from the syndrome of the same name in the dog. Cauliflower-like masses form on the vertebrae, ribs, and bones of the skull that have an aggressive appearance with indistinct lesion margination. While the lesions often involve the axial skeleton, the appendicular skeleton may be affected as well. A tendency for symmetry between lesions is lost if a single lesion achieves rapid growth potential resulting is the formation of a prominent bony mass.

The presence of the lesions appears to be driven by a virus similar to that found in feline leukemia and transmissible feline sarcoma. The lesions increase in size rapidly and are associated with clinical signs that lead to the death of the patient.

Feline Spondylosis Deformans

Bony spurs that form at intervertebral disc spaces have been described frequently in the cat (Jones 1932, Pommer 1933, Glenney 1956, English and Seawright 1964, Seawright and English 1964, Read and Smith 1968; Read 1966; Beadman et al 1964). These vertebral osteophytes originate on the ventral and lateral margins of the vertebral end plates and range in size from the smallest identifiable spur or cuff to complete bony bridges. They are single or multiple around a given disc space and are found at one or many disc spaces. In the cat, the frequency of distribution is seen as a bell-shaped curve extending from C1 to the LS junction with the peak at T7-8.

The frequency and size of the vertebral osteophytes in spondylosis deformans increases with age and all cats over 10 years of age have some degree of spondylosis deformans. Often the vertebral osteophytes are found in conjunction with narrowing of the disc space and sclerosis of the end plate, both of which are associated with the instability caused by a slowly degenerating disc. However, vertebral osteophytes are found around discs with gelatinous nucleus pulposus complicating an understanding of the etiology (King and Smith 1960). The cranial edge of the vertebrae is more frequently affected than the caudal edge. Male and female cats are similarly affected (Reed and Smith 1968). While ventral disc protrusions are noted in association with osteophyte development, there is no evidence that the osteophytes are secondary to the ventral protrusions (King and Smith 1960).

The bony osteophytes of spondylosis deformans grow slowly and have a characteristic shape with a smooth ventral border and a curved beak-like appearance. While most spurs are solitary, other develop to the point of interdigitating ventrally and lateral to the disc space, and other form solid bony bridges. The osteophytes usually are seen as "spurs" on the lateral radiographic projections. Actually, they form from the lateral and ventral periphery of the end plate and are more of a "collar" of bone.

The clinical significance of spondylosis has been exaggerated partially because of the assumption that what appear to be dorsally projecting bony spurs are placing pressure on the spinal cord. These spurs are, in fact, large dorsolaterally positioned spurs that, when seen on a lateral radiograph, incorrectly appear to extend dorsally into the vertebral canal (Reed and Smith 1968).

The term spondylosis deformans is best reserved for the generalized formation of osteophytes throughout the vertebral column secondary to generalized disc degeneration. The bony osteophytes that form secondary to more acute causes of vertebral disease, such as congenital instability, trauma, or infection, are more appropriately referred to as reactive spurring or vertebral osteophytes.

A Brachial Plexus Tumor

Case Description

"Rusty" is a 6-year-old male retriever with chronic progressive lameness of the right forelimb for the past 6 months. Muscle atrophy is evident. The right cutaneus trunci reflex is depressed to right and left stimulation. The left cutaneus trunci reflex is normal following right and left stimulation. Right pupil miosis is present. Rusty was thought to have a brachial plexus tumor. Noncontrast spinal studies and a myelogram were performed.

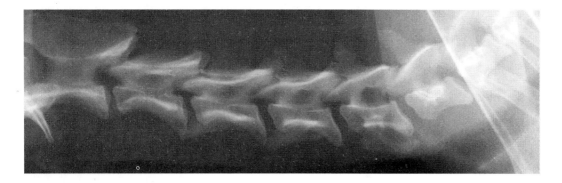

Radiographic Findings

The spinal changes in the noncontrast study (above) are limited to minimal spondylosis deformans.

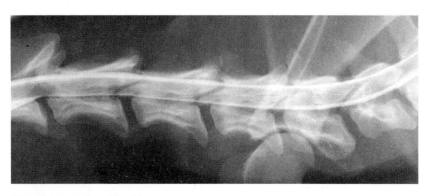

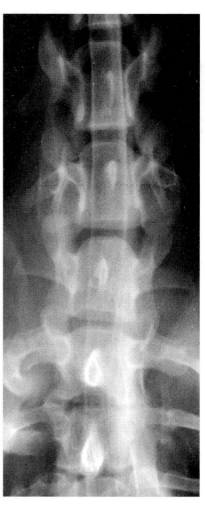

Myelographic Findings

The lateral and VD views from the myelogram are radiographically normal.

Comment

"Rusty" is an example of a patient with a progressive disease that ultimately caused his death and yet the radiographic studies were normal. A Schwannoma (tumor arising from a Schwann cell) was located just outside the spinal cord, and failed to cause any bony changes secondary to tumor expansion or myelographic changes due to tumor invasion into the spinal cord. An understanding of what type of lesions can be identified radiographically is important so that you know which lesions have not been ruled out by these studies.

"Rusty's" lesion may well have been detected by contrast-enhanced magnetic resonance imaging.

Question #1

Describe the pathway for the cutaneus trunci reflex.

Question #2

Some Schwannomas do cause radiographic and myelographic abnormalities. Can you describe these abnormalities?

Answer #1

The cutaneus trunci reflex is a long, intersegmental, spinal reflex. The pathway is as follows: dorsal cutaneus branch of spinal nerve innervating the skin where the stimulus is applied, spinal nerve and dorsal roots, synapse in dorsal horn, ipsilateral and contralateral fasciculus proprius, synapse with lower motor neurons in ventral horn at C8 and T1 spinal cord segments, C8 and T1 ventral roots and spinal nerves, lateral thoracic nerve, and cutaneus trunci muscle.

Answer #2

Noncontrast radiographs - Enlargement of the intervertebral foramen or enlargement of the vertebral canal due the slowly increasing mass may be seen.

Myelogram - Any one or any combination of the three mass myelographic patterns may be seen. A combination pattern is very suggestive of Schwannoma, because the nerve fibers are located both extradural and intradural. At its juncture with the spinal cord, a Schwannoma may undermine the arachnoid and the pia and therefore appear myelographically as an intramedullary mass. A multilobulated mass is also possible because the tumor may involve multiple spinal nerves and nerve roots and cause an extradural pattern.

Diagnostic Approach for Lameness

Overall, the most common cause of lameness is musculoskeletal disease, not neurologic disease. Therefore the recommended diagnostic plan for these animals is:

1. Acquire a complete history and perform a general physical examination.
2. Perform an orthopedic examination of the affected limb(s).
3. If any musculoskeletal abnormalities are detected, perform indicated diagnostic procedures (radiographs, biopsy, etc).
4. If an orthopedic cause for the lameness cannot be identified, do a complete neurologic examination of the animal, including cutaneous sensory testing of the affected limb(s).
5. If neurologic disease is detected or suspected, localize the lesion.

6. Construct a list of differential diagnoses.
7. If a radiculopathy, meningopathy, or myelopathy is on the differential list, do noncontrast spinal radiographs.
8. If spinal radiographs do not show a cause for the lameness, do a CSF analysis.
9. If CSF analysis does not determine the cause, perform contrast radiographic studies as indicated by the location of the lesion (e.g., myelogram, epidurogram, discogram).
10. If contrast radiography does not detect the cause, consider special radiographic procedures such as CT or MRI, or surgical exploration.

Motor Accidents

Dogs are hit by cars so often, and frequently incur multiple, serious and often life-threatening injuries, that these patients deserve special attention. Most of the dogs involved are young, and often they are larger dogs that are permitted to run freely.

Dogs that are hit by a car should be handled very carefully (preferably restrained in lateral recumbency on a rigid surface) until a survey radiographic study of the spine can be examined. Often a diagnosis can be made from the noncontrast study. A myelogram can add useful information, however, particularly if surgical intervention is contemplated. The newer contrast agents do not seem to be particularly harmful to a traumatized spinal cord; therefore the procedure is much safer than earlier. All of the dogs below were presumed to have been struck by automobiles. Examine the radiographs and make your diagnosis.

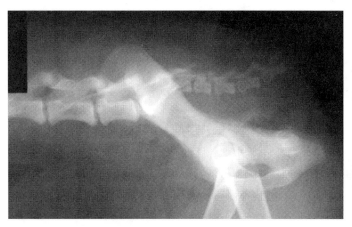

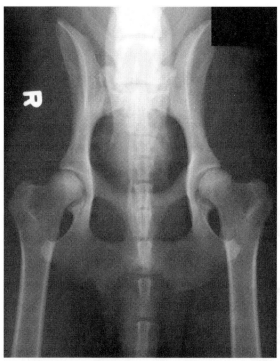

Case Description

"Shane" is a 2-year-old male mixed-breed dog who was hit by a car 1 week ago and now has pain in the hindquarters when sitting down. He shows pain on movement of his tail and when you attempt to perform a rectal examination.

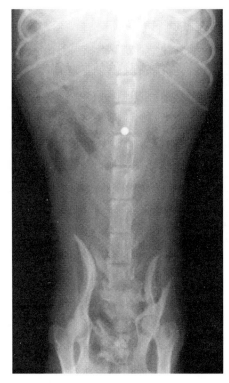

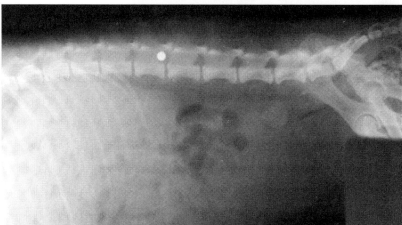

Case Description

"Sue" is a 3-year-old female mixed-breed dog who has upper motor neuron paraplegia and apparently is anesthetic in the pelvic limbs. The owner's are unable to provide any relevant history other than they found her in this condition. Thoracic and abdominal radiographs are made. The abdominal study is above.

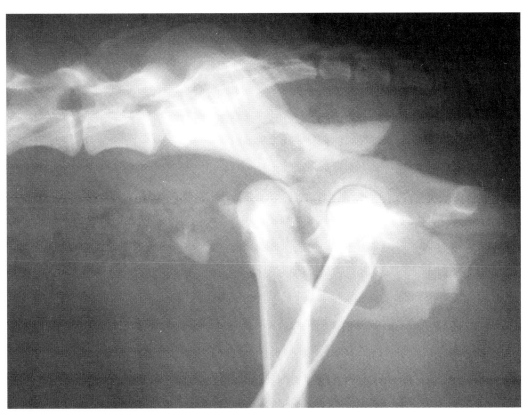

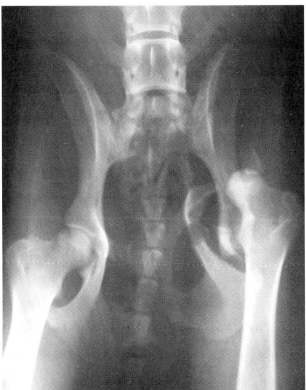

Case Description

"**Suzie**' is a 1-year-old female pointer who was hit by a car 11 days ago and was just referred because of suspected pelvic injuries. A detail lateral view is seen below..

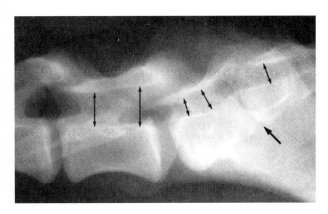

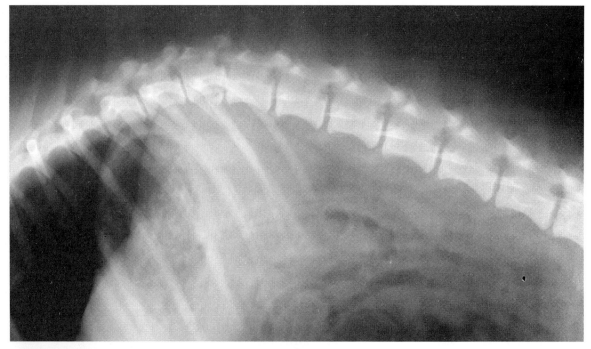

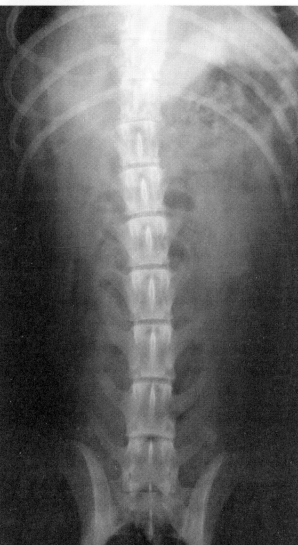

Case Description

"BC" is a 1-year-old female collie who is paraplegic after being injured. She has upper motor neuron signs in the pelvic limbs. Pain perception in the pelvic limbs appears to be decreased.

Question #1

Can you discern the status of the spinal cord from this study?

Question #2

Does this dog have a diaphragmatic hernia with gastric herniation as seen on the lateral view?

Question #3

Did you note the transitional LS segment?

"Shane" - Radiographic Findings

"Shane's" pelvic radiographs show a sacral fracture with fragment separation. The minimal prostatic enlargement is noted and can be evaluated later.

Comments

Sacral lesions can be overlooked on the lateral view if the film is underexposed, and not seen on the ventrodorsal view because of fecal material and gas within the rectum. While not life threatening, their detection explains the clinical signs demonstrated and eliminates the need for additional costly diagnostic procedures.

"Shane" has bilateral hip dysplasia. The hip joints have an early arthrosis and may be more susceptible to trauma than normal hips and may play a role in the pain he is exhibiting.

"Sue" - Radiographic Findings

"Sue's" thoracic radiographs are normal; however, the abdominal study is confusing to say the least. She has bilateral luxation of the sacroiliac joints, which has permitted the pelvis to displace cranially. She also has a displaced left ilial fracture. Both hip joints appear normal. Only with careful examination can you ascertain that the bony fragments are modeled, have some callus formation, and represent a nonunion/malunion fracture.

Then, the real problem becomes apparent—the air gun pellet in the vertebral canal at the level of L2-3. (Note that both lateral and ventrodorsal views are necessary to identify the pellet's location within the vertebral canal.) No evidence of vertebral fracture is seen indicating the pellet must have gained entrance to the vertebral canal through an intervertebral foramen. While this appears to be an unlikely event, the authors have seen several other dogs as well as cats in which this has happened.

"Suzie" - Radiographic Findings

"Suzie's" pelvic radiographs show an acute left acetabular fractures with a femoral head luxation, and right pubic and ischial fractures resulting in pelvic canal narrowing. Of equal clinical importance is the transitional lumbosacral vertebra with a marked decrease in the height of the vertebral canal (double-headed arrows). The separation between the transitional segment and the sacrum is identified on the detail view (large arrow). This congenital anomaly is seen frequently with the suggestion of either immediate or potential clinical importance.

Comments

The diagnosis of pelvic fractures with femoral head luxation attracts the immediate attention of the surgeon. However, the vertebral canal stenosis associated with the transitional vertebral segment is extreme and the trauma may have caused injury to the LS disc and thus accentuated the development of a cauda equina syndrome.

"BC" - Radiographic Findings

"BC's" radiographs show a fracture-luxation with spinal malalignment at T13-L1 with a chip fracture from the body of T13.

Answer #1

No

Answer #2

No. "BC" is laying on her right side and the gas filled fundus of the stomach on the left side is "pushed" so it appears cranial to the right crus of the diaphragm.

Answer #3

We hope so. The spinous process of the transitional segment is separated from the sacral processes as seen on the VD view.

Radiography of Spinal Trauma

With a known trauma patient, lateral radiographs should be used as a survey technique before additional radiographic examinations are performed that require extensive movement of the spine. If no evidence of fracture-dislocation is identified on the lateral projection, the patient may be positioned carefully in dorsal recumbency and ventrodorsal radiographs can be made. In trauma cases, it is always important to obtain a radiographic evaluation of the entire vertebral column in the event of multiple fractures or dislocations that may be unsuspected on physical or neurological examination.

Physeal fractures occur in young patients with separation of the end plate. Skeletally immature patients have bony trabeculae that lack strength and compression fractures are common. Little or no displacement of fragments is seen other than the collapse. Oblique fractures are most common in the thoracic and lumbar regions of mature patients and the radiolucent fracture lines extend through the vertebral body causing a resulting malalignment of vertebral fragments. Injuries that center on the disc space and dorsal vertebral joints cause narrowing of the disc space, minimal vertebral malalignment, and fracture of the articular processes and are often evaluated as luxations rather than fractures.

Separation of the odontoid process is a special type of physeal fracture usually recognized by the ventral displacement of the axis and marked narrowing of the vertebral canal. Use of a lateral view with the head flexed and a ventrodorsal open-mouth projection may more clearly demonstrate the free fragment.

Fractures involving only the dorsal arch of the vertebra without major fragment displacement are difficult to detect. Caudal to the anticlinal segment, the caudally projecting articular processes fit snugly inside the cranially directed articular processes from the next caudal vertebra and normally provide a repeated radiographic pattern that can be interrupted by trauma.

The degree of vertebral displacement seen radiographically does not tell the degree of displacement at the time of the injury and, hence, the maximal injury to the spinal cord. In patients with marked fracture-dislocation, the injury to the spinal cord is assumed to be severe. However, the arch of the vertebra may be broken free resulting in minimal canal stenosis and adequate space for the spinal cord exists due to the "traumatic dorsal laminectomy."

Differential Diagnosis

Differential diagnosis in most cases of acute vertebral trauma is limited. The rapid onset of neurological signs plus the clinical history are strongly supportive of a history of acute trauma. Pathological fracture is the most difficult to separate from a trauma-induced fracture

Radiographic features in spinal fracture-luxation

1. lateral view
   a. disruption of the line indicating the floor of the vertebral canal
   b. kyphosis
   c. shortening of a vertebral body
   d. separation of an end plate
   e. fracture lines
   f. vertebral displacement
   g. canal stenosis
   h. disc space collapse
2. ventrodorsal view
   a. disruption in the line drawn between adjacent spinous processes or pedicles
   b. scoliosis
   c. shortening of a vertebral body
   d. separation of an end plate
   e. fracture lines
   f. vertebral displacement
   g. disc space collapse

Clinical Signs of Spinal Trauma

Spinal injuries in dogs and cats result most commonly from direct physical trauma such as an automobile accident, falling, or a bite wound. Following injury, the spinal cord may undergo sustained compression and/or distraction. The severity of a spinal cord injury as determined by the eventual quality of recovery is related to three factors: (1) the velocity with which compressive force is applied, (2) the degree of compression (transverse deformation), and (3) the duration of the compression. Unfortunately, these factors cannot accurately be evaluated on the radiographs.

Neural tissue may be physically disrupted and fail on a mechanical basis, however, more commonly the spinal cord remains physically intact but is functionally deranged. A profound ischemic or hypoxic insult follows and the neuronal population subsequently undergoes coagulative necrosis. The adjacent white matter is relatively less affected

There are three levels of spinal cord injury to consider as you consider the findings from the physical and neurological examination and the radiographic studies. Spinal cord concussion is a clinical syndrome caused by an immediate and transient impairment of neuronal functions due to a mechanical force. It can result in neurologic dysfunction which is usually temporary. Spinal cord contusion is a syndrome resulting from bruising and necrosis, with hemorrhage and edema. When malacia of neurons has begun in this lesion, irreversible changes to the spinal cord ensue. Spinal cord laceration is due to spinal cord displacement or fracture fragmentation.

Clinical assessment

Dogs and cats with a spinal cord injury frequently have serious injuries of other organ systems. A major component of the clinical assessment of an animal's condition, therefore, is the determination of the relative urgency of need for treatment of non-neurogenic injuries versus the need for early treatment of spinal cord injury.

At the time of presentation, the animal should be placed in lateral recumbency and should remain in that position during subsequent clinical and radiographic examinations. A thorough assessment of the animal's general condition must be made, looking for major problems such as hemorrhage, shock, airway obstruction, or limb fractures. Immediate treatment is limited to those problems that are life-threatening. Treatment of other conditions is often deferred until initial management of the spinal cord injury is underway.

A complete neurologic examination is performed to localize the site of the injury and to determine severity of the injury. Careful palpation of the vertebral column may aid in identification of a vertebral fracture or luxation. It is important that administration of tranquilizers or analgesics be delayed until completion of a neurological examination, as these agents may alter an animal's responses. A neurologic examination should be done with minimal movement of the animal in order to prevent further injury resulting from vertebral instability.

Extent of a spinal cord injury usually can be assessed accurately at the time of initial examination, as most spinal injuries are nonprogressive and as spinal shock (a phenomenon resulting in loss of physiologic functions caudal to a spinal cord injury) is not of clinical significance in animals.

Several aspects of the neurologic examination are of special importance in the assessment of a cat or dog with a spinal injury. Attention should be given to the animal's posture which may aid in determination of location and severity of a lesion. For example, Schiff-Sherrington syndrome, which results from a severe lesion caudal to T2, is of great localizing value and must be differentiated from other postures such as decerebrate rigidity or decerebellate rigidity.

Motor function, muscle tone, and spinal reflexes must be carefully assessed. These functions are utilized to localize a lesion to one of four major regions of the spinal cord: cervical (C1-C5), brachial enlargement (C6-T2), thoracolumbar (T3-L3), and lumbar enlargement (L4-Cy5).

Multiple spinal fractures may occur, and the clinical signs of a more caudal lesion may mask those resulting from a second lesion located further cranially. For example, the lower motor neuron signs caused by a lesion at L5-6 may mask the hyperreflexia that would be caused by a second injury at T13-L1.

The most important factor in neurologic prognosis is pain perception. Pain perception is assessed by applying a painful stimulus and observing the animal for a brain-mediated response. The stimulus applied to a foot may result in withdrawal of the limb by a spinal reflex mechanism (the flexion reflex), even though the spinal cord may have been severed. It is essential to distinguish these spinal reflex movements from brain-mediated responses. Two types of pain perception are sometimes distinguished in animals. "Superficial" pain perception is manifested by a response to pricking or pinching of the skin, and "deep" pain perception is shown by response to pinching of the toes or tail with a hemostatic forceps. The loss of "superficial" pain perception occurs with less severe lesions than those resulting in loss of "deep" pain perception.

Previous Radiographs Can Be Helpful

In some patients, the availability of previous radiographic studies makes a diagnosis easier. These patients all have earlier spinal studies that can be used in comparison.

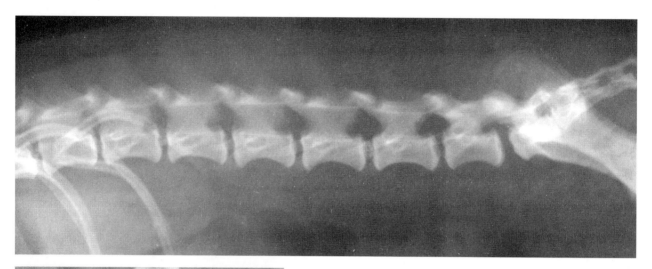

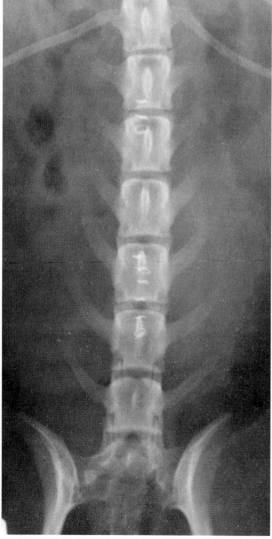

Case Description

"**Blossom**" is a 5-year-old female Pekingese with a long history of back pain. Recently, she developed a mild paraparesis with an area of increased sensitivity over L4-6. The spinal reflexes appear normal. You examine radiographs made 3 years ago before looking at today's study.

Radiographic Findings - (3 years ago)

The radiographs from 3 years ago (seen on this page) show heavily calcified disc tissue at L4-5. You note that "Blossom" has only 6 typical lumbar-type vertebrae and an LS transitional segment with asymmetrical transverse processes. Neither of these was thought to be causing clinical signs at that time.

At the time of this earlier study, "Blossom" had upper motor neuron signs in the pelvic limbs. She was assumed to have a TL lesion. The discs from T11-12 through L2-L3 were fenestrated. It was hoped this would prevent further disc disease.

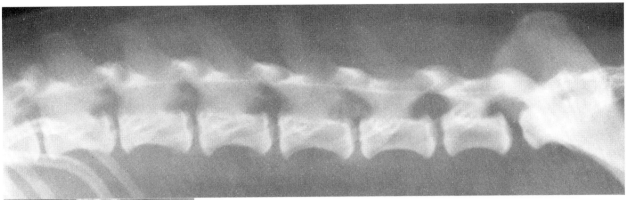

Radiographic Findings (today's study)

The radiographs of "Blossom" that were made today show calcified disc tissue positioned over the L4-5 disc space (see enlargement view below). The transitional LS segment with asymmetrical transverse processes appears stable as earlier without development of reactive spondylosis deformans. The diagnosis is herniation of a previously noted calcified disc.

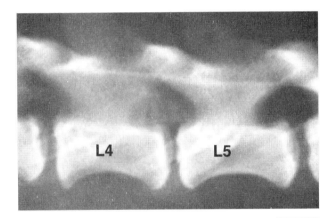

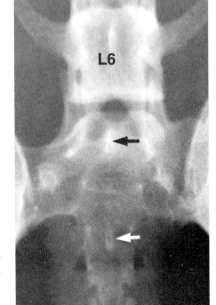

Comments

It is unfortunate that the status of the L4-5 disc was ignored earlier. The rule that determines how many discs are to be fenestrated at the time of the first detection of neurologic signs is not clear.

The spinous processes from the sacrum are almost absent suggesting a tendency toward an incomplete arch formation or a spina bifida. The spinous process of the transitional segment is identified (black arrow) as is the spinous process of the sacrum (white arrow). The congenital anomaly shows good vertebral alignment and is probably stable and without vertebral canal stenosis and requires no treatment at this time.

Case Description

"**Fritzi**" is a 4-year-old male dachshund with paraparesis. The upper motor neuron signs in the pelvic limbs began on the left side 12 days ago and became bilateral 9 days ago. Progression of neurological signs is always an indication of a clinically important lesion. You have three studies to examine. The first 23 months ago, the second study 9 months ago, and the study made today. Try to plot the changes within the cervical discs during the past 2 years.

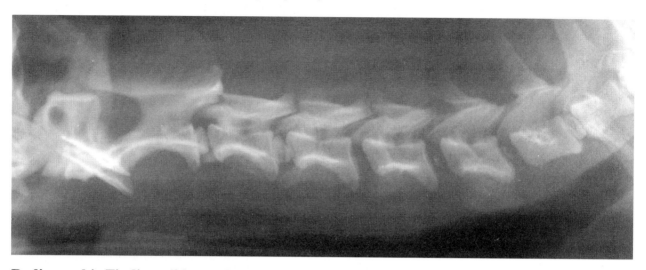

Radiographic Findings (23 months ago)

"Fritzi" had a herniated disc at T13-L1 at the time of the first study that was treated with a TL hemilaminectomy. The radiographs also demonstrated calcified cervical discs without evidence of herniation. The cervical discs were not treated because the dog did not show any clinical signs of cervical disc herniation.

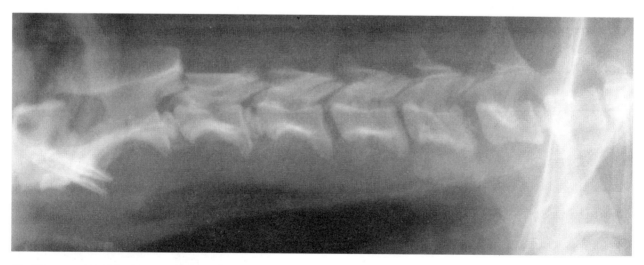

Radiographic Findings (9 months ago)

"Fritzi" began to show cervical pain and became anorexic 13 months after the first study, or 9 months ago, and radiographs made at that time show collapse of C5-6 with probable dorsal herniation of the disc. He was treated at that time by confinement and recovered satisfactorily.

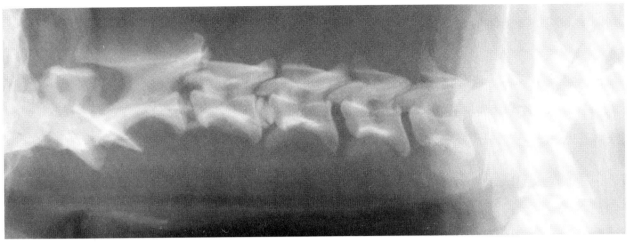

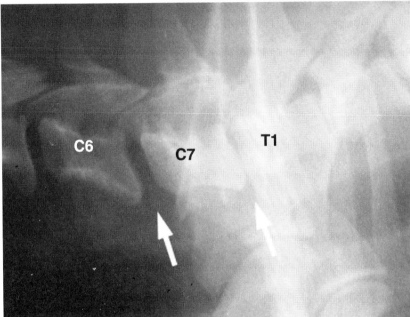

Radiographic Findings (today's study)

At the time of the study today, "Fritzi" has cervical pain with limping on one forelimb. This third set of radiographs show persistent narrowing of C5-6 and probably narrowing of C6-7. In addition, the calcified disc tissue at C7-T1 that has been present since the first study has herniated into the vertebral canal. A detail radiograph of the cervicothoracic area shows more clearly the narrowing of C6-7 (arrow) and the narrowing and empty appearance of C7-T1 (arrow).

Comments

"Fritzi" is an example of a patient who from the age of 4 to 6 years is in the veterinary clinic on three separate episodes with disc disease. The role of prophylactic fenestration in a dog of this type needs to be strongly considered.

The goal of disc fenestration is prevention of disc herniation by removal of disc material from the disc space and by provision of an alternate, non-harmful, "herniation" path for any remaining disc material. Most neurosurgeons believe that disc fenestration does have prophylactic benefit, but some surgeons disagree and the subject is quite controversial. If fenestration is performed, usually all the discs that can be reasonably reached and that have a high probability of protrusion are fenestrated. In the cervical region, the discs commonly fenestrated are C2-3 to C6-7. In the thoracolumbar region, the commonly fenestrated discs are T11-12 through L3-4. If C7-T1, T10-11 or L4-5 are heavily calcified, an attempt may be made to fenestrate, but these three discs are more difficult to expose surgically than are the others.

Because disc disease usually involves many discs in a single dog, and because all the discs in any one dog cannot be fenestrated, the probability always exists that one of the unfenestrated discs could herniate at a later time and cause clinical problems. Careful education of the pet's owner is imperative in dealing with this disorder so they understand the generalized nature of disc disease.

Case Description

"**Lobo**" is an 11-year-old male shepherd that had weight loss for 1 month. A non-specific prostatic disease was diagnosed. Two earlier abdominal studies had been made. The first was made in July (8 months ago) and the next in the following November (4 months ago). The most recent study was made in February (at the time of the most recent admission). The studies were all abdominal studies and only the lumbar spine as seen on those studies is included in the figures.

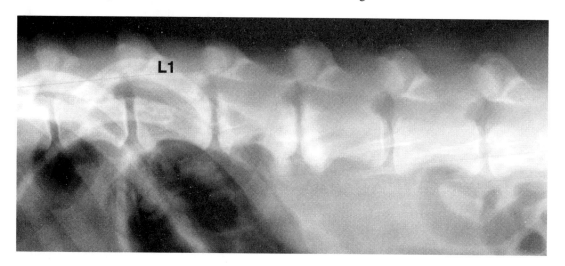

Radiographic Findings (8 months ago)

The first radiographic study made in July shows minimal end plate destruction at L1-2 and L2-3 that has an indistinct margin suggesting an acute destructive process. Disc space narrowing is noted. Reactive vertebral osteophytes are present at T13-L1 and L2-L3.

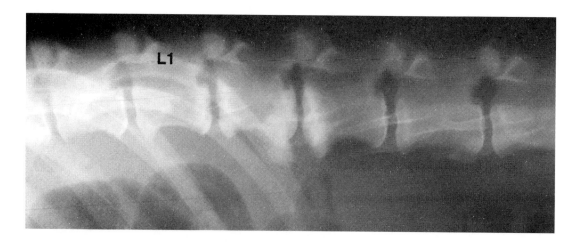

Radiographic Findings (4 months ago)

The second radiographic study made 4 months later in November shows the progression of the end plate destruction with persistent disc space collapse. The vertebral osteophytes are larger and more dense.

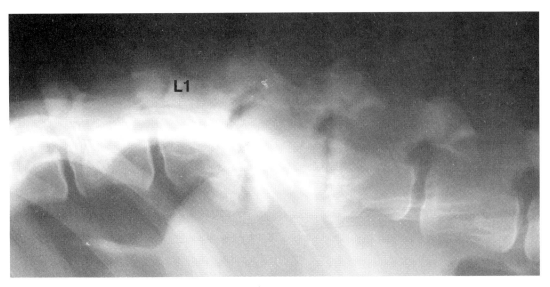

Radiographic Findings (today's study)

The third radiographic study was made 3 months later in the following February at the time of latest admission and shows marked progression of the end plate destruction with shortening of the vertebral bodies and disc space collapse. Note the resulting kyphosis. Destruction is now present within the vertebral joints as well.

The diagnosis of a progressive discospondylitis was delayed because it was thought the clinical signs were due to a prostatic lesion. The rather minimal nature of the destructive lesions as seen radiographically on the early studies was ignored. The progression of change radiographically called attention to the bony lesions that are typical for an inflammatory, hematogenous discospondylitis with a resulting malalignment present on the last study.

Comments

Migrating grass awns (seed heads) are a common cause for a spondylitis in the lumbar region, but they typically cause a periosteal new bone response and uncommonly affect the disc spaces until later in the course of the disease. In "Lobo", the lesions center in the disc spaces with end plate destruction suggesting instead, a hematogenous method of spread. Staphylococcus sp. grew repeatedly from blood cultures despite antibiotic therapy.

The bony collapse and malalignment of the vertebral bodies suggests the possibility of an instability and "Lobo" would have needed to be confined to avoid potentially serious spinal cord injury.

At necropsy shortly after the last study, endocarditis, meningoencephalitis, poliomyelitis, myocarditis, pancreatitis, hepatitis, enteritis, nephritis, splenitis and adrenalitis were identified, all due to a generalized Staphylococcus sp infection and confirmed the hematogenous method of spread of the infection.

Case Description

"**Max**" is an 8-year-old male dog with a chronic history of urethral obstructions that required repeated cystotomies. Cystic calculi were palpated today. After being in the clinic for 1 week, the dog developed a painful gait. Radiographs of the lumbosacral region were made. These were followed by additional studies made 1 month and 2 months later. The first of the three studies of the lumbosacral region is shown below. You should be able to make a tentative diagnosis from these films.

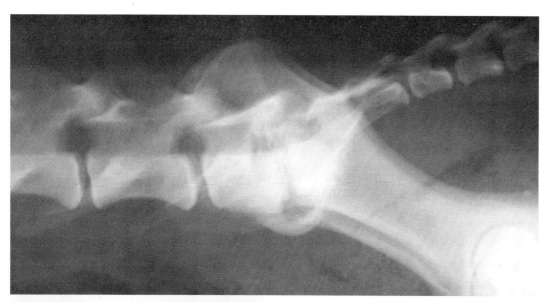

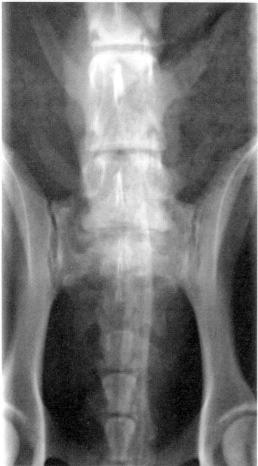

Radiographic Findings (first study)

The first radiographs show changes at the LS disc space characterized by: large sequestra in the end plates, collapse of the LS disc space, sclerosis of the end plates, and a reactive spondylosis deformans. No evidence of vertebral canal stenosis, vertebral instability, or malalignment is present. These changes suggest an acute LS discospondylitis superimposed over a chronic LS disc disease. This is a common sequence with hematogenous infection superimposed over a degenerating LS disc.

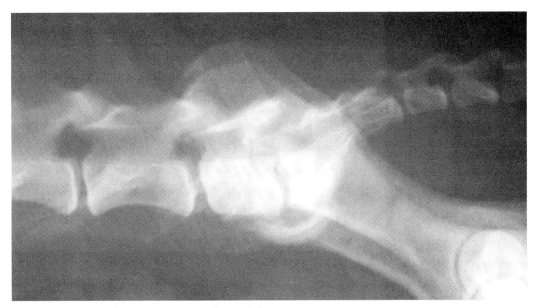

Radiographic Findings (second study)

A second radiographic study made 1 month later shows a progressive bony destruction at the LS junction. The end plates have an undulated margin resulting in shortening of the body of L7 as well as the sacrum. Malalignment between the vertebrae is indicated by ventral displacement of the sacrum. This study is diagnostic of a progressive discospondylitis.

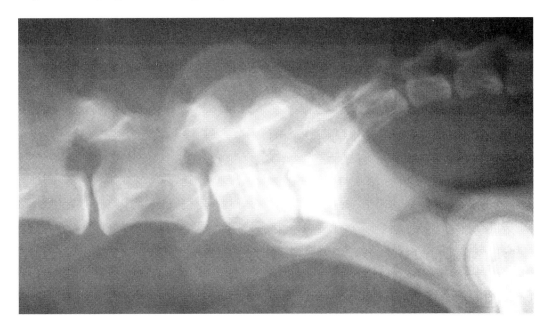

Radiographic Findings (third study)

The third radiographic study was made 1 month after the second study and shows the further collapse of the LS disc space. "Max" now has pain on elevation of the tail probably associated with the resulting vertebral canal stenosis secondary to instability or projection of diseased disc tissue into the vertebral canal.

Comments

The radiographic studies show a progression of change but a single study does not provide information on whether the LS lesion is active or is in a stage of healing.

"Max" was castrated and chronic, necropurulent to pyogranulomatous epididymitis was found. E.coli was grown from the surgical biopsy specimen. In an older male dog with chronic disc disease, LS discospondylitis in conjunction with pelvic inflammatory disease is often found.

What Is Your Diagnosis?

These are a series of cases that are somewhat unique and will require your careful attention in reaching the correct diagnosis. Not all of the lesions are of equal clinical importance. The diagnoses are discussed on the following pages.

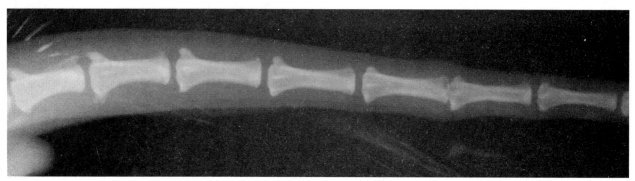

Case Description

"Sam" is a 4-year-old male Labrador retriever who has a small swelling on his tail that was painful when palpated.

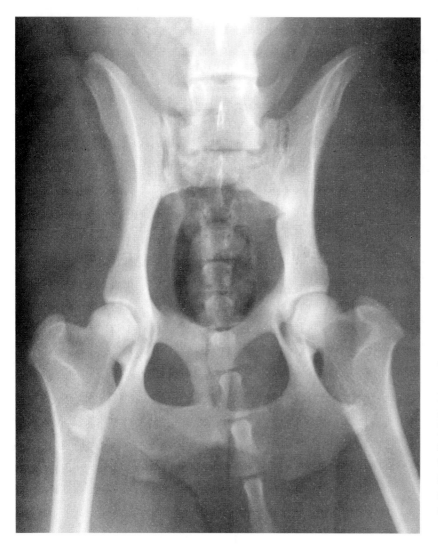

Case Description

"Chica" is a 2-year-old female Labrador retriever who was playing and suddenly developed right hind limb lameness after running into a fence. The owner thought she had been lame in that limb for 4 to 5 weeks. An earlier radiograph is shown at the end of the section along with a discussion of the diagnosis.

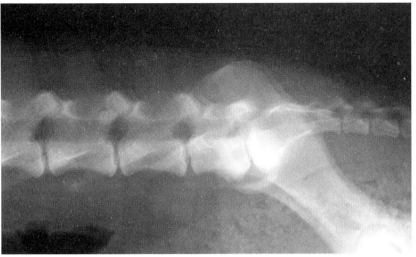

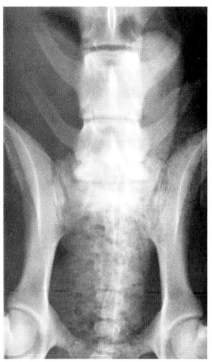

Case Description

"**Shandy**" is a 4-year-old male terrier who was referred with a 5-week history of clinical signs suggestive of prostatitis. He is noted to have pelvic limb lameness on physical examination. Noncontrast pelvic studies were made.

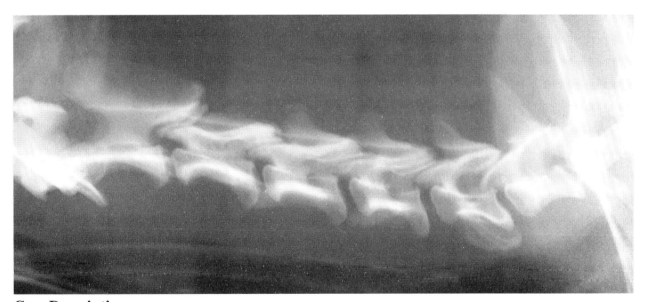

Case Description

"**Fred**" is a 5-year-old male Basset hound with cervical pain. Examine the radiograph from the current cervical studies. After you have made a tentative diagnosis, examine the cervical radiograph at the end of the section that was made 1 year earlier.

"Sam" - Radiographic Findings

The single radiograph of the tail shows a focal soft tissue swelling, collapse of the disc space, and lucency in the end plates. The diagnosis is a discitis and early spondylitis most likely associated with a bite wound.

Comments

The prominent marks on the radiograph around the tail are the result of a wet hair coat.

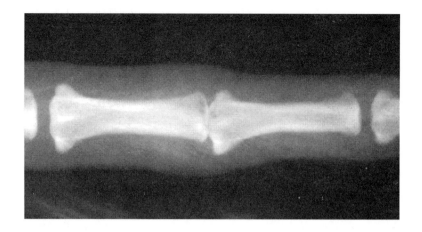

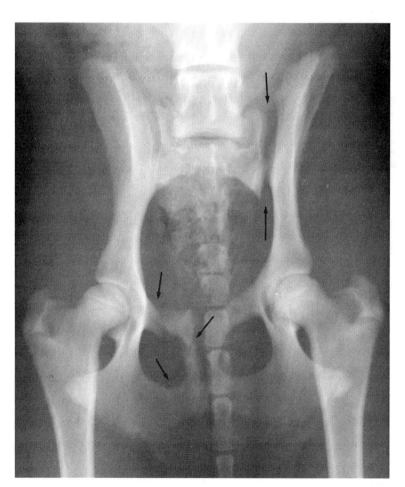

"Chica" - Radiographic Findings

The current radiographs show new bone formed around the left sacroiliac junction and midshaft of the left ilium. The pelvis seems to be malpositioned with atypical fusion of the left sacroiliac joint. These abnormalities are most likely post-traumatic. This assessment is based on the mature appearance of the new bone featuring a smooth, complete margin and the absence of reactive periosteal new bone and destructive bony features. Fortunately an earlier radiograph was found that confirmed the results of the earlier trauma (arrows).

Comments

Post-traumatic changes can be confusing because they appear productive and suggest either an inflammatory or a neoplastic lesion. Earlier radiographs always make the radiographic interpretation easier. On further physical examination, the cause of the acute lameness was found in the stifle joint.

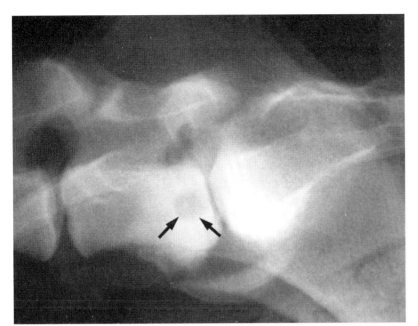

"Shandy" - Radiographic Findings

The noncontrast radiographs show: (1) a cystic lesion in the caudal aspect of L7 (arrows), (2) a collapsed lumbosacral disc space, (3) end plate sclerosis, and (4) reactive spondylosis deformans. No evidence of malalignment or canal stenosis is present. The spondylosis deformans suggests chronic instability. A discogram is shown below.

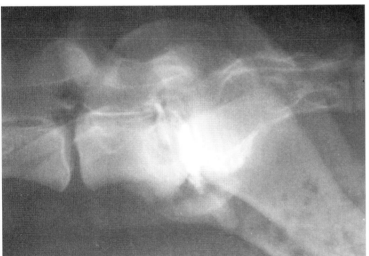

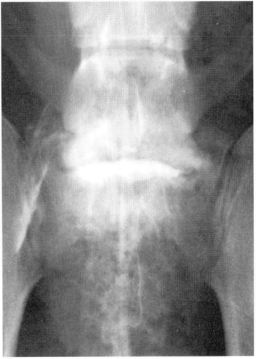

Discographic Findings

To study the cystic lesion in "Shandy" more closely a discogram was performed that showed cavitation of the lumbosacral disc with spread of contrast medium ventrally and laterally. The contrast agent did not spread dorsally and did not flow into the cystic lesion. The contrast medium did escape into the internal vertebral venous plexus. The diagnosis was an abscess cavity associated with a chronic discospondylitis, but without vertebral canal involvement.

Comments

Abscess cavities such as this are seen in chronic inflammatory lesions but are uncommon. They may be referred to a Brodie's abscess. A bone biopsy was done under fluoroscopic control but did not provide sufficient tissue on which to base a diagnosis.

Movement of the LS region was painful and the owner was advised of the likelihood of continued degeneration of the LS disc and the possibility of development of a cauda equina syndrome.

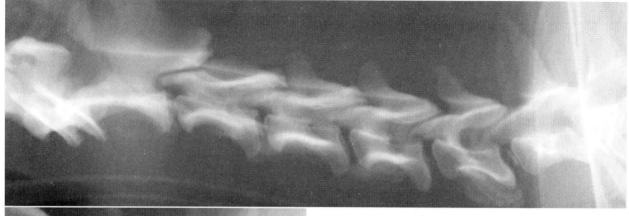

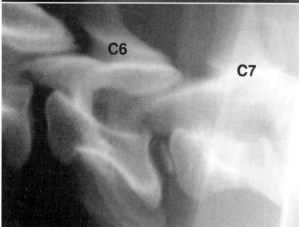

C6

C7

"Fred" - Radiographic Findings

The radiograph made at 4 years of age shows calcification of C6-7 (see the adjacent enlargement) while the radiograph made at 5 years of age shows the C6-7 disc has herniated, emptying the calcified nuclear contents dorsally into the vertebral canal.

Comments

Notice how incompletely you are able to evaluate the disc space at C7-T1 because of the overlying heads of the first ribs.

Disc Degeneration in the Dog

An intervertebral disc is located between every vertebral body except C1 and C2 and the sacral vertebrae. The disc is composed of an amorphous, gelatinous center (the "nucleus pulposus") and a lamellar, fibrous outer ring (the "anulus fibrosus") that attaches firmly to adjacent vertebrae. The dorsal portion of the anulus is reinforced minimally by the dorsal longitudinal ligament, which extends along the floor of the vertebral canal. In the thoracic region (T1-2 to T10-11), intercapital ligaments extend transversely from one rib head across the floor of the vertebral canal to the opposite rib head. These ligaments blend with the anulus fibrosus dorsally, and help to reinforce it. The intervertebral disc, particularly the semifluid nucleus, serves as a shock absorber, whereas the tough anulus distributes the stresses and strains of movement. If the retaining anulus ruptures or degenerates, the gelatinous nucleus can shift in position or extrude.

Pathogenesis of disc degeneration and rupture

Hansen described, in 1952, two morphologically distinct forms of disc degeneration: one in chondrodystrophoid dogs (e.g., Dachshund or Pekingese) at a comparatively early age, and the other in aged dogs of all breeds. The first form is preceded by a chondroid metamorphosis of the nucleus pulposus. At the age of one year, 75 to 100 percent of all nuclei have undergone this change. Thirty to 60 percent of these nuclei eventually calcify. The second form of disc degeneration (seen typically in nonchondrodystrophoid breeds) is preceded by a fibroid metamorphosis of the nucleus, which develops more slowly than the chondroid metamorphosis. Calcifications are much less common.

Because degeneration affects all the discs of the vertebral column, the disease can be considered to be systemic. Certain breeds, and perhaps certain dogs, seem to be in an intermediate position in which some discs calcify, but not at as early an age or in the large numbers as seen in a typical chondrodystrophoid breed. Beagles belong in this group and certain Doberman Pinschers also frequently have calcified nuclei.

Following the nuclear degeneration of either type, the anulus begins to degenerate and nuclear material can begin to protrude. If a total rupture of the anulus occurs, there is a massive extrusion of nuclear material into the vertebral canal. This type of disease is Hansen's Type 1 and is particularly characteristic of discs undergoing chondroid degeneration. This occurs in the younger dog in which the water content of the nucleus remains high. If the anulus remains intact and the nucleus looses a part of its water content, Hansen's Type II lesion results with a bulging of the anulus without nuclear extrusion.

Although these two distinct forms of disc degeneration do occur, there is considerable overlapping. Fibroid degeneration and Type II protrusions occur mostly in the middle-aged to older, nonchondrodystrophoid dog. However, nonchondrodystrophoid dogs may also have a heavily calcified nucleus and Type 1 protrusions. Type II disease may be seen in all dogs as they age. If the dog survives a Type 1 lesion a third type of lesion results. This occurs when the protruded material becomes a fibrotic mass within the vertebral canal causing chronic cord compression and is thought of as a Type III lesion. It is an extradural mass and because of its chronicity, lacks the clinical importance of an explosive Type 1 disease.

Disc ruptures or protrusions can occur ventrally, laterally, or dorsally. Dorsally located lesions are clinically important because they can cause meningeal irritation and spinal cord compression.

Although chondroid and fibroid degeneration takes place in all discs, nuclear herniations have a regional distribution. This distribution is apparently due to both mechanical and anatomic factors. The T11-L3 region has the greatest mechanical load and, therefore, the largest number of prolapses. The cervical spine bears the second heaviest load of stresses and strains. Protrusions in the region from T1-2 to T10-11 are relatively rare, probably because of the light mechanical load and the protection offered by the intercapital ligament. LS disc degeneration is frequent in certain breeds and is often associated with a transitional LS vertebra. These patterns of distribution are influenced by the breed type.

Clinical features

Typically, the Type 1 disease occurs rapidly as a result of sudden rupture of the anulus; consequently, the clinical signs develop quickly, usually within minutes or hours. A slower onset can occur in the older dog as the water content of the nucleus decreases and sometimes the clinical signs may develop in stepwise fashion, as though small amounts of nuclear material were being released at intervals. Sometimes clinical signs develop, then disappear, then develop again days or weeks later. This can occur many times ending in complete or irreversible paralysis. TL herniations occurs more quickly while cervical herniations are slower in development.

Type II disease is generally gradual in development. The onset may be subtle, with progression over weeks or months. Often, the initial onset and early progression is so insidious that it is not noticed by the owner. Typically, these dogs are presented with a several-month history of progressive hindlimb or forelimb weakness or both. Type III lesions have a similar clinical picture to the slowly progressive Type II lesion, however, the owner may report earlier signs suggestive of a Type 1 disease that proceeded the Type III disease.

The clinical signs of intervertebral disc disease are varying degrees of pain and neurologic deficit dependent on the amount of extradural tissue, the rate of herniation or protrusion, and the force of the nuclear tissue as it strikes the spinal cord. The pain arises from meningeal or nerve root irritation or both, and the neurologic deficit results from nerve root or spinal cord compression or both. Cervical Type 1 disease, even massive in nature, often produces only pain. Clinically, those cases are indistinguishable from cervical meningitis. With thoracolumbar Type 1 disease, neurologic deficit without pain is common, although pain may have been an early sign. The clinical picture of Type II disease differs from that of Type 1, primarily in that pain is not an outstanding feature and the onset of paralysis is generally slower. Type II disease and Type III disease are indistinguishable clinically from spinal cord tumor or the degenerative myelopathy of German Shepherd Dogs.

In essence, the syndrome of disc disease of any type is one of spinal cord trauma, and usually a transverse myelopathy is the result.

"Felice"

Case Description

"**Felice**" is a 7-year-old female Labrador retriever with a history of difficulty in walking. Cervical pain is evident on the neurological examination and a C1-5 myelopathy is suspected. On the noncontrast radiographs, the caudal portion of the roof of the vertebral canal at C2 appears displaced dorsally, perhaps the result of an expanding lesion within the vertebral canal.

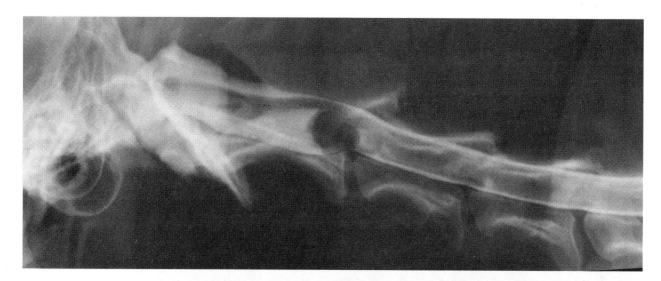

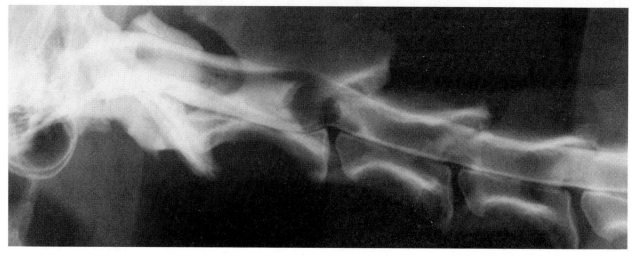

Question #1

What are the neurologic abnormalities indicative of a C1-5 myelopathy?

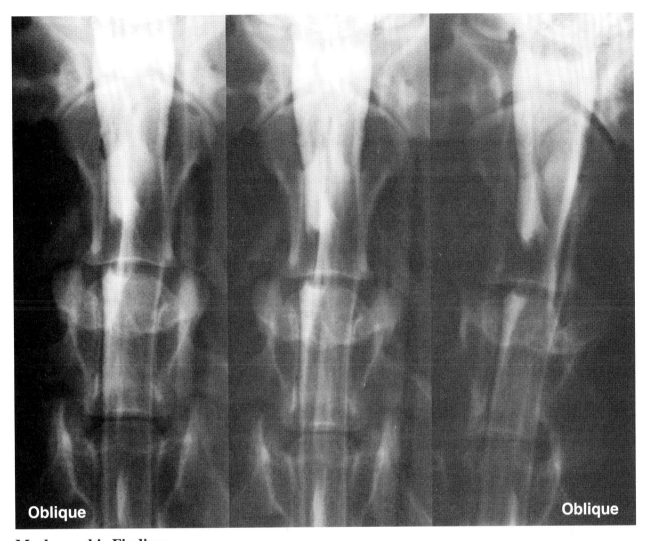

Oblique

Oblique

Myelographic Findings

Both lateral views demonstrate a focal mass at C2-3 that causes an increase in the height of the spinal cord with thinning of the contrast columns. The VD and oblique views show a right-sided mass at the same site with an increase in the width of the contrast column on the right just cranial and caudal to the mass ("tee" sign). The cord is shifted to the left and the contrast column on that side is thinner.

The manner in which the mass lesion alters the appearance of the contrast columns is diagnostic of an intradural-extramedullary lesion. The "tee" sign is present both cranial and caudal to the mass.

Comments

The mass was excised via a right hemilaminectomy and was identified as a meningioma.

Answer #1

Tetraparesis/ataxia with upper motor neuron signs in all 4 limbs. No brain or cranial nerve abnormalities present.

"HBC"

Each of these dogs has been hit by a car ("HBC"). Owners of such dogs can rarely provide specific information about the accident. In fact in many instances being struck by a car is only surmised, based on the dog's proclivities or finding it injured alongside the road. Regardless, the fact that the dog has been traumatized is usually evident because of its wounds. Any animal so traumatized should be assumed to have a spinal fracture until proven otherwise, even if the animal can walk! The radiographic findings and answers to the questions are on the following pages.

Other injuries may arise from "HBB" (hit by a bicycle), "HBT" (hit by a truck), or "HBBT" (hit by a big truck). All result in a similar pattern of injury differing only in the severity of the injury..

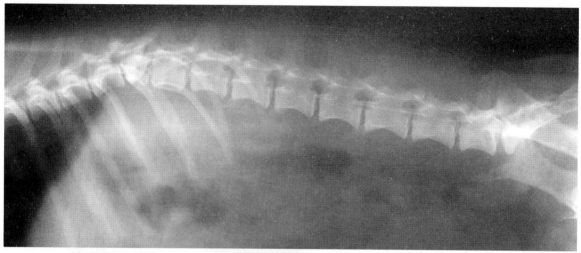

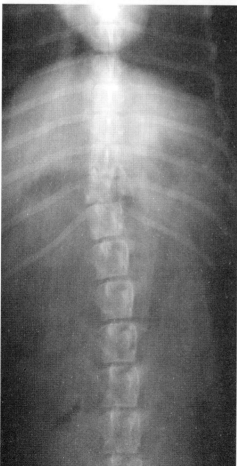

Case Description

"Cy" is a 1-year-old male mix breed who was hit by a car and was brought to the hospital because he was paraplegic. Examine the radiographs on this page.

Question #1

A technical question, what was the length of time of the radiographic exposure?

Question #2

Is a myelogram helpful in this patient?

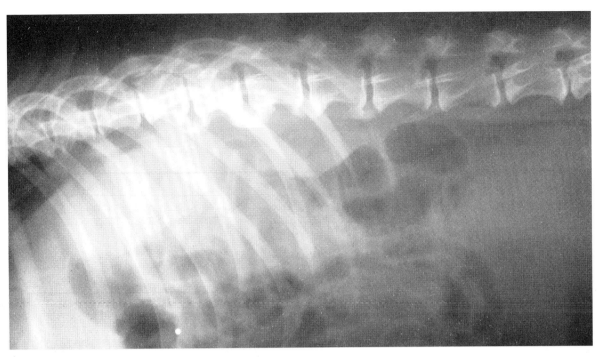

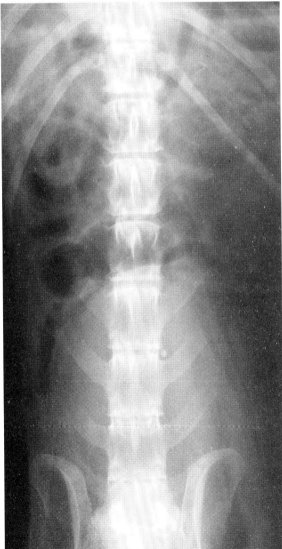

Case Description

"**Cobb**" is a 14-year-old male setter who was struck by a car yesterday. After the accident the dog walked home but does not have use the pelvic limbs today. Abdominal radiographs were made.

Question #3

What role does the spondylosis deformans play in this injury? in the radiographic interpretation?

Question #4

What is the small density on the left side of L4-5?

Case Description

"Jeremyah" is a 3-year-old male Labrador retriever who was hit by a car and was immediately paraplegic. He had upper motor neuron signs in the pelvic limbs. When lying on his side, his thoracic limbs were held stiffly in extension. He could move the thoracic limbs, however, and spinal reflexes and pain perception in them were normal. A survey radiographic study used only lateral views.

Question #5

In what area of the spinal cord is "Jeremyah's" lesion located? What is the cause of his forelimb stiffness?

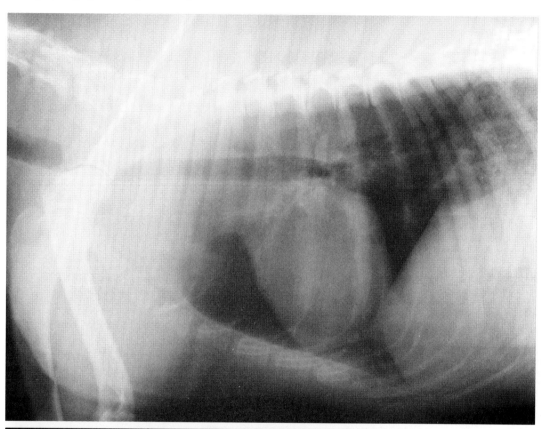

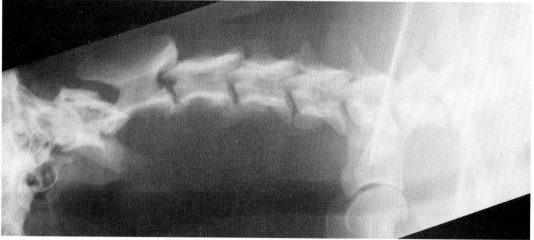

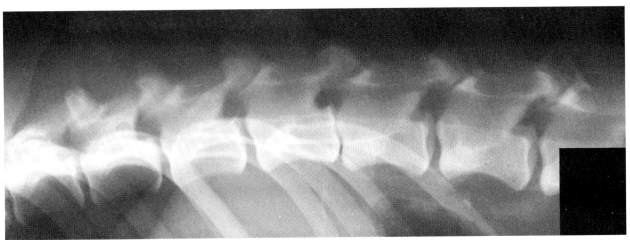

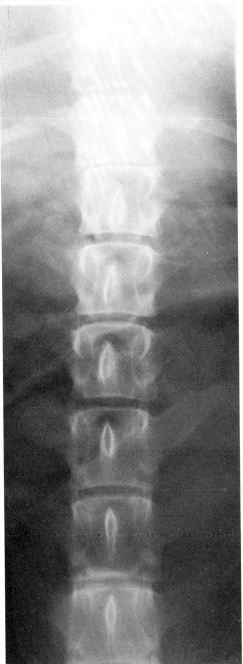

Case Description

"**Justice**" is a 7-year-old male Labrador retriever who was hit by a car and was treated for shock at an emergency clinic. The dog was returned later for treatment of a tarsal fracture. The spine was radiographed 20 days after the original injury because the clinician detected neurologic deficits at that time.

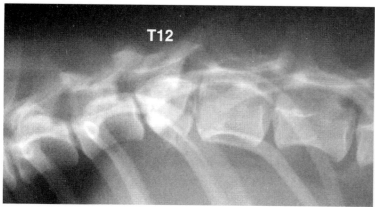

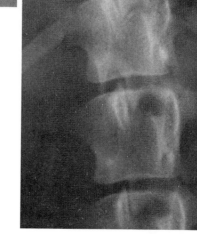

"Cy" - Radiographic Findings

The radiographs show a shortening of the body of T12 and angulation at T12-13 resulting in kyphosis and scoliosis. The diagnosis is a compression fracture with vertebral dislocation. Marked rotation of the spine is evident on the lateral radiograph by noting the lateral projection of the thoracic vertebrae and the oblique projection of the lumbar vertebrae (note rib attachment). Rotation is evident on the VD view by noting the difference in projection of the spinous processes.

Question #6

What is the most important radiographic feature of the fracture-luxation?

Question #7

The urinary bladder was distended. Does this have any clinical importance?

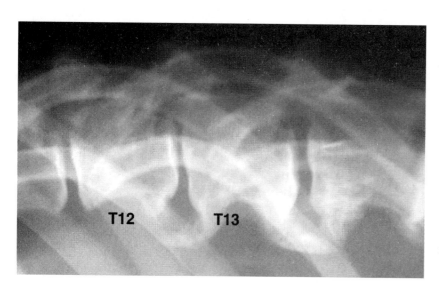

"Cobb" - Radiographic Findings

The radiographs show malalignment and collapse of the disc space at T12-13. The diagnosis is fracture-luxation with traumatic disc rupture.

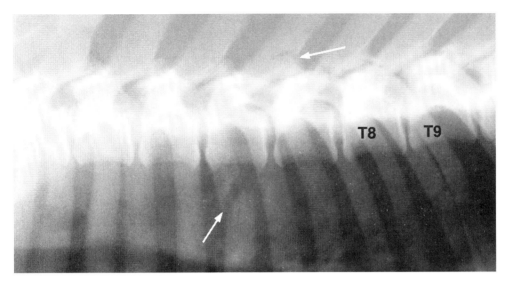

"Jeremyah" - Radiographic Findings

The radiographs show: (1) collapse of disc space at T8-9, (2) vertebral malalignment at T8-9, (3) fractures of the spinous processes of T6, T7, and T8 (arrow), (4) fracture of one of the 5th ribs (arrow), and (5) increase in fluid in the dorsal lung fields. The diagnosis is a spinal fracture-luxation with rib fractures and pulmonary contusion. The cervical spine is radiographically normal.

Comments for "Jeremyah"

Disc space narrowing without end plate sclerosis and spondylosis deformans is assumed to indicate an acute collapse in "Jeremyah" probably due to trauma.

You can confirm your interpretation of the increased density within the dorsal lung fields by noting that you cannot identify the aortic arch.

"Justice" - Radiographic Findings

The radiographs show a collapse of the T13-L1 disc space and rotation of the caudal spine at T13-L1. The injury seems to be limited to a spinal luxation.

Comments for "Justice"

This is a common problem—an obvious fracture in a limb interfering with a complete neurological examination and a spinal injury going undetected until later. If the spinal injury causes marked instability and remains undetected, the spinal cord may be badly injured by routine hospital care or by normal activities at home after the accident. In this patient, the vertebral column remained stable and the injury resulted in only minimal neurologic signs that were not detected until he became more ambulatory with his limb fracture. Alternatively, the injury may have weakened the T13-L1 disc, which then collapsed and protruded slowly over the ensuing 20 days, eventually causing the noted clinical signs.

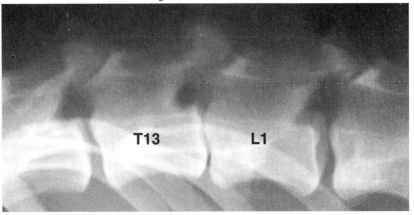

Answer #1

It is long, probably in excess of 0.1 second as indicated by the movement of both thoracic and abdominal organs on the radiographs.

Answer #2

Yes. The presence and degree of cord compression cannot be determined on the basis of noncontrast radiographs. Although the prognosis for recovery is based on the neurologic status of the dog, the myelogram would likely provide information helpful in determining the necessity for and the type of decompressive surgery to be used.

Answer #3

The vertebrae from T13 caudally are at least partially fused by the spondylosis deformans creating a rigid portion of the spine. It is interesting that the fracture-luxation occurred just at the cranial edge of that rigid section. The only possibility of error in radiographic diagnosis is to assume that the bony spurs at T12-13 are fractures and area post-traumatic. Usually the osteophytes only reach out and interdigitate without forming a solid bridge.

Answer #4

The density is a fragment of laterally-positioned, herniated, fragment of calcified nucleus.

Answer #5

T3-L3. Schiff-Sherrington syndrome, which is caused by an acute, severe spinal cord lesion caudal to T2.

Answer #6

The ventral displacement of the T13 vertebra indicating malalignment, possible vertebral instability, and possible severe cord injury.

Answer #7

Yes. It could be the result of urinary tract obstruction, inability to posture, neurologic dysfunction (e.g., reflex dyssynergia or detrusor areflexia), or overdistention with or without neurologic dysfunction.

Malalignment of Vertebrae

Malalignment of vertebrae may be associated with: (1) congenital or developmental anomaly, (2) trauma, (3) acute or healing discospondylitis, (4) pathologic fracture, and (5) acute or chronic disc degeneration. The malalignment is identified on the lateral radiograph by drawing a line along the floor of the vertebral canal and observing any offset. The same type of observation can be made using the ventral aspect of the vertebral bodies that normally create a continuous line or series of shallow segmental arcs. Similar shadows are created by the pedicles as seen on the VD views and can normally be joined in a continual line. Vertebral alignment can also be determined by observing the position of the spinous processes on the VD view where they normally lie in a straight line separated by an equal distance. All of these features are seen more clearly in the dog, but may be noted in a cat as well.

Vertebral malalignment can be directed laterally creating a scoliosis in which the radiographic evaluation must be made on a VD or DV radiograph or the malalignment is directed dorsally or ventrally causing a kyphosis or lordosis identified on a lateral view. Instability between adjacent vertebrae in either plane can be accentuated by the careful use of stress radiography. Width of the disc space can be helpful in the determination of malalignment with the space of the disc being either widened, narrowed, or being wedge shaped and varying from the appearance of the disc cranially or caudally.

Lesions resulting is malalignment can create angulation, slippage, or a combination of these features. Early lesions or those that are minimal in deformity can cause only a "slippage" between two vertebrae without angulation. This can occur with acute or chronic disc disease, some fractures, some tumors, and some inflammatory lesions. With time, more prominent deformity may result with the diagnosis much easier to make.

In determination of the clinical importance of these lesions, the change in size and shape of the vertebral canal needs to be evaluated as well as the presence of vertebral malalignment and instability. The vertebrae may be badly malaligned, however, if the vertebral canal is not made stenotic, clinical signs may be absent and the lesion discovered as an incidental finding. Instability often converts a vertebral canal of adequate size to one that is stenotic with a resulting myelopathy.

However, malalignment can exist between two vertebrae and be more in the form of an instability that requires stress radiographic techniques to identify. Cervical spondylopathy in its varying forms causes a malalignment of this type or may result in a prominent malposition that is evident on routine radiographic studies. The breed and age of the dog at the time of the study may influence the strength of the intervertebral disc and thus, how the malalignment or instability is seen. Malalignment is also present in many lumbosacral lesions associated with congenital transitional vertebral vertebrae. Lesions in these two locations can be profitably studied through the use of carefully used stress radiography.

Congenital vertebral anomalies such as hemivertebra, "butterfly" vertebra, fused dorsal spinous processes, and block vertebra may cause a kyphosis, scoliosis, and less commonly, a lordosis. Healing fractures or healing discospondylitis may result in a kyphosis or scoliosis because of principle involvement at the level of the intervertebral discs with preservation of the true vertebral joints. With chronic spinal or nerve root lesions that are unilateral, muscle atrophy may occur with a resulting scoliosis with the concavity on the side opposite the muscle atrophy. It is possible for an inflammatory lesion to cause muscle contraction resulting in a similar appearing concavity on the side of the injury.

Another error in alignment may result in a rotational deformity and is evident in trauma cases on the VD view where the tips of the spinous processes do not form a line when connected. Acute intervertebral disc disease may cause minimal instability between two vertebrae and a change in size of the dorsal interarcuate space. The resulting minimal change in position of the articular facets is seen on the lateral view. Chronic intervertebral disc degeneration may cause malalignment and instability after destruction of the disc with complete herniation of the disc material, and destruction of the end plates with shortening of the vertebral bodies. This creates a kyphosis often evident at the thoracolumbar junction but restricted to geriatric patients.

In the post-operative patient following aggressive fenestration or an enlarged decompressive procedure, weakness may result between the vertebrae and a sharp lateral scoliosis occurs that borders on a subluxation. This type of lesion can also be seen with a severe discospondylitis. The patient with a healed vertebral fracture or a healed discospondylitis may have a malalignment, the importance of which is determined by presence of canal stenosis.

Cats show a unique kyphosis at the TL junction as they age with wedging of the vertebral bodies ventrally and prominent disc degeneration. Malalignment of this type is also seen in older members of the smaller toy breeds of dog.

Larger breeds of dogs may have DISH (disseminated idiopathic skeletal hyperostosis) and cause a malalignment in which the vertebrae are fused in a too-perfect alignment. This may be found throughout the vertebral column, but is often in the lumbar region. Excessive movement bordering on malalignment can be seen at either end of these fused vertebra ("domino" effect)..

Great clinical importance is seen with lesions at the LS junction that cause malalignment that may cause a canal stenosis leading to a clinical pattern of cauda equina syndrome. This has such a frequent occurrence that it is often described separately. Another potential site of malalignment that is clinically devastating occurs at the OAA region where a resulting acute canal stenosis may result in tetraplegia or death.

Causes of vertebral malalignment
1. Kyphosis
   a. hemivertebrae
   b. "butterfly" vertebrae
   c. block vertebrae
   d. compression fracture
      1. acute
      2. healed
   e. spondylitis
      1. acute
      2. healed
   f. discitis
   g. chronic disc degeneration
   h. pathologic fracture
2. Lordosis
   a. fused dorsal arches
   b. hemivertebrae
   c. "butterfly" vertebrae
   d. block vertebrae
3. Scoliosis
   a. hemivertebrae
   b. "butterfly" vertebrae
   c. block vertebrae
   d. compression fracture
      1. acute
      2. healed
   e. spondylitis
      1. acute
      2. healed
   f. discitis
   g. post-surgery
   h. pathologic fracture
4. Rotational malalignment
   a. fracture
   b. postsurgical instability
5. Unique conditions
   a. OAA congenital anomalies
   b. LS degenerative lesions
   c. rigid spine associated with DISH
   d. LS transitional vertebral vertebrae

Four Traumatized Dogs

We expect the clinical signs caused by trauma to be apparent immediately and to resolve with time. However, sometimes this is not what happens and instead the signs develop later or are progressive over the days following the injury. Note the histories of these dogs who all had spinal trauma. The questions are answered at the end of the section.

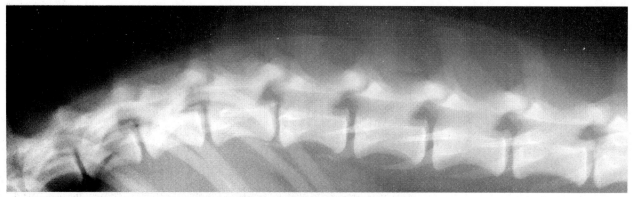

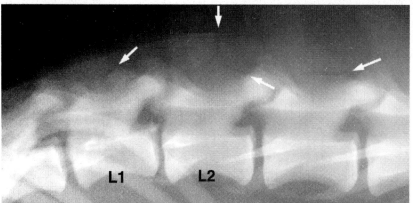

L1   L2

Case Description

"**Pax**" is a 1-year-old retriever who fell in the mountains. He was immediately paraparetic and progressed to paraplegia over the next few days. He has upper motor neuron signs to the pelvic limbs.

Radiographic Findings (today's study)

The radiographs above were made following the injury and show: (1) malalignment at L1-2, (2) ventral displacement of L2, and (3) fractures of the spinous processes of L1, 2, and 3 (arrows). All of these are features of a fracture-luxation centered at L1-L2.

Radiographic Findings (3 weeks later)

Radiographs made 3 weeks later continue to show the unstable relationship of L1 and L2 with a progressive collapse of the disc space (lines mark the vertebral canal floor).

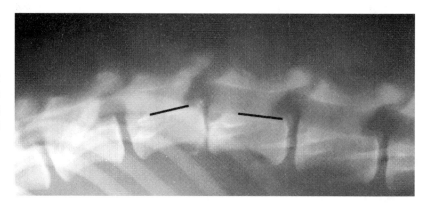

Comments

Note on the first study how the diaphragm causes a line that extends across the body of T12 that could be confused as a "fracture line". This is a type of "Mach" line.

Note the persistent stability of the vertebrae as seen on the lateral radiographs but rotation of the vertebrae caudal to the fracture site was evident on the VD view. This suggests that the injury was not as stable as it might appear if only the lateral radiographs were evaluated.

Case Description

"Joe" is a 1-year-old male mixed breed dog who was in a dog fight yesterday. This morning he is paraparetic with upper motor neuron signs in the pelvic limbs.

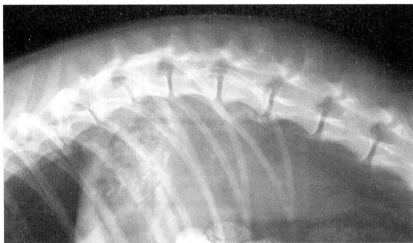

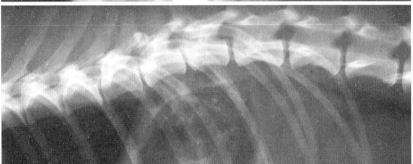

Radiographic Findings

Lateral survey radiographs show a shortened body of T12 and malalignment at T11-12. The diagnosis is a fracture-luxation. Radiographs of the thorax were made because of respiratory distress.

Comments

Note on a second lateral view how the spine has been extended and straightened making the diagnosis of the fracture-luxation more difficult.

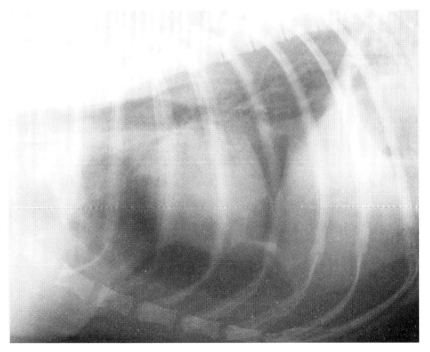

Question #1

What are the artifacts over L1-2?

Question #2

Does "Joe" have a diaphragmatic hernia?

Question #3

Does "Joe" have a pneumothorax or just hyperinflation of lung lobes?

Question #4

Does "Joe" have pleural effusion?

Question #5

Should you consider stress views on a patient of this type?

Case Description

"Mitzi" is a 9-year-old female shepherd who was kicked by a horse. She was able to walk after the injury but became paraplegic 24 hours later.

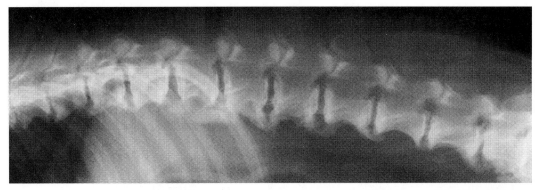

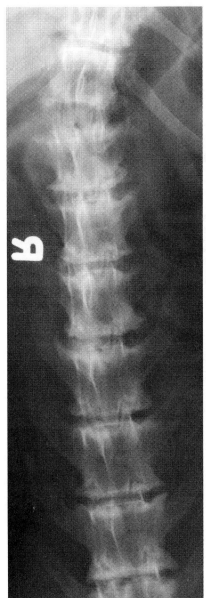

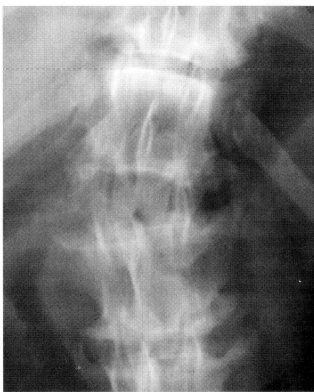

Radiographic Findings

Radiographs show marked chronic degenerative changes in the form of spondylosis deformans and end plate sclerosis centering on all disc spaces. However, the widening of the disc space at T13-L1 and lateral angulation of the spine at T13-L1 as seen on the VD view are more acute and diagnostic of a fracture-luxation at T13-L1.

Comments

Note the productive changes around the true vertebral joints and the degenerative changes at the lumbosacral junction. Positioning of this type of patient with a spinal malalignment and suspected instability for a radiographic study is always done with some risk to the patient.

Case Description

"Shom" is a 5-year-old male sheltie who had a sudden onset of pain 3 days ago while running. He was immediately paretic in the pelvic limbs. His tail is paralyzed and his anal sphincter is dilated. Bladder control is normal. (The owner reports that the dog has not moved the tail in the two years that the owner has had the dog.)

Radiographic Findings

Radiographs show a luxation at the sacrocaudal junction. The osteopenia of the last sacral segment and tapering of the first coccygeal segment are features noted today that suggest that the injury is chronic. The diagnosis is a long-standing sacrocaudal separation. (see the enlarged views)

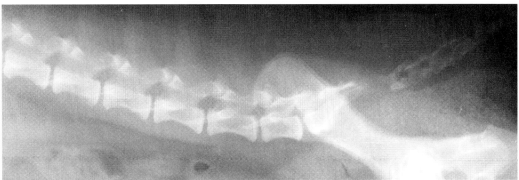

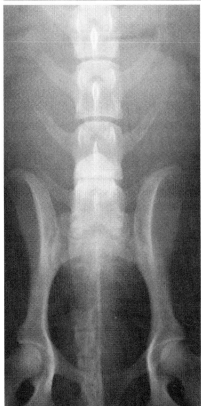

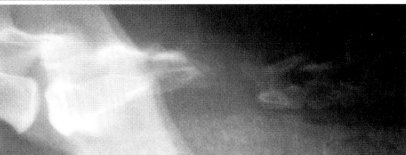

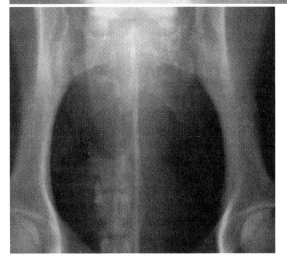

Comments

Note that the clinical history does not appear to match the severity of the bony lesion. It is important to note the change in shape and size of the first caudal vertebra and the tapering of the sacrum and absence of the caudal end plate of the sacrum.

It is likely that the features noted represent bone atrophy associated with a nonunion fracture-luxation that occurred several years ago, and the clinical signs today only represent a new trauma subsequent to a chronic injury. Another possibility is that the signs that developed 3 days ago are not related to the old fracture at all. Fibrocartilagenous embolism is one disorder that characteristically causes a peracute onset of neurologic deficits, often associated with exercise. This syndrome is more common in nonchondrodystrophic dogs than in chondrodystrophic dogs and causes no diagnostic radiographic changes on either noncontrast or on a myelogram.

Answer #1

The artifacts over L1-2 are the result of a wet hair coat.

Answer #2

"Joe" does not have a diaphragmatic hernia.

Answer #3

"Joe" has a pneumothorax. Note the elevation of the cardiac silhouette.

Answer #4

"Joe" has a pleural effusion as indicated by the collection of fluid ventrally in the thoracic cavity.

Answer #5

Stress views on a patient of this type should not be considered because the lesion is most likely unstable.

Spondylosis Deformans in the Dog

Large bony spurs that bridge or almost bridge intervertebral disc spaces have been described in the dog (Morgan 1967), cat (Read and Smith 1968, Read 1966, Beadman et al 1964), and bull (Thomson 1965, Bane and Hansen 1962). Vertebral osteophytes are single or multiple and originate on the ventral and lateral margins of the vertebral end plates, and range in size from the smallest identifiable spur to complete bony bridges. These osteophytes when associated with degenerative disc disease are referred to as spondylosis deformans.

The incidence and size of the vertebral osteophytes increases with age and all dogs over ten years of age have some degree of spondylosis deformans. In the dog, vertebral osteophytes form frequently near the anticlinal vertebra and at the lumbosacral junction. However, pattern of distribution are breed dependent. Osteophytes are less common in the cervical region and in the cranial portion of the thoracic region. The distribution of the osteophytes on the margin of the end plate in the dog assumes a specific pattern. The majority of spurs in the cervical region are on the ventral midline. In the thoracic region, cranial to the anticlinal segment, approximately two-thirds of the spurs are equally divided to the right and left of the midline. From the anticlinal segment caudally until L4-5, the location is on the midline, with a more lateral location noted at the lumbosacral disc. Often the vertebral osteophytes are found in conjunction with narrowing of the disc space and sclerosis of the end plate, which are associated with the instability caused by a slowly degenerating disc.

The bony osteophytes (spondylosis deformans) that form, associated with degeneration of the discs, have a characteristic shape with a smooth ventral border and a curved beak-like appearance. The spurs may grow so large that the osteophytes projecting cranially and caudally from a given vertebral body join in the mid-portion of the vertebral body increasing its height so that the thickness of the new bone nearly equals the original dorsoventral dimension of the vertebral body. The osteophytes may develop to the point that bony spurs forming from adjacent vertebral end plates interdigitate ventrally and lateral to the disc space, but they rarely form solid bony bridges. The more extensive is the growth of the osteophyte, the greater the modeling of the vertebra with disappearance of the original cortex.

While the osteophytes are usually seen on the lateral projections, it is important to realize that they form from the lateral and ventral periphery of the end plate and are more a "collar" of bone than a "spur" of bone. Only rarely do the spurs ever form in such a way that they encroach dorsally upon the vertebral canal.

The clinical significance of the vertebral osteophytes has been exaggerated partially because of the assumption that dorsal projecting bony spurs could place pressure on the spinal cord. This has been shown to be incorrect (Morgan 1967). What were assumed to be dorsally projecting spurs were, in fact, large dorsolateral spurs that, when seen on a lateral radiograph, appeared to extend dorsally, putting pressure on the spinal cord. Presence of the osteophytes confounds the detection of calcified disc material so a patient with disc disease may be misdiagnosed because of the prominent vertebral osteophytes. It is fortunate that spondylosis deformans occurs most prominently in members of the nonchondrodystrophoid breed where the incidence of calcified disc disease is less common. Conversely, dogs of the chondrodystrophoid breeds with frequent disc disease rarely produce large vertebral osteophytes until older.

Osteophytes can also form from the periphery of the vertebral end plates in the face of instability between adjacent vertebral vertebrae from causes other than disc degeneration. The vertebral instability if often more acute and can be secondary to: (1) vertebral fracture, (2) vertebral luxation with destruction of the intervertebral disc, (3) congenital anomaly such as hemivertebra or cleft vertebra, (4) healed discitis or discospondylitis, or (5) postsurgical status following disc fenestration. The appearance of the bony response varies with each of these causes of instability. The term spondylosis deformans should be used to describe the generalized formation of osteophytosis throughout the vertebral column when the apparent cause is that of generalized disc degeneration. The bony osteophytes that form secondary to the other more acute causes of vertebral instability form more quickly dependent on the nature of the lesion and are usually focal in distribution depending of the etiology.

Unique Myelographic Patterns in a Group of Dachshunds

Myelography is a dynamic radiographic examination. A liquid radiopaque contrast agent is injected into the subarachnoid space where it mixes with the cerebrospinal fluid. Thus, the appearance on the radiograph is dependent on the flow and pooling of the contrast agent and the manner in which the mixing occurs. The appearance on the radiograph is controlled in part by: (1) the rate at which the agent is injected, (2) the quantity of agent injected, (3) the site of injection, cerebellomedullary or lumbar cistern, (4) the presence of a partial or complete blockage of flow of the agent, and (5) leakage of the agent from the subarachnoid space into the epidural space.

These cases illustrate some of the rules of contrast agent behavior in myelography. Examine both the noncontrast radiographs (NCR) and myelograms (Myel) of these dachshunds and answer the specific questions that are posed. All of these dogs have neurologic deficits in the pelvic limbs. Try to determine the cause of the unusual myelographic pattern in each dog.

The radiographic findings and answers to the questions are discussed following the case descriptions of the 9 cases.

Case Description

"**Heidi**" is a 4-year-old female dachshund. Examine views from both the noncontrast and contrast radiographs.

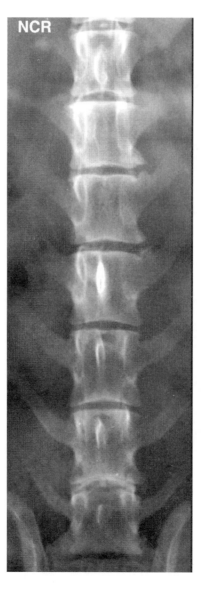

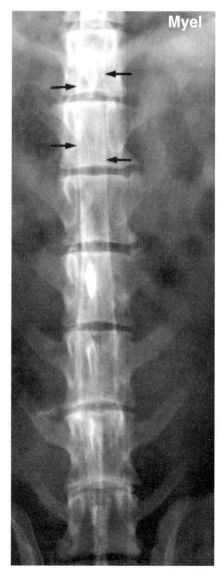

Question #1

Why was "Heidi's" myelogram unique (arrows)?

Case Description

"**Rip**" is a 4-year-old male dachshund. The heavily calcified disc herniation blends with the body of L3 (white arrows). The myelogram is diagnostic but some of the contrast agent enters the central canal of the spinal cord cranial to the site of the lesion (black arrows). The spinal needle remains in position at L4-5 during the making of the first radiograph. Note the location of the needle bevel and consider the effect of this position.

Question #2

What is the importance of filling of the central canal?

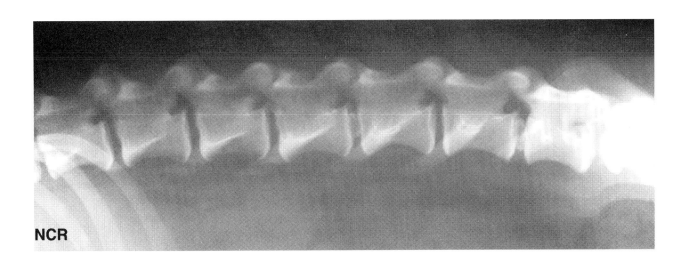

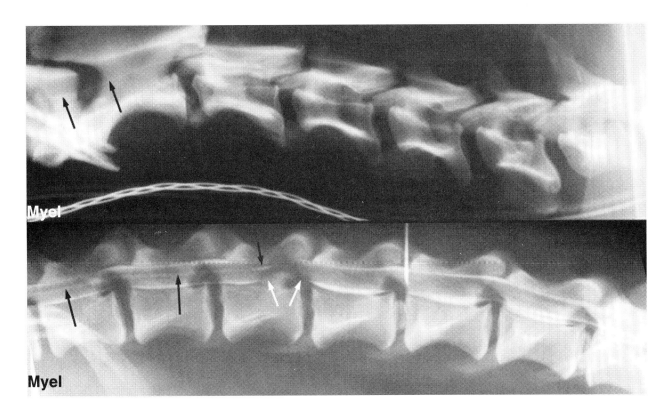

Case Description

"**DeeDee**" is a 12-year-old female dachshund with a damaging disc herniation at T12-13 as seen on the myelogram.

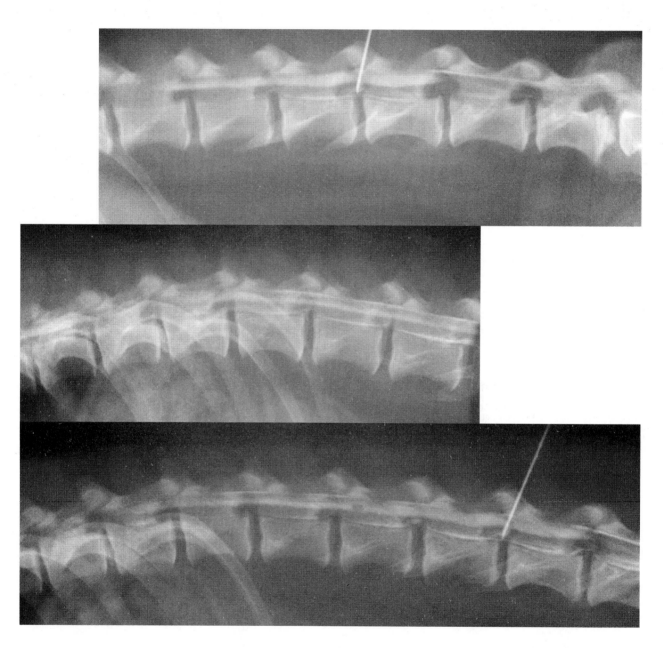

Question #3

Explain the unusual pattern of the contrast agent.

Case Description

"**Sam #1**" is a 10-year-old male dachshund. Examine views from both the noncontrast radiographs and the myelogram.

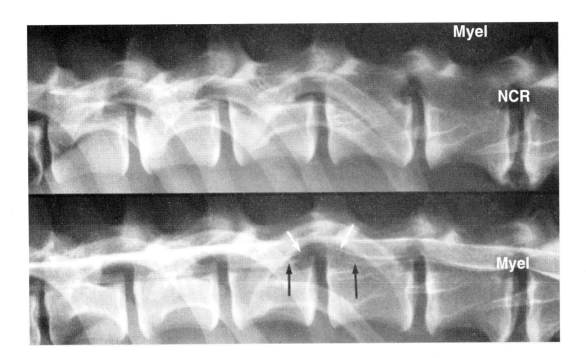

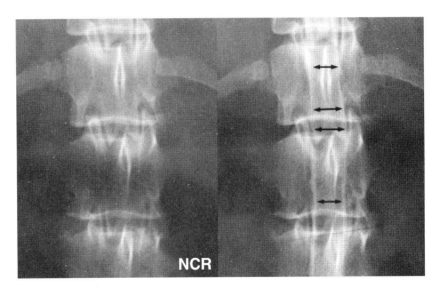

Question #4

Why are the subarachnoid columns at the site of the disc herniation unique?

Case Description

"Hansi" is a 5-year-old male dachshund examined with a myelogram.

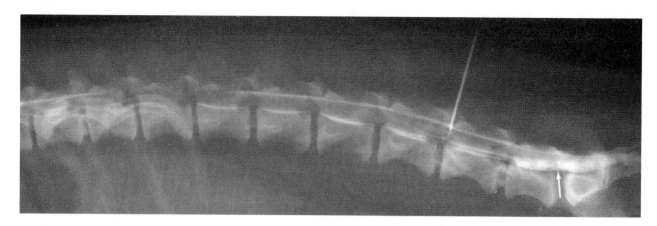

Question #5

Explain the accumulation of contrast agent in the caudal portion of the subarachnoid space.

Case Description

"Wally" is a 10-year-old dachshund. Myelography often identifies more than one lesion.

Question #6

Can you find a second, smaller lesion in "Wally's" studies?

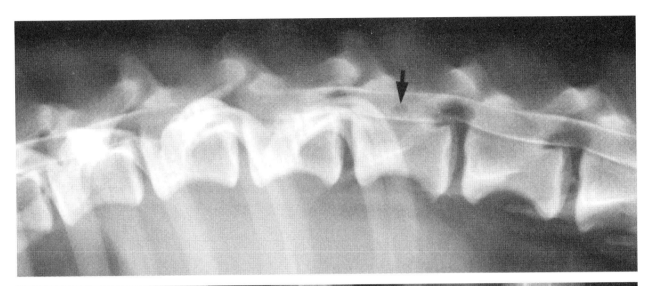

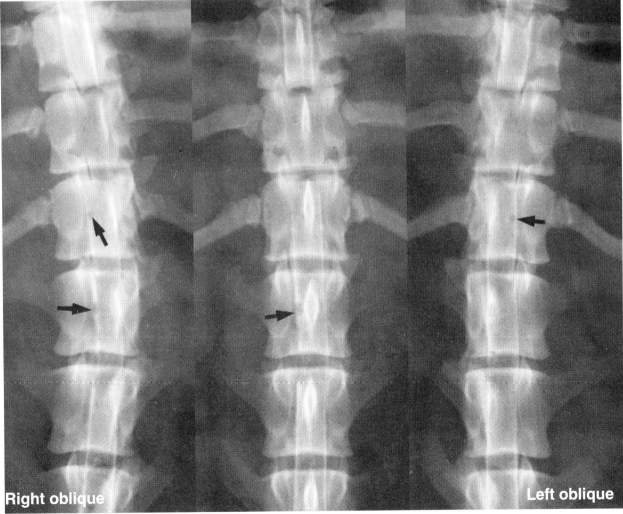

Right oblique   Left oblique

Case Description

"**Ginger**" is a 6-year-old female dachshund with noncontrast and myelographic studies.

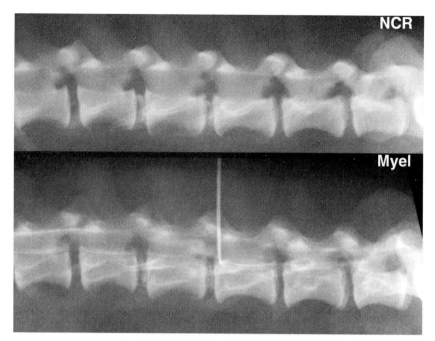

Question #7

Why is this a non-diagnostic myelogram?

Case Description

"**Sam #2**" is a 10-year-old male dachshund. Evaluate the noncontrast and myelographic studies.

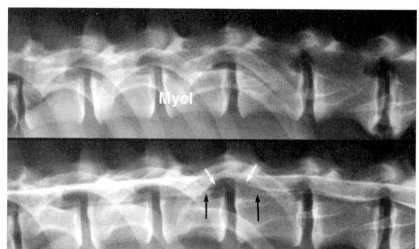

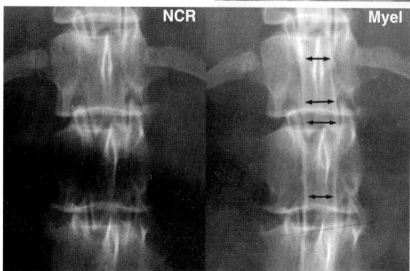

Question #8

Why is the cord widened at T13-L1 on the VD view?

Case Description

"Calahan" is a 5-year-old male dachshund. Evaluate the noncontrast and myelographic studies.

Question #9

Does the unusual filing of the caudal portion of the subarachnoid space have any clinical importance?

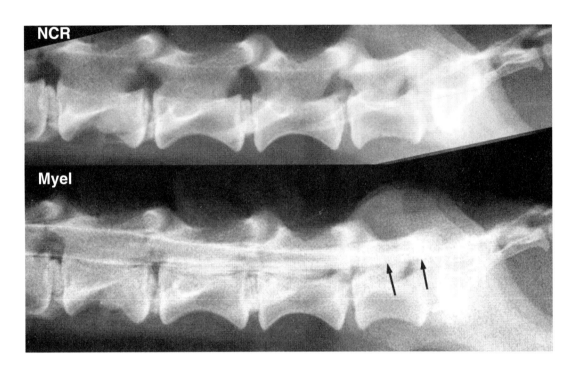

"Heidi" - Radiographic Findings (Question #1)

"Heidi" is unique because she had an earlier hemilaminectomy. As a result, the spinous processes of L2 and L3 are missing and the pedicles on the left side of L3 and L4 are altered surgically.

On the ventrodorsal view of the myelogram, the cord is slightly widened at L1-2 (arrows). On the lateral view of the myelogram the narrowing and displacement of the spinal cord are seen without narrowing of the subarachnoid contrast columns. The cord is atrophic and draped over the scar that represents the remnants of the disc herniation. No evidence of a dorsal surgical scar was evident.

Note how much further caudally the spinal cord and lumbar extension of the subarachnoid space extends in chondrodystrophic breeds. The lumbar enlargement is located at the L5 segment.

"Rip" - Radiographic Findings (Question #2)

"Rip" has central canal filling on the myelogram (black arrows), a pattern that is not uncommon. It may relate to the location of the needle tip within the cord and represent injection of contrast agent directly into the central canal. It may also relate to injury to the cord from the disc herniation (white arrows) and represent an aberrant flow of CSF because of compression of the subarachnoid space. Necrosis of the cord may allow contrast fluid access to the central canal at the site of the lesion. The blockage of CSF flow may also cause hydromyelia. Normally, little CSF "flows" in the central canal so the filling identified in this patient has clinical importance suggesting more severe cord injury. Note that the elevation of the central canal matches the elevation of the subarachnoid columns and helps to identify the protruded disc at L3-4.

The needle through which the injection was made for the myelogram remains in position.

"DeeDee" - Radiographic Findings (Question #3)

"DeeDee" has apparently suffered severe cord injury caudal to the site of the disc protrusion that has caused a marked widening of the central canal. Cord injection at the lesion site that has malacia/central necrosis within the cord may alter the expected flow of the contrast agent. Cranial to the disc protrusion, the contrast agent fills a central canal that is still larger than normal. Note an air bubble within the central canal at the level of L3.

"Sam #1" - Radiographic Findings (Question #4)

"Sam #1" has a Type II disc protrusion at T13-L1. The disc material is located on the right side, causing "splitting" of the contrast columns with one column resting on the floor of the vertebral canal (black arrows) and the other column elevated away from the floor of the vertebral canal (white arrows) by the disc material.

"Hansi" - Radiographic Findings (Question #5)

"Hansi" has a Type 1 disc protrusion at T13-L1 that is causing cord swelling and resistance to cranial flow of the contrast agent. Consequently, a large amount of the contrast agent flows caudally and fills the caudal portion of the subarachnoid space, providing an excellent study of the slightly protruding LS disc (arrow). A potential obstruction to flow explains why it is appropriate to inject the contrast agent slowly to permit its flow cranially. Note that the needle tip is placed in the dorsal subarachnoid space rather than placing the tip through the cord to the floor of the vertebral canal. Injection made with the needle tip in this position is less traumatic to the spinal cord.

"Wally" - Radiographic Findings (Question #6)

"Wally" has as Type 1 disc lesion at T12-13. A second smaller lesion is present on the right side ventrally at L1-2 and appears to be an older lesion. Air bubbles were injected accidentally and are located at T13 and L1 where they interfere with interpretation (arrows). Notice how the oblique views are helpful in evaluation of the location of an extradural mass.

The possibility of multiple spinal lesions must be considered in a patient such as "Wally". Other categories of disease also need to be considered: congenital anomalies, neoplasia, trauma, inflammatory diseases, and vascular disorders. After localizing a neurologic lesion, the clinician must then decide if additional lesion sites might be present, and if so, where those lesions might be.

"Ginger" - Radiographic Findings (Question #7)

"Ginger" unfortunately had a disc protrusion at L4-5, just at the site of needle placement. The contrast agent was injected into the injured cord where it caused further injury and was absorbed into the malacic cord, creating patches of increased density. An injury of this type is unusual because of the less common location of disc protrusion. "Ginger" had neurological signs that indicated a lower motor neuron lesion in the pelvic limbs that should have suggested that this might be a possible problem. To prevent this problem, a radiograph should have been made after a trial injection of only 0.1 cc. That radiograph would have shown the early pooling of the contrast agent in the injured cord.

"Ginger" had lower motor neuron signs in the pelvic limbs. The other dachshunds in this group had T3-L3 myelopathies and should have had upper motor neuron signs in the pelvic limbs. Consider the following in the separation of upper and lower motor neuron signs in the pelvic limbs.

The L4-L6 spinal cord segments mediate the patellar tendon reflex. The L3-L4 vertebrae house these cord vertebrae in the average chondrodystrophic dog. The withdrawal and gastrocnemius reflexes are mediated by the sciatic nerve that is located in the L6-S2 cord vertebrae within the L4-L5 vertebrae.

"Sam #2" - Radiographic Findings (Question #8)

"Sam #2" has a Type II disc protrusion at T13-L1 that elevates the cord and causes it to appear widened on the VD view (arrows). Note that as the cord widens, the subarachnoid columns become narrow. An intramedullary mass also causes the cord to appear widened; however, it should appear widened on both views. This is the same dog as the one named "Sam" that you looked at earlier in the series. Did you note the splitting of the subarachnoid columns?

"Calahan" - Radiographic Findings (Question #9)

"Calahan" has prominent cord tethering that results in elevation of the cord and nerve roots at their caudal attachment. This anomaly protects the cauda equina from injury from a mass on the floor of the vertebral canal. He remains, however, a candidate for extensive disc fenestration.

Achondroplasia

Achondroplasia is usually thought of as a short-limbed dwarfism and not recognized as the most frequently encountered condition that is associated with spinal stenosis. As early as 1925, Donath and Vogl, demonstrated the relative shortness of the vertebral pedicles and the shortness of the length of the vertebral bodies of these unique people. On the other hand, the shape and length of the spinal cord and cauda equina in this condition is normal, emphasizing that it is this disproportion between the dimensions of the vertebral canal and the volume of its contents that may lead to neural deficits. The normal length of the spinal cord within a shortened spine positions the termination of the cord further caudally and alters the relationship between the vertebrae and the emerging spinal nerves.

This form of dwarfism was first described by von Soemmering in 1791. In 1878, Parrot coined the term "achondroplasia" for the condition which literally means "without cartilage formation". It was Kaufmann who in 1892 substituted this name for the more adequate term "chondrodystrophia fetalis". Unfortunately, the term achondroplasia remains the one that is most frequently used.

There is the question of whether during the postnatal growth period there is excessive periosteal bone formation resulting in thickening of the pedicles, laminae, and articular processes in the achondroplastic patient. The edges of the vertebral bodies project into the vertebral canal more dorsally than the middle portion of their dorsal surfaces, resulting in scalloping of the dorsal aspects of the vertebral bodies that is most pronounced in the lumbar region. This deformity of the vertebral bodies gives them the scalloped appearance seen radiographically.

The comparative size of the vertebral canal was studied in the German Shepherd Dog and the dachshund showing that the vertebral canal was much smaller in the chondrodystrophoid breed. Also, the cauda equina terminated much further caudally in the dachshund. The canal stenosis in the dachshund explains why the disc protrusion or nuclear extrusion is so much more of a traumatic event when it is recognized that there is little extradural space in the canal and, thus, no place for the new tissue to locate. Consequently, the cord is compressed.

Hansen clearly described the clinical importance of disc disease in the chondrodystrophoid dogs. In the chondrodystrophoid dwarf, the disc degenerates through the process of chondroid metaplasia and calcification of the nucleus is readily identified on the radiograph. The radiographic identification of disc tissue that has herniated or protruded into the vertebral canal is much easier if it is calcified.

Other radiographic changes in the chondrodysplastic dwarf include the shortened rib with costal cartilage that calcify early and show a bizarre "ladder" pattern of mineralization. Tracheal and bronchial rings calcify as they degenerate providing an airway pattern that is prominent on the thoracic radiograph.

Contraindications for Myelography

Contraindications for myelography are uncommon, but need to be considered. The most important is in a patient in which the clinical signs are in agreement with changes that can be adequately visualized on noncontrast radiographs and surgery is not considered in treatment. If this patient does not progress as expected following medical management, the case can be re-evaluated and myelography may be advised.

If the patient has specific diseases, it is thought that the contrast agent can cause inflammation or increase already present inflammation in the cord or meninges which may lead to seizure activity or even death. These diseases include: (1) any inflammatory process causing a meningitis or myelitis, (2) hematomyelia, (3) myelomalacia, or (4) recent myelography.

The recommendation concerning recent myelography may be questioned in light of newer contrast agents. Few studies have been performed to evaluate how often a myelographic procedure can be repeated. In one study using normal Beagle dogs, repeated cervical myelograms were performed weekly for 4 weeks without any difficulty detected clinically or on CSF evaluation. It is recommended that a week between studies be used as a conservative guide in clinical practice.

Four Young Dachshunds with Thoracolumbar Myelopathies

A group of young Dachshunds had acute signs of a TL transverse myelopathy causing paraparesis or paraplegia. Three had upper motor neuron signs to the pelvic limbs, one had decreased patellar reflexes. All had deep pain perception in the pelvic limbs. All were suspected of having an acute Type 1 disc disease with escape of nuclear tissue into the vertebral canal. Only the radiographs near the TL junction are shown.

On the noncontrast radiographs (NCR), identify the disc you believe is causing the clinical signs. Compare these findings with those seen on the myelogram (Myel) and determine whether you selected the correct disc. Determine what additional information you gained from the myelogram that would be helpful in treatment of the dog. Descriptions of the radiographic findings are on the pages following the case descriptions.

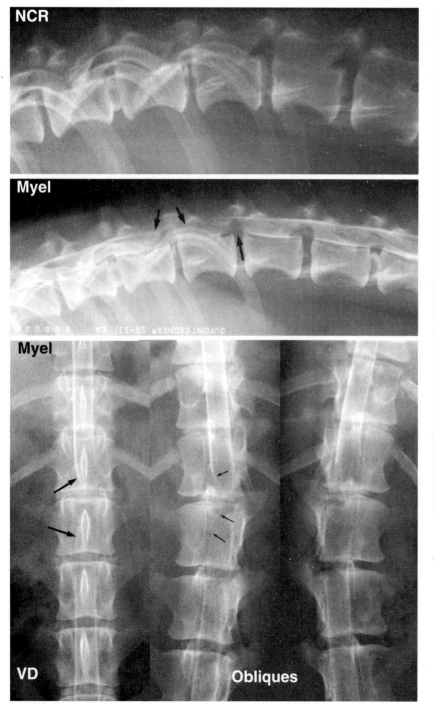

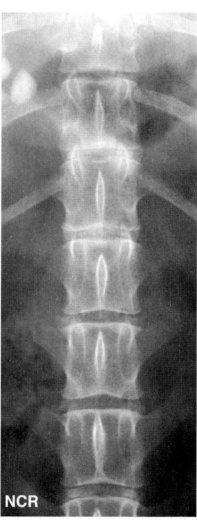

Case Description

"**Howler**" is a 5-year-old male.

Case Description

"**Ginger**" is a 2-year-old female.

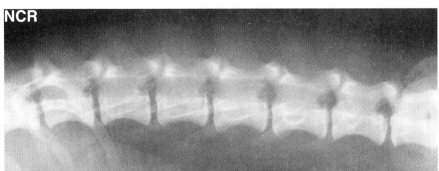

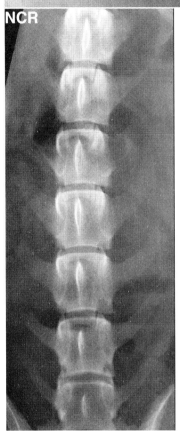

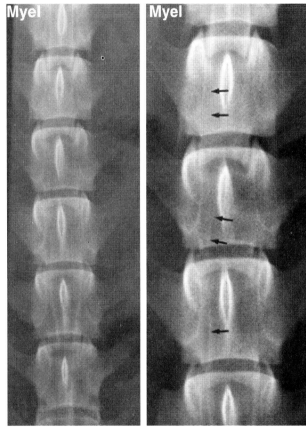

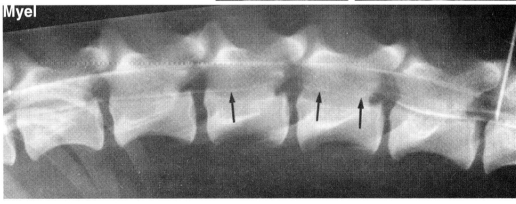

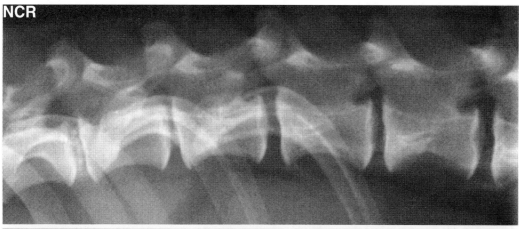

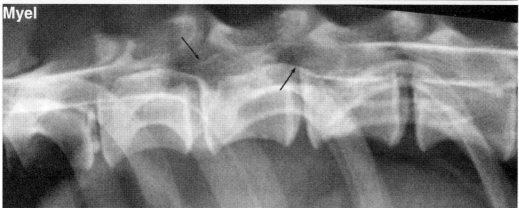

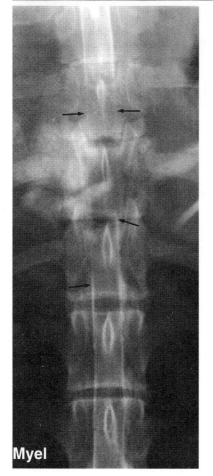

Case Description
"Cecil" is a 4-year-old male.

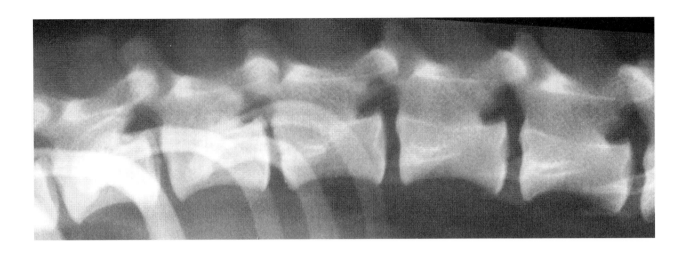

Case Description
"Ricky" is a 6-year-old male.

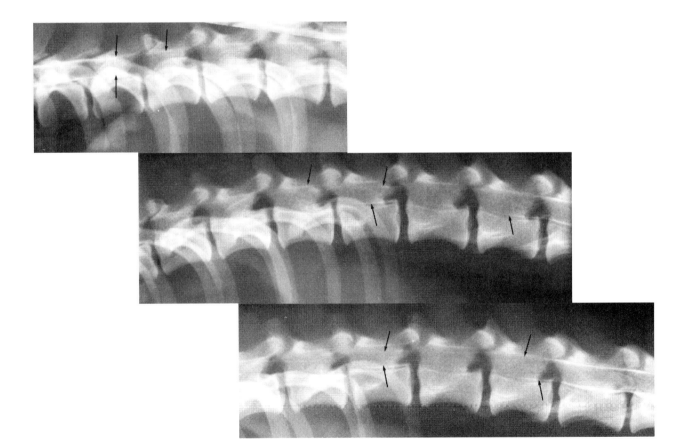

"Howler" - Radiographic Findings

T13-L1 is partially calcified with a cloud of calcified tissue dorsal to the disc space. This is difficult to evaluate because of the overlying rib shadows. L1-2 has an arch of more dense calcified tissue just dorsal to the disc space. T12-13 has a large calcified disc with no signs of dorsal protrusion. No secondary changes are identified around the disc spaces. The ventrodorsal view is not particularly helpful. It is difficult to speculate which of these discs most likely is causing the clinical signs.

The myelogram outlines a ventral extradural mass at T13-L1 which elevates the spinal cord and compresses the dorsal subarachnoid space (arrows). In addition, the mass occupies the right side of the vertebral canal as seen on the VD views causing marked shifting of the spinal cord to the left (arrows). The oblique views show the calcified mass ventrally on the right side with displacement of the cord dorsally and to the left (arrows). The opposite oblique view is of less value. The cord swelling extends the length of a single vertebra. In addition, a smaller disc protrusion is seen at L1-2 (arrow) with cord elevation and narrowing of the subarachnoid columns.

"Ginger" - Radiographic Findings

On the noncontrast study, L3-4 and L4-5 both have a thin pattern of calcified nuclear tissue located dorsal to the slightly narrowed disc spaces. The ventrodorsal view furnishes no additional information.

The myelogram confirms that both discs appear to have prolapsed nuclear tissue. In addition, the myelogram offers additional information that the disc tissue is principally ventral (arrows) but also on the right side as indicated by a shifting of the contrast column to the left (arrows) as seen on the VD views.

"Cecil" - Radiographic Findings

On the noncontrast study, T11-12 is calcified and the disc space is slightly narrowed. Only a slight amount of calcified nuclear tissue remains in T12-13 and that disc space is slightly narrowed. Both are considered possible sites of disc protrusion.

The myelogram confirm your suspect diagnosis and provides additional information. The extradural mass at T11-12 is dorsal (arrow) and the extradural mass at T12-13 is ventral (arrow). Both could be a part of a single disc protrusion or could represent protrusions of both discs. The ventrodorsal view shows the cord swelling that causes compression of the contrast columns (arrows).

Comments

The quality of the ventrodorsal myelogram is badly compromised. The problem is the presence of what appear to be bones mixed within the gastric contents, which interfere with interpretation of the ventrodorsal views.

"Ricky" - Radiographic Findings

The disc space at T13-L1 is narrowed without any secondary bony changes, suggesting an acute disc space collapse. The remainder of the disc spaces are without evidence of nuclear calcification and are of normal width.

The myelogram confirms your suspicions. Spinal cord swelling and narrowing of the subarachnoid spaces extends from T11 to L1. In addition, a second lesion is present at L1-2 with a dorsal extradural mass and a third lesion at L2-3. The subarachnoid columns are identified (arrows). The last two patterns may result from the same nuclear herniation. The length of the cord swelling plus the finding of a second and possibly third lesion are helpful in planning a surgical decompression.

Question #1

Which dog had decreased patellar reflexes? (answer next page)

Comments

Following degeneration of the nucleus pulposus of the disc, the anulus begins to degenerate and the nucleus can begin to herniate or protrude. If the anulus ruptures completely, an acute, massive extrusion of nuclear material into the vertebral canal may occur, traumatizing and compressing the spinal cord. Hansen termed this a Type 1 protrusion. Type 1 protrusion is characteristic of discs undergoing chondroid degeneration and calcification, and therefore occurs most commonly in the chondrodystrophic dogs. In contrast, Hansen's Type II herniation is a bulging of the anulus without extrusion of the nuclear tissue. Type II herniations generally develop more slowly and slowly compress neural tissue. Type II disc disease is more common with discs undergoing fibroid degeneration, and is therefore more common in nonchondrodystrophic dogs. However, calcified discs may develop Type II protrusions if the degenerated anulus bulges but does not completely rupture.

Disc material in a Type 1 disease may migrate from the point of herniation and create a focal mass or spread out in the epidural space as a "sandy sheet". Myelography can help locate the displaced material. Location of the disc material within the vertebral canal is important in planning surgical decompression and it is especially important in enabling the surgeon to determine the proposed length of the hemilaminectomy as well as the laterality of the surgery. The craniocaudal location of disc material or the craniocaudal extent of cord swelling determine the length of the laminectomy. The location of compressive material within the vertebral canal is actually more important information than is the identification of the offending disc.

Multiple areas of spinal cord compression may be the result of herniations of more than one disc (old and/or recent). Hematomas forming from internal vertebral venous plexus hemorrhage may also produce a compressive mass lesion. The hematoma may be part of the compressive mass of disc material, or form a mass separate from the mass of disc material.

Answer #1

"Ginger" has a protrusion at L3-4, L4-5 that apparently injured spinal cord segments L4-6 that mediate the patellar reflex.

A Thoracolumbar (TL) Transverse Myelopathy in "Spooky"

Often patients present with upper motor neuron signs in the pelvic limbs and signs of pain that suggest the lesion is at the thoracolumbar area. Disc disease is prominent at this location; therefore, this disease is usually first on the list of differential diagnoses and often the only disease considered in these patients. Review this case and see what other lesions can be present at this location.

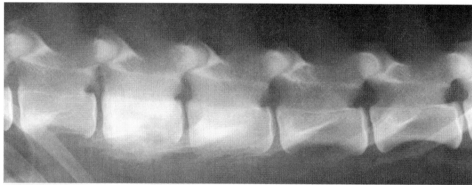

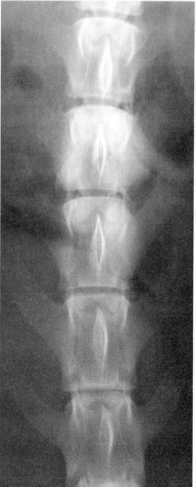

Case Description

"Spooky" is an 8-year-old male Labrador retriever with a 4-month history of inability to rise on the pelvic limbs without help by the owner. The dog was thought to have a ruptured cranial cruciate ligament in the right pelvic limb. On examination, he had decreased proprioception in the pelvic limbs and hyperesthesia over the lumbar region of the back. A spinal radiographic study was made.

Radiographic Findings (day 1)

The radiographic study shows new bone production on the body of L3 and L4 with slight narrowing of the interposed disc space. The end plates are well preserved without signs of bone destruction. The changes are primarily in the vertebrae, however, with the disc space narrowing, the diagnosis is a discospondylitis probably secondary to a migrating grass awn (seed head).

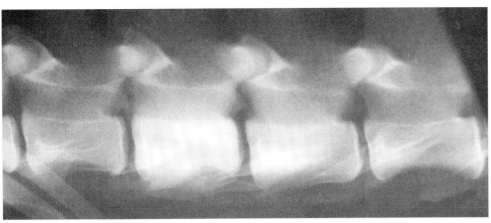

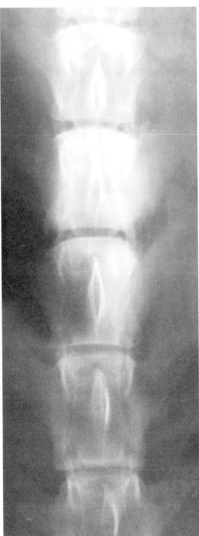

Radiographic Findings (day 30)

Radiographs made 1 month later suggest that the new bone production is more dense and mature with a more distinct margin. The disc spaces appear to be more nearly normal in width and the discospondylitis is thought to be in a healing phase.

Comments

The clinical signs of developing spondylitis and discospondylitis precede the bony radiographic changes of the disease by approximately 2 weeks at the minimum. Resolution of the clinical signs may also precede apparent resolution of the radiographic changes. Nonetheless, serial radiographs are important in following the disease as it is being treated since they establish the direction of change. Often other discs become infected even while the disease is being treated. This seems particularly true of hematogenous discospondylitis. Therapy should consist of specific antimicrobial drugs (based on culture and sensitivity of blood, urine, disc aspirate, exudate from draining tracts, or bone biopsy) and usually needs to be continued for 4-6 months.

What to Do with "Moss"?

Case Description

"Moss" is a 16-year-old female shepherd with paraparesis for over 6 months that began with the right pelvic limb and extended to involve the left pelvic limb. Now she has obvious loss of proprioceptive placing. Urinary incontinence has also been noted. Both noncontrast spinal radiographs and a myelogram were ordered.

This case forces you to determine which of the many degenerative lesions in the spine of the older dog is of clinical importance.

Radiographic Findings

The noncontrast radiographs show arthrosis of the true vertebral joints (arrows) and pseudoarthroses that have formed between the spinous processes (arrows). Marked stenosis of the vertebral canal is present at the LS junction. An unusually prominent spondylosis deformans is present at C6-7, while most other disc spaces are free of this type of reactive bone. The lateral view of the cervical spine is oblique making interpretation of the canal contents difficult. Dural ossification is present. The apparent increase in width of the disc spaces at C5-6 and C6-7 maybe the result of traction placed on the head during the examination.

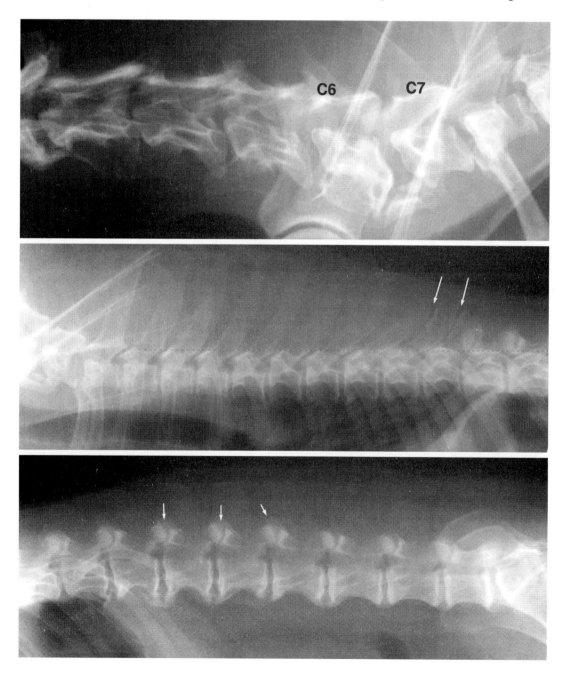

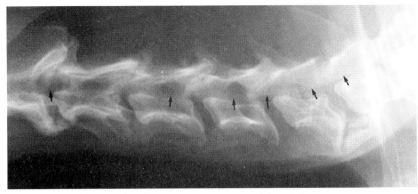

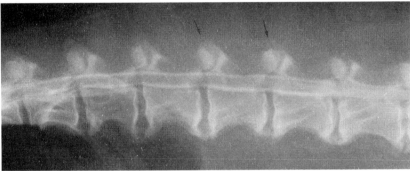

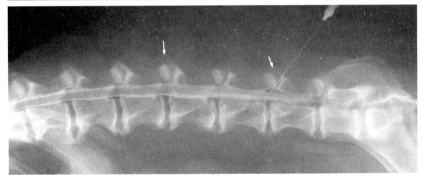

Myelographic Findings

Incomplete filling of the cervical subarachnoid space (arrows) makes evaluation of the several small Type II disc protrusions difficult. The cervical portion of the myelogram is unsatisfactory because the contrast columns do not extend into that region because the quantity of contrast agent injected was not sufficient due to her large size. Note that the cauda equina ends at L6-7 making the myelogram an unsatisfactory study to evaluate the LS junction. (Myelography is typically unable to fully illuminate the lumbosacral vertebral canal especially in large breed dogs.)

Question #1

What would be the next diagnostic test to utilize?

Question #2

What would you do to attempt to visualize the cervicothoracic region on the myelogram?

Comments

A myelogram can detect a mass lesion within the vertebral canal but cannot detect any type of disseminated lesion within the spinal cord (intrinsic myelopathy) unless the lesion causes a change in the size or shape of the cord. Degenerative changes seen on the noncontrast radiographs of older dogs such as "Moss" are usually treated as less important than if detected in young dogs. The clinical importance of the arthrosis in the true vertebral joints (arrows) in the midlumbar region is especially difficult to ascertain in the older patient.

"Moss" died 5 days later and the cause of her neurological signs, or the cause of her death, were not determined from the necropsy examination. No mass lesions were identified in the spinal cord or within the vertebral canal.

Answer #1

Analysis of lumbar CSF

Answer #2

When a dog is in lateral recumbency, the shoulders are at a higher point than the thoracolumbar spine. Consequently, the contrast agent pools in the thoracolumbar region and enters the cervical region only when enough liquid is present to flow over the cervicothoracic "hump". When this happens, the contrast agent flows quickly to the next low point which is at the cranial cervical region, leaving the middle cervical and cervicothoracic region with a nondiagnostic amount of contrast agent (arrows). To overcome this problem, try positioning "Moss" by using what is termed a "bucket position" with the head and hindquarters elevated thus making the cervicothoracic region dependent. It is possible that the injection of additional contrast agent may assist in filling the cervical region. If the myelogram remains nondiagnostic consider doing CT myelography or MRI.

Three Dachshunds with Unusual Disc Disease

In chondrodystrophic dogs, most disc disease occurs in the T11-12 to L3-4 region. In the younger, chondrodystrophic dog, the disease is characterized by Type I nuclear herniation while in the older, nonchondrodystrophic dog Type II protrusions are more common. Occasionally, varieties are found that differ from the expected and some of these are presented in this series. All are dachshunds and have upper motor neuron signs in the pelvic limbs. You are asked to explain the cause of the clinical signs after examining the radiographs.

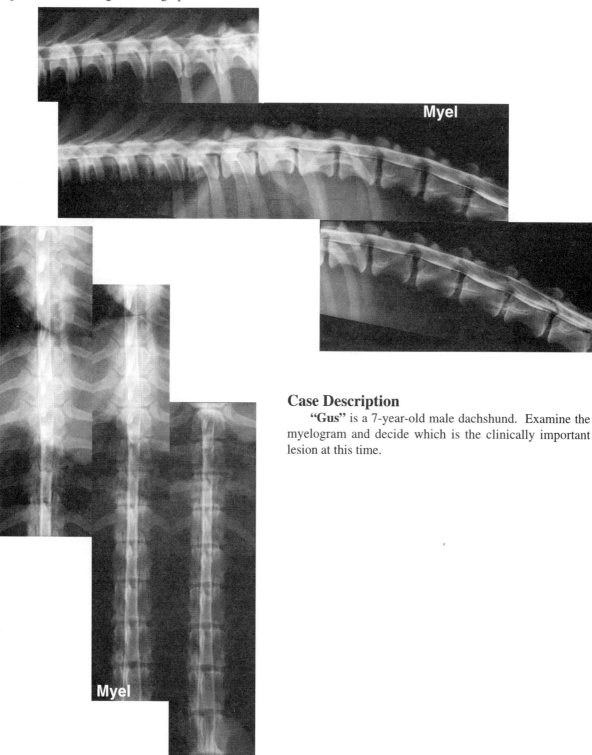

Case Description

"Gus" is a 7-year-old male dachshund. Examine the myelogram and decide which is the clinically important lesion at this time.

Case Description

"**Schnapps**" is a 5-year-old male dachshund. Examine the lateral views of the thoracic spine from the noncontrast study and from the myelogram. After you find the disc lesion, decide what to do with the lesion in the body of T7.

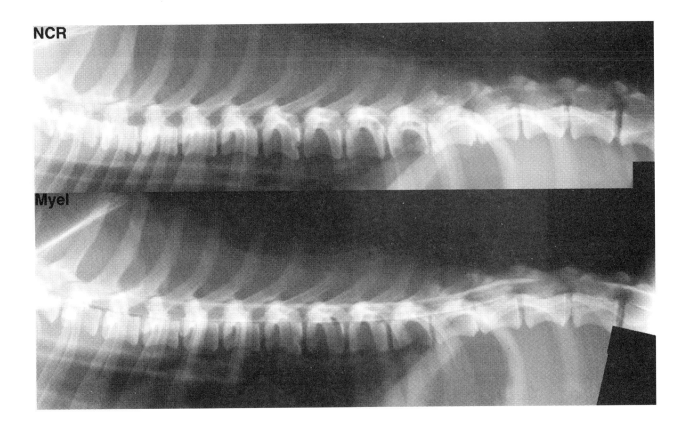

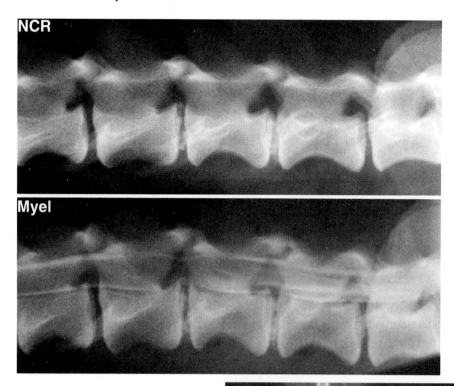

Case Description

"**Maxie**" is a 5-year-old female dachshund. The extradural lesion is seen on both the noncontrast and myelographic studies. Describe it completely.

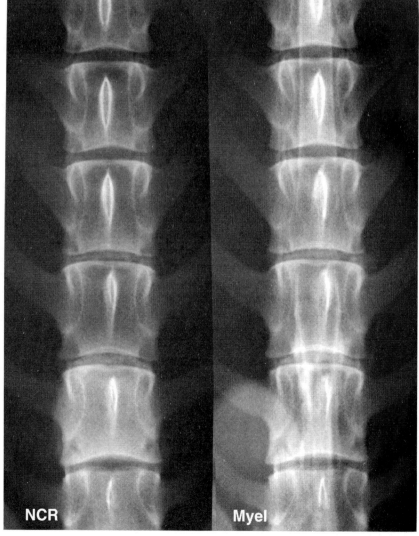

"Gus" - Radiographic Findings

"Gus" has an unusual type of disc disease because of its location. A Type II disc protrusion is located at T9-10 and is characterized by elevation of the cord that causes narrowing of the dorsal subarachnoid contrast column. On the ventrodorsal view, the cord appears widened with narrowing of the lateral contrast columns. Draw a cross-section of this lesion from the information provided on the two views.

The next lesion is more difficult to see because of its small size and because it is located at the lumbar intumescence. The lesion causes a splitting of the ventral contrast column at L4-5 on the lateral view and a roughening of the left contrast column on the ventrodorsal view.

The C7-T1 disc was heavily calcified and the dorsal anulus protrudes slightly. This is the indication of a potential lesion with clinical importance in a dog the age of "Gus". "Gus" was discharged after medical treatment.

Question #1

On what clinical and myelographic basis did you decide which of the two lesions was important at this time and which myelographic feature did you decide was most important clinically.

"Schnapps" - Radiographic Findings

"Schnapps" has as typical Type I disc protrusion at T13-L1 with the cord swelling causing collapse of the contrast columns. Note the central canal filling cranial to the lesion.

"Schnapps" has a bony lesion in addition to the disc disease. The lesion in the caudal end plate of T7 is interesting, but probably not of clinical importance and probably not related to disc disease. Repair of this lesion seems to be complete with a dense margin around the small defect in the end plate. A differential diagnosis should include: (1) a fracture of the corner of the end plate that has healed, (2) a healed discospondylitis, or (3) a type of vertebral osteochondrosis that has undergone repair. The bony protrusion ventrally looks more like a malunion fracture fragment. An active discospondylitis or bone tumor would not look as orderly as this lesion does.

"Maxie" - Radiographic Findings

"Maxie" has a chronic Type I disc protrusion at L4-5 suggested by the dorsally protruded calcified nucleus on the noncontrast study (see arrows on enlargements below). On the myelogram, the contrast columns are displaced medially on both views. This unusual circular pattern usually indicates cord compression by a circumferential, extradural mass. Some extradural tumors assume this pattern of growth and are said to have a "napkin ring" or "hourglass" pattern. It is uncommon for disc material to completely encircle the cord as in this case.

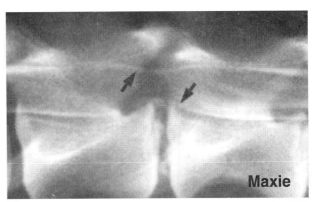

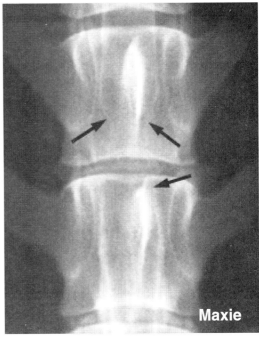

Answer #1

Because "Gus" has upper motor neuron signs in the pelvic limbs, the T9-10 lesion is more likely to be the cause of his problem than the L4-5 lesion. An L4-5 lesion should cause lower motor neuron signs, which would override the upper motor neuron signs. Even if both lesions were causing a myelopathy, the effects of the L4-5 lesion should be evident clinically. The C7-T1 lesion would be expected to cause lower motor neuron signs in the thoracic limbs which were missing in this dog. The T9-10 lesion is the one that causes the greatest cord compression on the myelogram and is most likely the one of most clinical importance.

A Group of Dogs Involved in Motor Accidents

Each of these dogs was suspected of being involved in a traffic accident. Locate and describe the radiographic abnormalities in each case.

Case Description

"**Cassandra**" is a 5-month-old female shepherd who was hit by a car and sustained a humeral fracture. She was also paraplegic with exaggerated pelvic limb spinal reflexes.

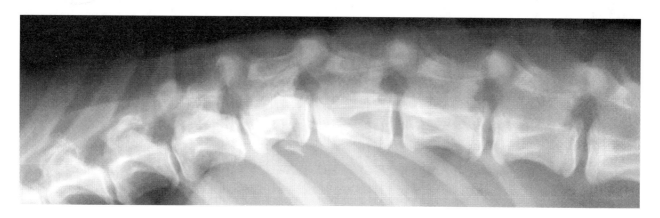

Spinal Radiographic Findings

A lateral spinal radiograph shows a collapse of the body of T12 and a collapse of the disc space T12-13. The diagnosis is a physeal fracture of the vertebral body with minimal fragment displacement (However, we do not have the other view to ascertain this completely,)

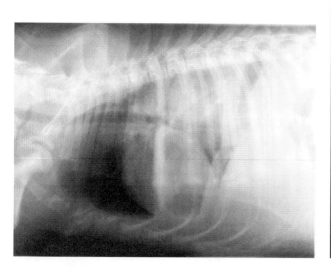

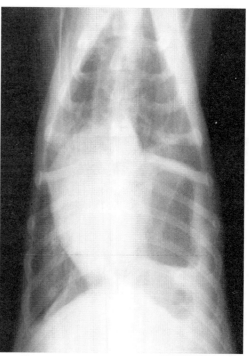

Thoracic Radiographic Findings

Spinal cord compression was relieved via a hemilaminectomy performed on the day of entry. The humeral fracture was not reduced immediately. The dog began to vomit 7 days after admission; however, radiographs of the thorax were not made until 13 days after admission. They show a left-sided mass with pleural fluid and cardiac shift ventrally and to the right. The diaphragm is not identified dorsally and on the left. There is a gas filled structure in the left caudal thorax.

Comments

Despite the diaphragmatic hernia, "Cassandra" survived the spinal surgery. The hernia was finally repaired 22 days after admission. At the same time the humerus was plated and the spinal fracture was plated. Although "Cassandra's" additional surgeries were delayed, she recovered quite nicely.

Question #1

Considering the neurological signs, where is her neurologic lesion located? Could she have more than one spinal lesion contributing to her myelopathy? If so, where could the second lesion be?

Case Description

"**Heidi**" is a 9-year-old female boxer who was struck by a car. She has paraparesis and her tail is flaccid.

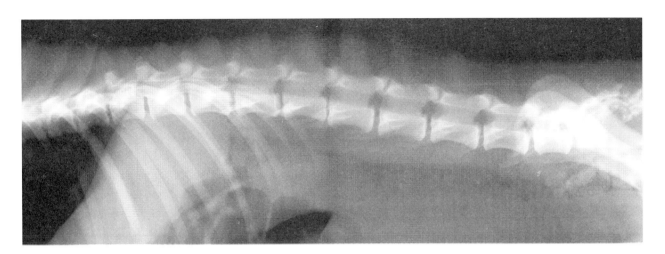

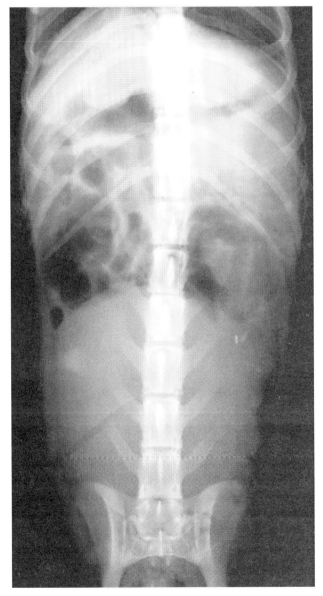

Radiographic Findings

The radiographs show a collapse of the L2-3 disc space with vertebral malalignment in addition to ventral displacement of the caudal vertebrae (tail). The diagnosis is a lumbar vertebral luxation and sacral fracture. In addition, a form of transitional LS vertebra is characterized by large transverse processes.

Comments

Examination of the entire spine is necessary in trauma cases to detect all injuries that might influence the prognosis.

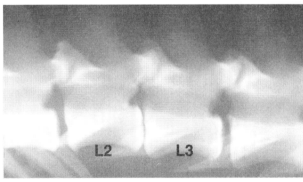

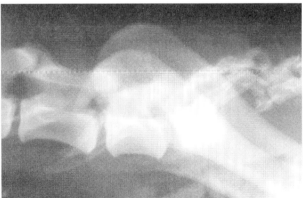

Case Description

"**Shep**" is an 8-months-old female shepherd puppy who was injured and could not walk properly.

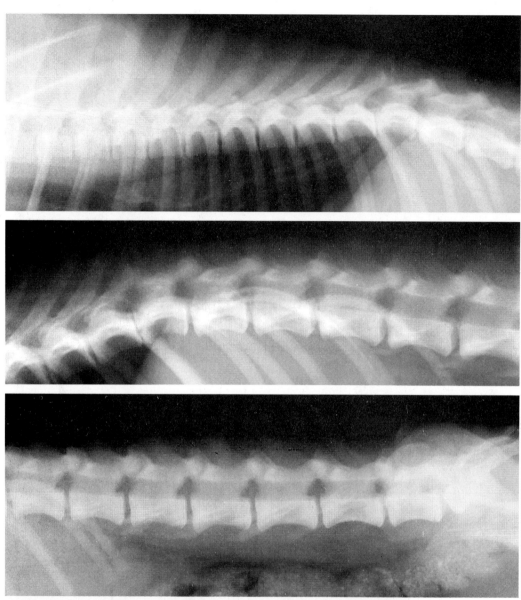

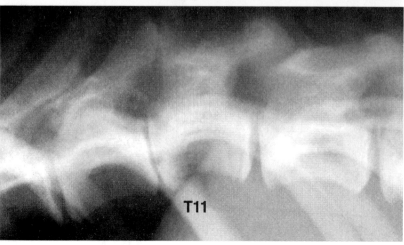

Radiographic Findings

The lateral views of the spine show: (1) shortening of the body of T11 with a fracture of the cranial end plate, (2) collapse of the disc space between T10-11, (3) a fracture of the spinous process of T10, and (4) a luxation of the true vertebral joints at T10-11 (see enlargement below). The diagnosis is a spinal fracture-luxation.

Case Description

"**Gay**" is an 8-months-old female puppy who was injured and is paraplegic. Pain perception appears to be normal in the pelvic limbs.

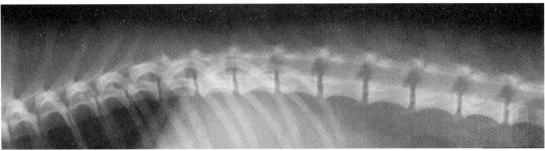

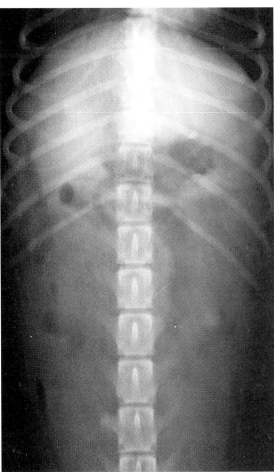

Radiographic Findings

TL radiographs show a collapse of the body of T10 and collapse of the disc space between T9-10. The diagnosis is a fracture-luxation.

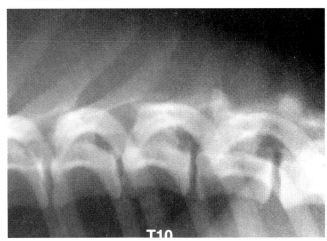

Comments

Use the width of the disc space, malalignment of the vertebrae, and the change in size and shape of the intervertebral foramina in making your diagnosis.

Question# 2

Should you recommend a myelogram on this patient and why? Where would you make the injection? What are the fine lines on the radiographs?

Answer #1

Her neurologic lesion is between T3-L3. Yes, a second or even third lesion could also be located in the T3-L3 area and she would still have upper motor neuron signs to the pelvic limbs. Trauma is one type of disease process that frequently causes multiple lesions.

Answer #2

Yes, a myelogram would help to assess the degree of cord compression at the site of the fracture-luxation and to look for additional spinal lesions. The injection site can be L4-5 or L5-6. The lines are from the use of a stationary grid.

Cauda Equina Syndrome

Examine the noncontrast studies of the following cases to determine the cause of the cauda equina syndrome. Decide if special radiographic studies are required to make a diagnosis or determine the prognosis.

Case Description

"Ginger" is a 4-year-old female Irish setter with a sudden onset of lumbosacral pain and weakness of the left pelvic limb. She has a history of migrating grass awns in the vulvar region.

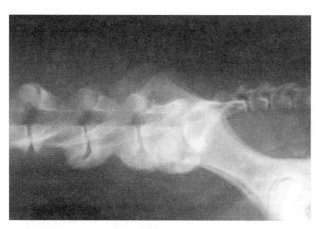

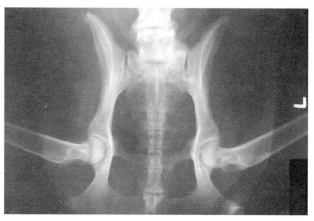

Radiographic Findings

The noncontrast radiographs show heavy new bone formation ventrally at L5-S1 but the width of the disc spaces is well preserved. The important feature is the destruction in the ventral portions of the LS end plates (arrows) that is supportive of a diagnosis of discospondylitis that appears

chronic (see enlarged views below). Note that the vertebral canal is of normal height without any evidence of stenosis, although a bony mass around the articular facets on the left side at the LS disc (arrows) could easily create a compressive mass that might not be identified on the radiograph.

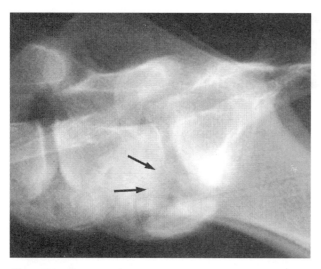

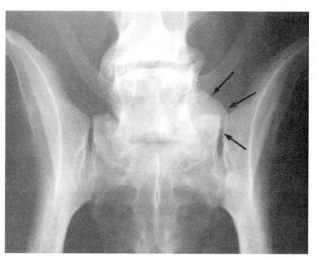

Comments

Spondylosis deformans around disc spaces with normal width may be better called DISH (disseminated idiopathic skeletal hyperostosis). The anomaly of the articular facets on the left side at the LS disc may be a component of DISH.

The radiographic diagnosis of discospondylitis is difficult to make because the destructive portion of the discospondylitis is hidden by the heavy overgrowth of bone associated with the DISH. At the time of a dorsal decompression, bone tissue was submitted for histologic

examination; the pathologic diagnosis was chronic, suppurative osteomyelitis.

Another feature that is difficult to understand is the manner of pelvic attachment. The size of the sacroiliac joint on the left is larger than on the right and the pelvis is rotated to the right. Often this type of pelvic attachment may cause an asymmetrical arthrosis in hip joints that are affected by hip dysplasia. In this dog the hip joints appear normal.

Case Description

"**Beauty**" is a 6-year-old female Labrador retriever with pelvic limb weakness and pain upon movement. Lately she has lost control of urination. On presentation at the clinic, a partial paralysis of the pelvic limbs with little motor control of the left pelvic limb was noted. The anal sphincter was dilated. The pelvic limb withdrawal reflexes seemed decreased, but the patellar tendon reflexes appeared exaggerated (pseudoexaggeration). Muscle atrophy was present over both the pelvis and hips. A 2 by 4 cm soft tissue mass was present on the left side of the rectum.

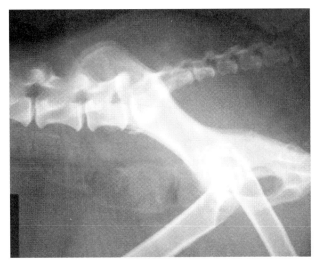
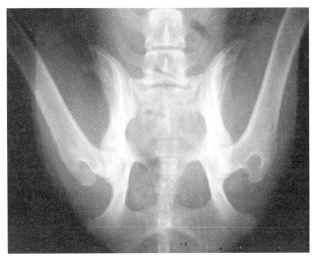

Radiographic Findings

The noncontrast radiographs show a productive-destructive lesion that extends dorsally from the sacrum (seen more clearly on the enlarged views below, white arrows) and a soft tissue mass that extends ventrally from the sacrum causing displacement of the fecal-filled rectum (black arrows). The soft tissue mass extends dorsally where it can be seen to contain a pattern of small calcified nodules. The minimal spondylosis deformans at the LS junction is expected in a dog of this age.

The diagnosis is a bone tumor originating from the sacrum with the characteristics of a chondrosarcoma.

Note how difficult it is to identify the tumor on the VD views where the most prominent change is osteolysis of the left sacroiliac joint at the site of tumor invasion (small black arrows). The chronic disc disease at the LS disc with secondary spondylosis deformans is unrelated to the primary bone tumor. The fecal material in the rectum serves as a contrast agent and makes detection of the rectal displacement relatively easy.

The lesion was biopsied thru the left perineum following the radiographic study and the pathologic diagnosis was a chondrosarcoma.

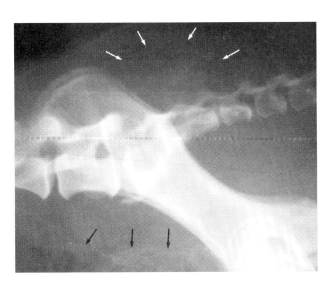
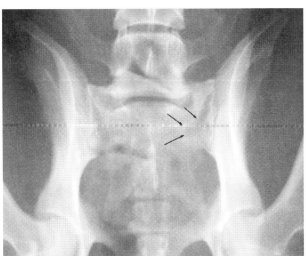

Case Description

"**Chico**" is a 7-year-old male Labrador retriever who has had "pain in the hips" for over a year according to the owner. Upon examination, pressure over the LS region or caudal extension of the pelvic limbs causes him pain. He was assumed to have arthrosis of the hips secondary to hip dysplasia.

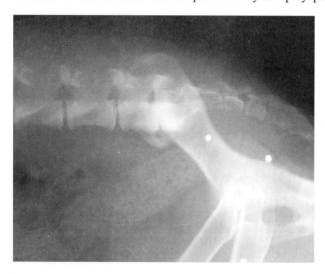
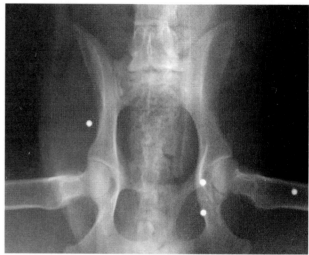

Radiographic Findings

The radiographs show prominent changes at the LS disc space including: (1) collapse of the disc space, (2) end plate sclerosis, (3) spondylosis deformans, and (4) sacral vertebral canal stenosis. No signs of instability or malalignment were noted. Some form of special procedure is required to evaluate for spinal cord compression at the LS disc space. The hip joints are normal.

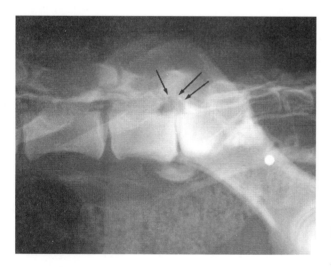

Venographic Findings

An intraosseous venogram (above) was used to show the soft tissue mass at the LS space, which represented the dorsal extrusion of disc material into the vertebral canal. When the contrast agent tried to flow around the spinal cord within the vertebral canal, the contrast filled veins were displaced dorsally over the mass (arrows). The protruded disc material plus the primary vertebral canal stenosis results in marked compression of the cauda equina.

Comments

Intraosseous venography is not a recommended procedure today because of difficulty in the injection into the marrow space of a caudal segment. Discography or epidurography is easier to perform at the LS space with more reliable results. It is difficult in this case to explain how a part of the intravenous contrast agent comes to be within the subarachnoid space but probably suggests leakage at the sight of injection in the caudal segment.

Pellets from a shotgun that show as white round shadows are commonly found around the hindquarters of hunting dogs.

Case Description

"**Digger**" is a 10-year-old male hound with chronic lameness, muscle atrophy, and neurologic deficits suggesting a cauda equina syndrome.

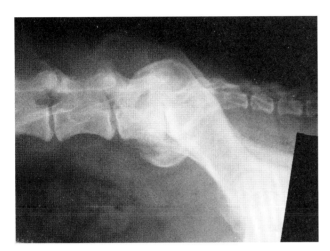

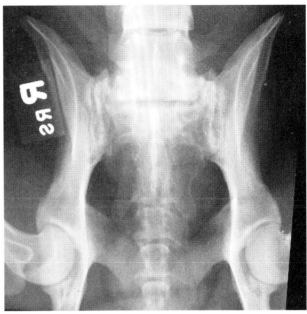

Radiographic Findings

The radiographs show: (1) LS disc space collapse, (2) end plate sclerosis, and (3) spondylosis deformans. No evidence of instability or malalignment is noted on these radiographs. Cauda equina syndrome can result from a mass in the vertebral canal or neural compression from either malalignment or instability. The use of stress radiographs is the quickest way to determine vertebral alignment and stability. Following a stress study, discography or epidurography can be used to detect a vertebral canal mass (below).

Digger's LS instability is identified by comparing the extended and flexed lateral views. The roof and the floor of the vertebral canal are identified (lines) and their closeness demonstrates the resulting canal stenosis. Since stabilization of the LS junction was required, further contrast studies were not pursued and the vertebral canal was visually examined at the time of surgical exploration.

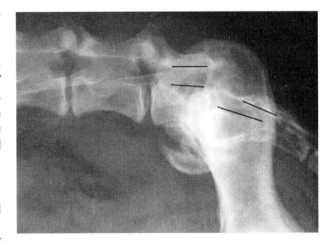

Comments

Surgery was performed to explore the LS vertebral canal and stabilize the LS spine. In addition to a herniated L7-S1 disc, a synovial cyst, 8 x 5 x 5 mm, was found on the left side adjacent to the L7-S1 vertebral joint.

Radiographic Diagnosis of the Lumbosacral Junction

The lumbosacral (LS) junction is a unique portion of the spine and can be evaluated radiographically using several different techniques. A routine radiographic study of the LS region includes ventrodorsal and lateral views and is often thought of as a survey study. Special techniques include: (1) stress radiography, (2) discography, (3) subarachnoid myelography, and (4) epidural myelography and assists in determining the specific cause of the cauda equine syndrome and the type of therapy indicated.

Survey radiography

Lateral radiographs of the LS junction are made with the dog on its side with the hindlimbs in a neutral position. The (1) width of the LS disc space, (2) character of the vertebral end plates, (3) height of the vertebral canal, and (4) nature of LS alignment can be determined. The status of the end plates can be determined from the VD view.

Chronic LS disc disease in dogs and less often cats have the following patterns on the survey radiograph: (1) collapse of the LS disc space, (2) end plate sclerosis, (3) vertebral osteophytes (spondylosis deformans), (4) vertebral canal stenosis, and (5) vertebral malalignment.

Stress radiography

A series of lateral radiographs of the LS region is made with the hips in a neutral, fully flexed, and fully extended position and graphically illustrates the range and nature of motion at the LS space. The motion is created by using the hind limbs as a lever and L7 vertebral body as the fulcrum. The range of motion permitted by the healthy LS disc is 30 to 45°. In a neutral position, the disc space with a healthy LS disc has minimal wedging with the apex dorsal. On full extension, the disc space with a healthy LS disc assumes a more prominent wedge shape with the apex remaining dorsal. On full flexion, the disc space with a healthy LS disc assumes a wedge shape with the apex ventral. The range of motion with a diseased LS disc may be limited because of secondary fibrous and bony changes (spondylosis deformans) that stabilizes the disc space or motion may be increased because of destruction of the anulus fibrosus within the disc.

Lateral views also permit evaluation of the relationship between the LS vertebrae. Normally, a continuous line that is drawn along the floor of the vertebral canal has a slight dorsal angulation of 20 degrees at the LS disc. With stress, the angle changes slightly. LS malalignment is indicated by a "stair step" in the line along the floor of the vertebral canal caused by an abrupt dorsal or ventral displacement of the sacrum. The malalignment may be stable or it may be altered by movement of the pelvic limbs and causes a fixed or variable stenosis of the vertebral canal. More commonly, the sacrum is displaced ventrally on flexion of the hip joint. Malalignment between L7 and S1 may be present without segmental instability.

Discography

Discography permits an understanding of the character of the intervertebral disc in the dog with a suspect cauda equina syndrome. A 20-ga spinal needle is positioned with the tip within the center of the LS disc and a contrast agent is injected into the nuclear portion of the disc. The location of the needle tip can be determined from a lateral radiograph prior to injection. Little or no contrast agent can be injected within a normal intervertebral disc or one with only early degeneration, whereas 2 to 3 cc or more of the contrast agent can be accommodated within a severely degenerated disc with cavitation. Radiographs are made following the injection of each 0.5 cc aliquot. This technique shows the progression of the flow of the contrast agent and the exact direction and extent of discal protrusion on both lateral and ventrodorsal views. The contrast agent may escape from the disc in a dorsal, ventral, or lateral direction through a partially torn anulus. The discogram is often combined with an epidurogram since both studies can be performed following slight repositioning of the tip of a single needle.

Epidurography

Epidurography is accomplished following the injection of a contrast medium between the bony wall of the vertebral canal and the outer sheath of the spinal cord (dura) and permits detection of a mass lesion within the epidural space. The epidurogram is used to detect a: (1) primary vertebral canal stenosis or a (2) secondary vertebral canal stenosis due to a thickened interarcuate ligament, thickened vertebral joint capsule, or dorsally protruded discal tissue. Uncommonly, the epidurogram detects other masses within the vertebral canal such as tumor mass or synovial cyst.

The injection is made through a 20-ga spinal needle with the tip placed within the epidural space at the LS junction or between the first caudal vertebrae. Complete filling of the epidural space is difficult to accomplish because the space is poorly defined, contains fat, and has multiple openings through the laterally positioned intervertebral foramina that permit drainage of the contrast agent. Usually, the study enables the clinician to outline the dorsal and ventral surfaces of the vertebral canal as seen on lateral radiographs. Repeated injections of additional contrast agent enable further visualization of a space occupying lesion within the vertebral canal. Radiographs are made following the injection of each 1.0 cc aliquot. Following removal of the needle, lateral radiographs can be made in stressed positions. The ventrodorsal view is of little value in epidurography. Epidurography can be utilized in combination with discography to demonstrate the thickness of the intact dorsal anulus of the LS disc.

Myelography

Myelography is the filling of the subarachnoid space, that lies between the inner two sheaths of the spinal cord, with a positive contrast agent through a cisternal or lumbar tap using a 20 or 22 ga spinal needle. This technique is usually not recommended as a technique for the evaluation of the LS canal because the subarachnoid space does not usually extend that far caudally and if it does, it often does not fill with the contrast agent. Another problem with the use of myelography in detection of an LS lesion is the normal elevation of the contrast-filled caudal extension of the subarachnoid space away from the floor of the vertebral canal that prevents detection of a mass lying on the floor of the vertebral canal. However, in the hands of some investigators, myelography is reported to be a valuable tool in the study of LS lesions. Myelography is a greater help in evaluation of the LS region in chondrodystrophoid breeds because the termination of the spinal cord and the caudal extension of the space are positioned further caudal. However, cauda equina syndrome is not common in chondrodystrophoid breeds and the need for the examination in those breeds is not frequent.

Examination protocol

Not all special radiographic procedures achieve their maximum diagnostic level in each patient. Therefore, a protocol should be used that utilizes the procedures in a correct sequence to insure that the diagnosis can be made with the least technically demanding study and with the studies that are of least risk to the patient. The routine survey study and stress series can be performed safely and with absolute accuracy on a cooperative or sedated patient and should be performed first. The discogram and epidurogram require experience to perform, are done on an anesthetized patient, are of high diagnostic value and are the next examination(s) to be considered. Myelography also requires anesthesia and, in addition, requires a particular needle tip placement to perform the study satisfactorily and often does not demonstrate the LS region in larger non-chondrodystrophoid dogs.

Protocol for study of LS lesions

1. noncontrast lateral and ventrodorsal radiographs in neutral position
2. noncontrast lateral stress radiographs with full extension and full flexion of the LS joint
3. discography with lateral and ventrodorsal radiographs following incremental injection of the contrast agent
4. epidurography with lateral and ventrodorsal radiographs following incremental injection of the positive contrast agent
5. myelography with lateral and ventrodorsal radiographs following positioning of the patient in a manner that fills the caudal extension of the subarachnoid space

Disseminated Idiopathic Skeletal Hyperostosis (DISH)

The radiographic changes in the spine may be prominent and yet not easily explain the cause of the clinical signs. This is the situation with "Sego". Both noncontrast radiographs and a myelogram are shown in part.

Case Description

"Sego" is a 2-year-old male Great Dane with mild paraparesis/ataxia for the past month. In his pelvic limbs, his proprioceptive placing is decreased, but his spinal reflexes are normal. Lumbar studies were made.

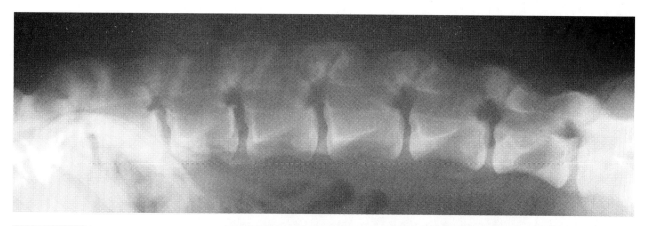

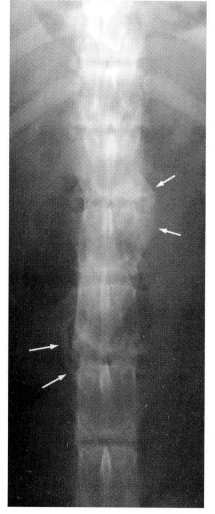

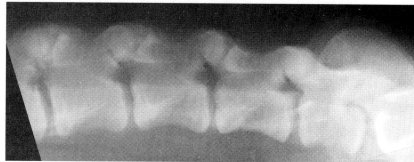

Radiographic Findings

The noncontrast radiographs show prominent new bone formation that results in bony fusion around the true vertebral joints as well as between vertebral bodies (arrows). A myelogram was performed (next page).

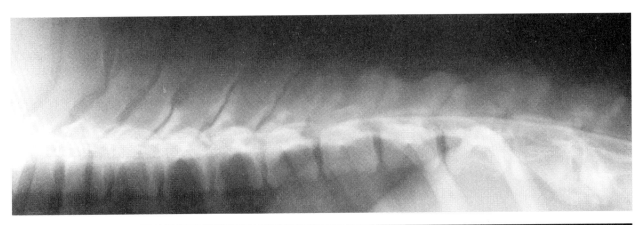

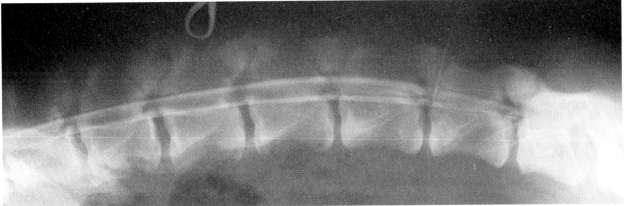

Myelographic Findings

The myelogram identifies the compression of the contrast columns at T10-11. In addition, note how the contrast columns shift ventrally at L7. Usually the cord is tethered at this level and in the dorsal portion of the vertebral canal. The ventral position suggests a dorsal mass. Note the spinal needle used in making the myelogram remains in position.

The diagnosis is midthoracic cord compression secondary to a form of DISH (disseminated idiopathic skeletal hyperostosis) with involvement dorsally instead of ventrally, causing vertebral canal stenosis. The possibility of a second stenotic lesion at L7 needs to be considered. Note the extensive amount of new bone formation in contrast to the paucity of neurological signs.

Question #1

What would you recommend next for "Sego"?

Question #2

Does a radiographic finding of "narrowing or collapse of the subarachnoid columns" mean the same as "narrowing or collapse of the spinal cord"?

Answer #1

The spinal radiographs do not provide an unequivocal diagnosis for Sego's T3-L3 myelopathy. The vertebral stenosis appears to compress the spinal cord as seen on the myelogram but does not positively identify the cause of the mass. Some other imaging procedure (such as MRI) as well as analysis of the CSF are indicated.

Answer #2

No. The subarachnoid spaces surround the spinal cord and can be collapsed without compression of the spinal cord. Change in the height of the spinal cord is a separate and more important radiographic feature.

Disseminated Idiopathic Skeletal Hyperostosis (DISH)

A limited study suggests that DISH in a rather common ossifying diathesis of large and giant breeds of dogs of rather young age and is characterized by bony hyperostosis at tendon and ligament attachments on both axial and extra-axial locations. Spinal osteophyte production is widespread and is the most extensive bony change with localized bony outgrowth in extra-axial location being less prominent. However, it is thought that both anatomical locations may represent different ends of the same disease spectrum. It is possible that all of the changes noted in DISH may be found in other sizes of dogs; however, they may be mild and localized. Lately, changes resembling DISH have been noted in aging cats and seems to present in a manner similar to that seen in the dog.

DISH may not represent a disease *per se*, but rather a vulnerable state in the patient in which extensive vertebral ossification results from some stimuli triggering an exaggerated response of the body in some patients that causes only modest new bone formation in others. In addition, these "bone formers" have a high incidence of associated extraspinal hyperostosis at the sites of ligament and tendon attachment. Hypotheses suggest that DISH in dogs may have a relation to other diseases including hypoparathyroidism, hyperthyrocalcitoninism (Krook et al 1971), hypervitaminosis A or D, fluorosis, and dietary calcium (Hazewinkel 1985) and need to be examined further. The possibility that DISH is one cause for cervical cord compression noted in cervical spondylopathy should be considered (Hedhammer et al 1974).

DISH is seem commonly in radiographic studies of the thorax and abdomen as well as in spinal studies in the presence of spinal pain or neurological signs. When noted as an incidental finding or when noted in the patient with spinal pain or neurological signs, it presents a dilemma in diagnosis as well as treatment.

Similar patterns of spinal hyperostosis have been described in man under various names such as spondylitis ossificans ligamentosa (Knaggs 1925, Oppenheimer 1942), spondylosis hyperostatic (Ott 1953), physiologic vertebral ligamentous calcification (Smith et al 1955), and generalized juxta-articular ossification of ligaments of the vertebral column (Sutro et al 1956). These conditions all referred to heavy bony formations in the spine that were basically thought to be ossification of paraspinal ligaments. Forestier and colleagues introduced the term "ankylosing hyperostosis of the spine," noting more prominent involvement of the anterior and right lateral aspects of the thoracolumbar region, uneven calcification and ossification, cortical hyperostosis, and large vertebral osteophytes (Forestier and Rotes-Querol 1950, Forestier et al 1969, Forestier and Lagier 1971). Differentiation from ankylosing spondylitis and osteoarthrosis was based on clinical, pathologic, and radiologic features. Further descriptions of the condition in the spine of man were made more recently (Resnick and Niwayama 1976) and extraspinal manifestations described (Resnick et al 1975, Utsinger et al 1976, Littlejohn et al 1981). These authors introduced the term "disseminated idiopathic skeletal hyperostosis" (DISH). DISH in people is usually found in older individuals and is found predominantly in males (Resnick and Niwayama, 1981). Since radiographic determination of ankylosis is often not apparent, terms using "ankylosis" may not in fact be accurate and they choose not to use that term. Also, extraspinal changes may be more extensive than vertebral changes in man, so the emphasis of a widespread nature of the condition was thought to be more appropriate.

Diagnostic criteria have been established for diagnosis of DISH in man and can be used in the dog and cat as well. They include: (1) presence of "flowing" calcification and ossification along anterolateral aspects of at least 4 contiguous vertebral bodies with or without localized pointed excrescences at intervening vertebral body-disc junctions, (2) relative preservation of disc height in involved areas and the absence of extensive radiographic changes of degenerative disc disease (intervertebral osteochondrosis) including vacuum phenomena and vertebral body marginal sclerosis, and (3) absence of apophyseal joint bony ankylosis and sacroiliac joint erosion, sclerosis or intra-articular bony fusion (Resnick et al 1975).

These criteria have been established in man to specifically eliminate from consideration other potentially confusing spinal disorders. A flowing pattern along at least 4 contiguous vertebral bodies is not found in typical spondylosis deformans. Preservation of disc height is not present in intervertebral disc disease. Changes across apophyseal and sacroiliac joints are characteristically found in ankylosing spondylitis. It must be appreciated that since DISH occurs in middle-aged to elderly people, an absolute lack of degenerative disc disease is not a constant. At the least, the presence of obvious disc disease is not a principle characteristic of DISH (Resnick and Niwayama 1981).

While descriptions of DISH in the dog may not be complete, vertebral hyperostosis has been strongly suggested (Wright 1982). Reference to a unique pattern of paraspinal new bone formation has been made in dogs (Reed and Smith 1968), especially in the Boxer dog (Morgan 1967. A recent report describes hyperostosis in the spine and extraspinal locations of a 4-year-old female Great Dane (Morgan and Stavenborn 1990). It is probable that cases of DISH in animals have been frequently described as a variant of spondylosis deformans.

The radiographic and pathologic features of DISH in the dog are distinctive and differ considerably from those of intervertebral disc disease (Hanson 1952) and more closely resemble extensive spondylosis deformans (Morgan 1967, Morgan and Biery 1985) but possess marked radiographic and pathologic differences. In chronic degenerative disc disease, sclerosis of cranial and caudal vertebral end plates is prominent and discs have moderate to severe decrease in width as a result of destruction of the anulus fibrosus. Vertebral osteophytosis associated with spondylosis deformans typically centers on individually degenerating discs and does not have patterns of flowing bone growth or dorsal periarticular changes. Hypertrophic osteopathy in dogs may produce periosteal new bone formation but its usual involvement of the diaphyseal portion of long bones and failure to involve the spine clearly allow separation of these conditions (Morgan 1972).

Radiographic criteria for diagnosis of DISH

1. Flowing calcification and ossification leading to segmental bony ankylosis
   a. along ventral and lateral aspects of contiguous vertebral bodies
   b. between vertebral articular facets
   c. between spinous processes
2. Formation of pseudoarthrosis between the bases of spinous processes
3. Periarticular osteophytes and calcification and ossification of soft tissue attachments (enthesophytes) in both axial and peripheral skeleton
4. Periarticular osteophytes, sclerosis, and ankylosis of sacroiliac joints
5. Bony ankylosis of the symphysis pubis
6. Absence of extensive radiographic changes of degenerative disc disease such as
   a. narrowing of disc width
   b. end plate sclerosis
   c. nuclear calcification
   d. localized spondylosis deformans

A Routine Thoracic Study with Spinal Changes

Often the changes within the thoracic spine that are seen on a routine thoracic study provide additional information of value to the clinician. That is the situation with "Pablo".

Case Description

"Pablo" is an 11-year-old male shepherd who was to be anesthetized for dentistry and because of his age had a pre-anesthetic thoracic radiographic study.

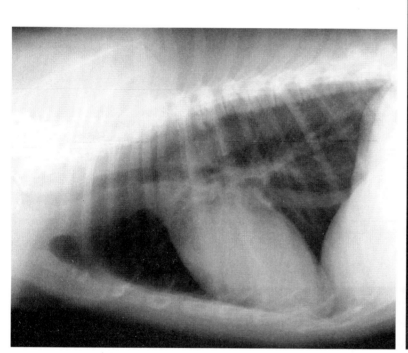

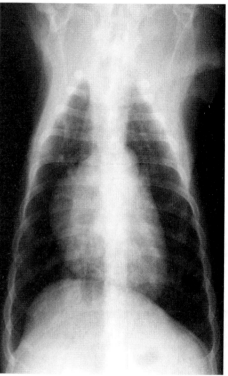

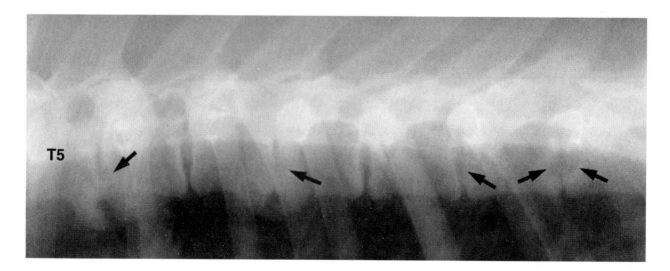

Radiographic Findings

The thoracic radiographs show: (see the enlargement of the thoracic spine)

1. collapsed disc spaces at T5-6, T7-8, T9-10, T10-11
2. end plate destruction (arrows)
3. reactive vertebral osteophytosis at T5-6 and T7-8 disc spaces
4. an elongated cardiac silhouette

The diagnosis is an extensive discospondylitis and generalized cardiomegaly.

Comments

Thoracic studies permit an evaluation of the thoracic spine and are often helpful in the detection of systemic inflammatory disease as well as degenerative changes that may be of clinical importance.

Chronic periodontal disease often serves as a focus for hematogenous spread of bacteria that may cause discospondylitis.

The presence of the osteophytes associated with spondylosis deformans shouldn't influence your diagnosis of discospondylitis.

The osteophytes can indicate:

1. an earlier disc degeneration with secondary neovascularity permitted the hematogenous infection to center is a certain disc space
2. an effort to correct vertebral instability following the discospondylitis
3. a condition totally unrelated to the inflammatory process

The heart is probably within normal limits for a dog this age but may suggest left ventricular enlargement and a possible endocarditis.

Different Etiologies for Thoracolumbar (TL) Lesions

All the dogs in this group have upper motor neuron paraparesis or paraplegia. Some had a recent, sudden onset of severe signs; others had a more protracted course of progressive signs. Based on the neurologic signs, the lesion in each was localized to the T3-L3 area of the spinal cord (thoracolumbar myelopathy) For each dog, interpret the noncontrast radiographs and decide if you need a myelogram to make or confirm a diagnosis.

Case Description

"Lucky" is a 4-year-old female dachshund cross who had an acute onset of paraplegia 2 days ago.

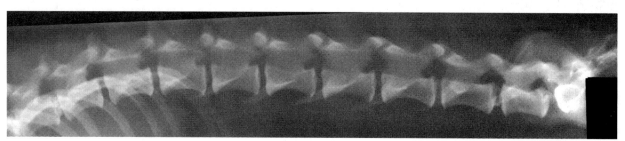

Radiographic Findings

The noncontrast radiographs (above and to the left) show a slight narrowing of the L1-2 disc with a suggestion of a "cloud" of calcified material within the vertebral canal dorsal to that disc. Additional calcified discs from L3 to the sacrum appear without evidence of disc herniation at this time. The radiographic signs are strongly suggestive, however you recommend a myelogram.

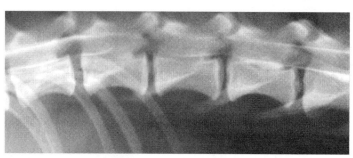

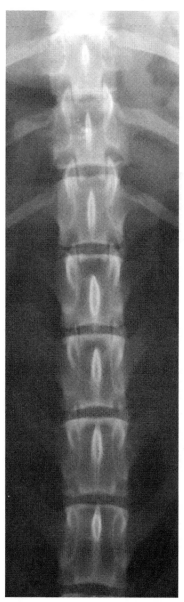

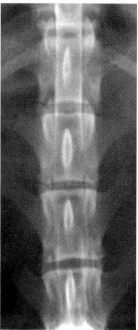

Myelographic Findings

The myelogram (above and to the left) shows an elevation of the spinal cord on the lateral view at L1-2 with compression of the subarachnoid columns. On the ventrodorsal view, widening of the spinal cord and compression of the subarachnoid columns can be seen. The myelographic features are typical for of a slowly herniating Type 1 disc disease with an absence of cord swelling and suggest an extradural mass probably associated with the previously suspected L1-2 herniated disc. Note the smaller degree of cord elevation and contrast column collapse at L2-3 suggesting a second site of disc disease.

Comments

The extent of the cord compression is remarkable and certainly indicates the need for immediate decompressive surgery and a search for more than one lesion.

Case Description

"Gabriel" is a 4-year-old male retriever with paraparesis for 1 month that progressed to paraplegia over the last 48 hours. A survey study of the spine was performed without anesthesia and only lateral views were made.

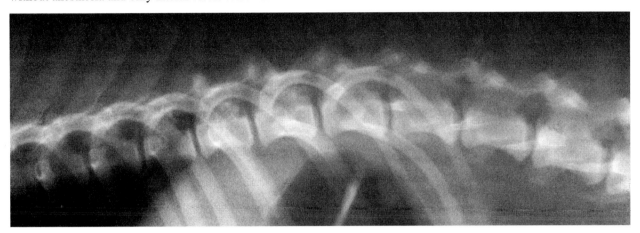

Radiographic Findings

The noncontrast lateral view (above) shows no evidence of abnormality in the spine. In particular, the disc spaces are of normal width without evidence of disc disease. A slight increase in the height of the vertebral canal at T13-L1 was detected but no importance was attached to that finding. No definitive diagnosis could be made; therefore, a myelogram was performed.

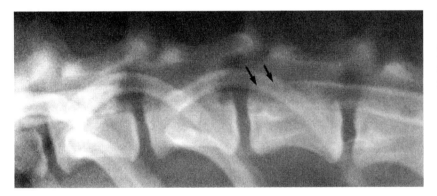

Question #1

Aside from neoplasia and disc herniation, what else may produce an extradural mass pattern on a myelogram?

Myelographic Findings

The myelogram (above) shows a dorsal extradural mass at T13-L1 causing ventral displacement of the cord (arrows). The subarachnoid columns are compressed. The dorsal mass is large and more suggestive of a tumor mass rather than protruding disc tissue. Again, an increase in the height of the vertebral canal is suggested.

Comments

At surgery, a 2 x 4 cm tissue section was removed from the mass in the vertebral canal at T13-L1 and was reported to be an undifferentiated sarcoma. At necropsy, additional tumor tissue was found in the perivertebral space with part of the mass extending into the vertebral canal at T13. Within the vertebral canal, the mass extended cranially for a length of 6 vertebrae and caudally for a length of 1 vertebra. The tumor was thought to be a sarcoma, specifically an anaplastic rhabdomyosarcoma. At necropsy, multiple metastatic nodules were located in the liver and neoplastic cells were found in the choroid plexus of the fourth ventricle of the brain.

An increase in height of the vertebral canal was confirmed at necropsy. This pattern is often associated with a tumor mass that is increasing in size and not associated with a disc herniation that is more stable and not increasing in size.

Case Description

"**Bambi**" is a 7-year-old female dachshund with a history of recurrent episodes of back pain and eventually paraparesis. Because the dog was not anesthetized, several views were made during the noncontrast study hoping for good patient positioning. Which is the most important lesion? Is it necessary to perform a myelogram?

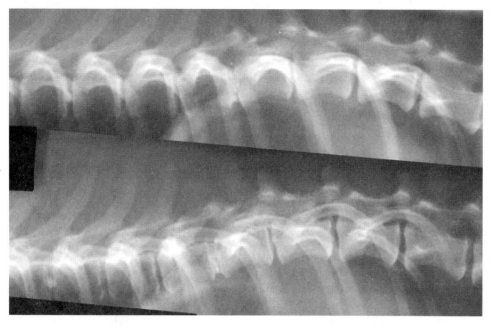

Radiographic Findings

"Bambi" has a large calcified mass within the vertebral canal at T11-12 on the midline (arrows on enlargement below). The noncontrast radiographs also show multiple calcified discs and narrow disc spaces at T12-13 and T13-L1.

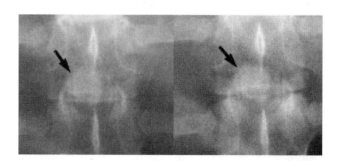

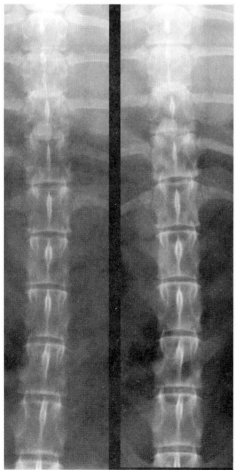

Comments

In an older dachshund, it is possible for several discs to have degenerated with dorsal herniations or protrusions. Sometimes it is possible to make a determination (guess?) of which disc is most likely to be the cause of the neurological signs. More often, a myelogram is necessary to insure the accuracy of your diagnosis. In "Bambi", the size of the herniated mass is so large and its density so great that it is relatively easy to center your attention on that lesion.

Question #2

How do you relate the slowly progressive clinical signs with the massive size of the disc protrusion?

Case Description

"**Rohrschac**" is a 9-year-old female Dalmatian who was hit by a car 2 weeks ago and has been non-ambulatory since that time. She has upper motor neuron signs in the pelvic limbs with good deep pain perception. A survey noncontrast study of the lumbar region was made.

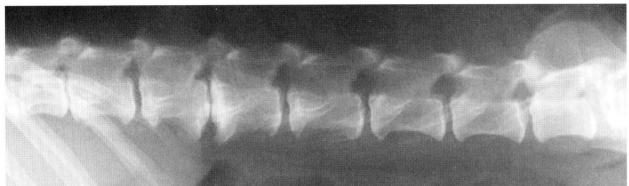

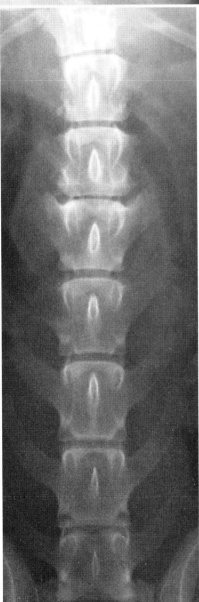

Radiographic Findings

The survey radiographs show a fracture-luxation of T13-L1 with lateral displacement of the caudal portion of the spine causing a focal scoliosis. The T13-L1 end plates are not parallel as seen on the VD view. Ventral displacement of the body of L1 is indicated by an interruption in a line drawn along the floor of the vertebral canal (see enlargement). Note the small chip fracture from the body of L1 (arrow). The chronic disc collapse at L2-3 with end plate sclerosis and spondylosis deformans is not thought to be clinically important at this time.

Comments

The lesion was at the edge of the radiograph on both views in the survey study and was identified only following a thorough examination of the radiograph. After the radiographic changes were noted, additional studies were made centering on the lesion.

Question #3

Do you assign clinical importance to the changes at L2-3?

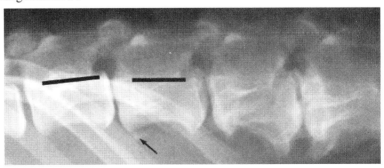

Answer #1

Hemorrhage/hematoma, abscess/exudate, foreign body, bone fragments, hypertrophic soft tissue, and cysts are all uncommon cause of an extradural mass pattern.

Answer #2

The severity of the clinical signs caused by spinal cord compression depends on several factors:

1. Degree of compression – the greater the compression, the more severe the signs.
2. Rate of compression – the more quickly the cord is compressed, the more severe the signs.
3. Duration of compression – the longer the period of time of compression, the more severe the signs.

In "Bambi's" case, the disc may have herniated very slowly and in small increments, therefore not causing a great deal of trauma (hemorrhage, edema) to the cord and allowing some time for neural or vascular compensation to the compression.

Answer #3

Probably not. The older the dog, regardless of the type of disc degeneration, the more difficult it is to correctly evaluate a degenerative lesion such as L2-3. However, end plate sclerosis and spondylosis deformans, especially if extensive, indicate a chronic lesion, one that is not thought to be the cause of the neurologic signs in a case such as this (acute onset of signs associated with trauma).

Osteoarthrosis

Reactive changes are seen dorsally surrounding the articular facets and are described as periarticular spurring or osteoarthrosis in the dog or spondylosis ankylopoetica in the cat. The diagnosis of arthrosis is difficult because of not being able to identify change affecting the articular surfaces. Consequently, we are limited to the identification of reactive bone which may appear as periarticular spurring which may actually be a form of enthesopathy. Clinical significance has not been routinely attached to the secondary changes involving these true vertebral joints. However, similar changes involving the articular facets in the cervical region cause new bone to protrude into the vertebral canal causing stenosis. This problem is found regularly in dogs with cervical spondylopathy.

Another form of arthrosis is seen with the creation of pseudoarticulations that form at the base of the spinous processes in the lumbar region and between the long spinous processes in the thoracic region and are identified in older and larger dogs as well as in older cats. Called "kissing lesions" in the horse, the clinical importance is not fully understood, however, these bony changes must limit movement between vertebrae and may be painful.

Secondary joint disease also frequently involves the costovertebral joints in both the dog and cat and may be noticed on the ventrodorsal projection by detection of periarticular spurring, sclerosis of the subchondral bone, and modeling of the articular surfaces. Clinical significance of this disease is poorly understood; however, rib motion would seem to be limited owing to the joint disease. It is also possible to see destructive changes in the articular surfaces associated with infectious inflammatory lesions and with noninfectious inflammatory lesions. These patterns all need further study.

Features of vertebral arthrosis

1. True vertebral joints
   a. spurring on articular facets
      1. prominent in all regions of the spine
      2. changes may be limited to periarticular tissues
   b. modeling of articular facets
   c. change in the size of the interarcurate space due to
      1. abnormal movement of the articular facets
      2. change in width of disc space due to disc disease
2. Costovertebral joints
   a. spurring on joint margins
   b. modeling of rib heads
   c. modeling of articular surfaces on the vertebral bodies
3. Pseudoarticulations between adjacent spinous processes at the
   a. base of the spinous processes in the lumbar region
   b. midportion of the spinous processes in the thoracic region
   c. midportion of the spinous processes in the cervical region

Calcified Discs

Chondroid metaplasia and calcification of disc tissue is the expected process of disc degeneration in chondrodystrophic breeds of dogs. However, calcified discs can also be found in nonchondrodystrophic breeds as well. The nucleus begins to calcify at an early age in both types of dogs and the process is progressive throughout life. As long as the calcified tissue remains within the disc, clinical signs are not noted. Even with protrusion or herniation of the nucleus, clinical signs may not be noted, particularly if the protrusion is lateral or ventral to the disc space. If the nucleus protrudes (Type II disease) or actually escapes from the disc (Type I disease) causing irritation, compression or trauma to the meninges, nerve roots, or spinal cord, then neurological signs may occur. If disc tissue is calcified and remains as a mass, it may be visible on the radiograph. Usually the greatest problem is to discern which of several calcified, degenerated discs is the current culprit. It is possible that another disc, not so readily identified on the radiograph, may be the problem today. Examine the radiographs of the following dogs and identify the offending disc.

Case Description

"**Mikko**" is a 4-year-old female Shi Tzu with progressive paraparesis over the past 4 days. Her spinal reflexes are normal. The noncontrast radiographs show 5 calcified TL discs. Your problem is to determine which is the most important.

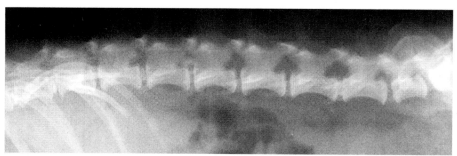

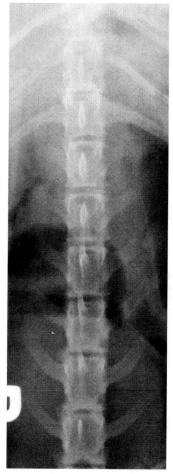

Radiographic Findings

"Mikko" has a large calcified herniated disc at L2-3 with a small tract connecting the nuclear area and the herniated mass within the vertebral canal (arrow on lateral view below). On the ventrodorsal view (below) it is not possible to determine laterality of the calcified nuclear tissue that has protruded into the vertebral canal at L2-3 (arrow). A calcified disc at L1-2 has herniated laterally to the left (arrow). Note also the transitional segment at T13 with transverse processes instead of articulating ribs.

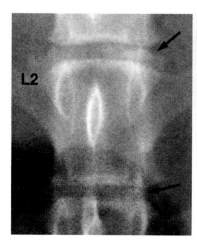

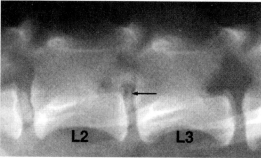

Question #1

Do you consider the radiographic study to be complete with consideration of the clinical signs and the dog affected?

Case Description

"Lobo" is an 8-year-old male beagle who wants to keep his head low and resents extension of his neck. He is lame in the left forelimb. Proprioceptive deficits are present in the right pelvic limb and his patellar reflexes are exaggerated, but his pain sensation is apparently normal. "Lobo" presented 18 months ago with typical signs of a TL disc. Evaluate a lateral view of the cervical spine made at that time first. That view is seen below.

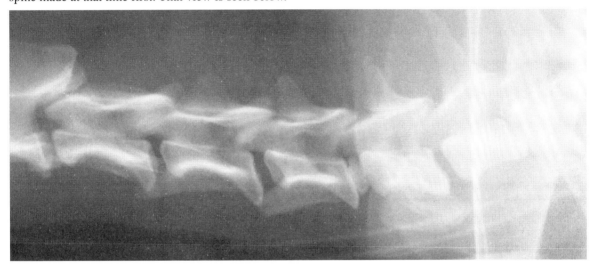

Radiographic Findings (18 months ago)

A heavily calcified disc is noted at C5-6 without evidence of protrusion. The lesion was not treated.

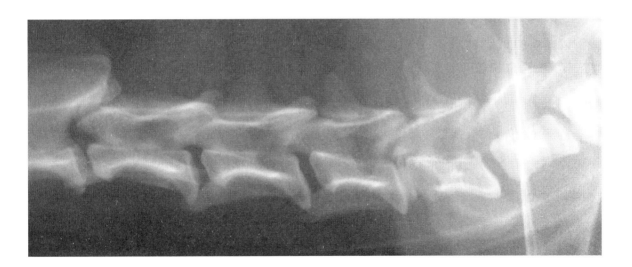

Radiographic Findings (today)

Comparison of the two radiographs made 18 months apart clearly shows the protrusion of the calcified nucleus at C5-6 into the vertebral canal (note the small "neck" connecting the calcified tissue in the nuclear space with the calcified tissue in the vertebral canal)

Comment

The pelvic limb proprioceptive deficit and exaggerated patellar reflexes may be residual effects of the TL disc problem that occurred 18 months ago. Both signs are consistent with a TL myelopathy (upper motor neuron lesion of the pelvic limbs).

Case Description

"**Rebel**" is an 8-year-old male poodle showing pain when handled for the past month. Now he is dragging the right fore limb and cannot elevate the right pelvic limb to urinate. He has decreased proprioceptive placing in both right limbs.

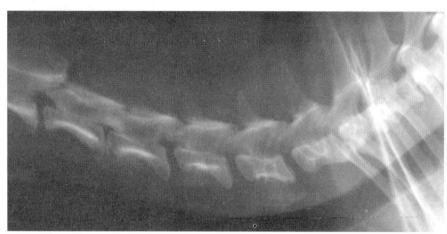

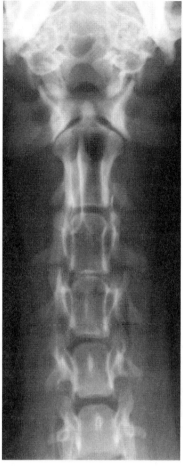

Radiographic Findings

The noncontrast radiographs show a large calcified herniated disc at C3-4. That disc space is narrowed without the features of end plate sclerosis or spondylosis deformans that would indicate a chronic collapse. A large herniated mass that is calcified can usually be identified on the ventrodorsal view (see the arrows on the enlarged view below). Note how the calcified mass occludes the intervertebral foramina on the lateral view.

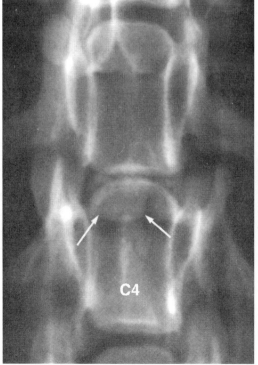

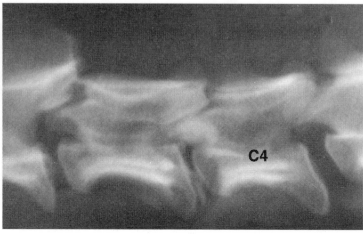

Case Description

"**Heidi**" is a 10-year-old female dachshund with intermittent thoracolumbar pain. She is reluctant to go up and down stairs.

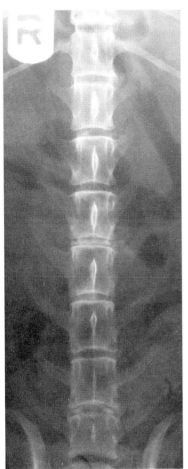

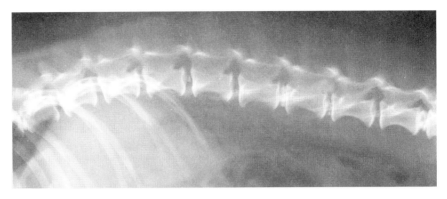

Radiographic Findings

The radiographic studies show the disc at L4-5 has herniated and the mass of disc material appears to almost fill the vertebral canal (arrows, best seen on the enlarged views below). Other discs are heavily calcified.

Comment

The disc at T11-12 had been fenestrated 4 years earlier but the calcified discs at L3-4, L4-5, and L6-7 were not included in the surgery.

Question #2

Can you determine if the calcified tissue is on the midline or located laterally?

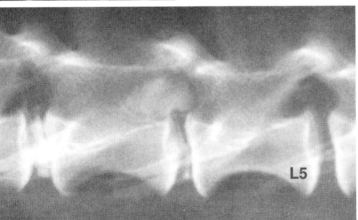

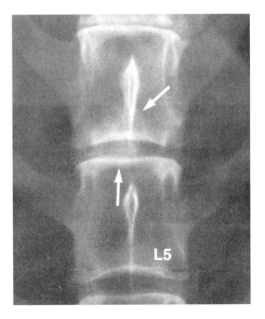

Answer #1

The disc space at L1-2 is between two calcified discs and could represent a disc that has recently emptied. Myelography is definitely indicated in this patient to determine between a definite chronic herniation and a potential acute herniation in another disc in which the calcified nucleus cannot be identified.

Answer #2

The disc material is located in the center of the vertebral canal extending toward the right side (arrows).

Trauma to Four Small Dogs

Typically, traumatized animals are brought to the hospital immediately for care. In some instances of trauma, however, the initial injury may not be particularly serious. Secondary problems may develop days or weeks later or the effects of the trauma may persist instead of resolving. These four patients are all male and all small breed dogs with known or suspected bite wounds.

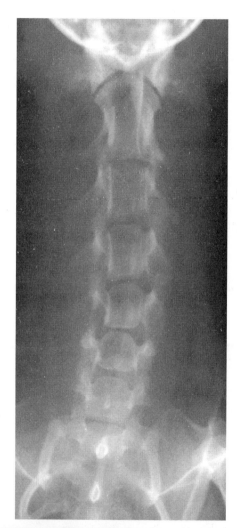

Case Description

"**Bandit**" is a small 7-year-old male poodle bitten in the neck 8 days ago and suffering multiple lacerations. He was immediately quadraparetic and has not shown improvement. Radiographs were not made until 1 week after the attack.

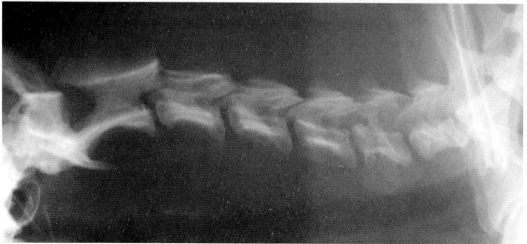

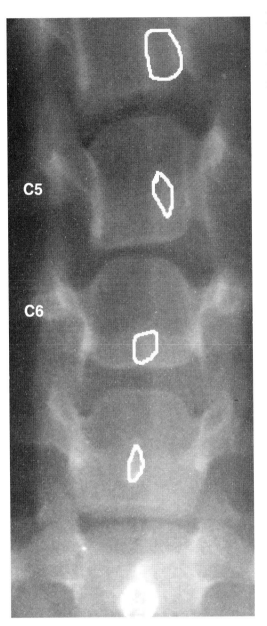

Radiographic Findings

The lateral radiograph shows collapse of the disc space C5-6 with dorsal displacement of the C6 vertebrae. The ventrodorsal view shows a minimal degree of vertebral rotation. Examination of the location of the tips of the spinous processes is a good technique for detecting this rotation (see circles on the enlarged views). These changes are indicative of a traumatic luxation.

Comments

End plate sclerosis and spondylosis deformans, changes suggesting disc disease, are not evident in this radiograph. A diagnosis other than traumatic vertebral luxation and disc rupture is difficult to support because the history suggests that the lesion is traumatic and the vertebrae are malaligned causing stenosis of the vertebral canal. Vertebral displacement is not a feature of acute disc disease. Fractures in the vertebral arch or articular facets are almost impossible to identify in the cervical spine in a case such as "Bandit".

The delay in the examination of "Bandit" until 1 week after his injury is very likely to be detrimental to his recovery. Any cord compression that occurred at the time of his injury is likely to still be present, and in the presence of vertebral instability, additional compression is likely to have occurred as he was cared for during the week. Persistent and recurring compression are both deleterious to eventual recovery.

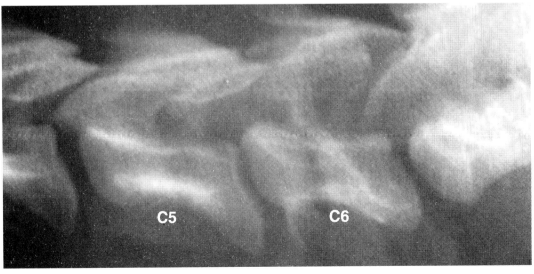

Case Description

"J-J" is a 2-year-old male terrier who was in a fight with another dog 2 weeks ago and has been paraparetic since that time. He also appears painful when his abdomen is palpated. Because of the clinical signs, abdominal studies were made.

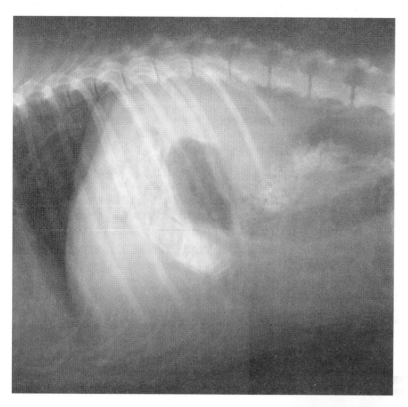

Abdominal Radiographic Findings

The abdominal radiographs show gastric foreign bodies. New bone production is identified on the ventral aspect of the bodies of T13-L2. Disc space width is difficult to determine on abdominal studies of a nonanesthetized patient. Because of the new bone, a lateral view was made of the lumbar spine (see next page).

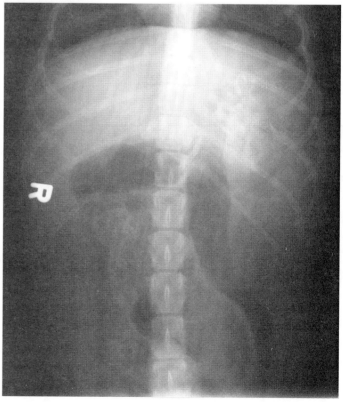

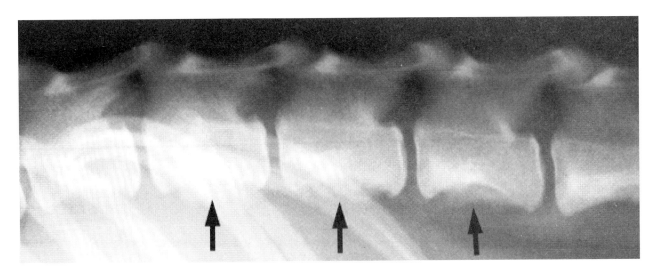

Spinal Radiographic Findings

The lateral radiographs of the TL spine confirm the bony changes on the vertebral bodies (arrows). The diagnosis is a spondylitis, probably secondary to a migrating grass awn (seed head).

Comments

The clinical history is misleading, that is, the bite wound is probably not the cause of the spondylitis. While it is possible for a penetrating wound to cause spondylitis, the location and appearance of the "J-J's" reactive bone, on the ventral aspect of the cranial lumbar vertebrae, are much more compatible with a migrating foreign body.

The gastric foreign bodies should receive continual evaluation. The material does not have the appearance of small bones but rather looks like plastic, glass, or rubber material, any of which could cause the clinical problem of bowel obstruction. The presence of some of the material in the colon suggests that some of the material has passed through the small bowel.

"J-J's" owner declined further diagnostic tests to determine if the bite wound and resulting spondylitis was the cause of the paraparesis. Typically, spondylitis does not result in acute paraparesis. A myelogram and CSF analysis might identify another cause for the clinical signs that "J-J" demonstrated.

Case Description

"**Prancer**" is a 7-year-old male miniature poodle who was bitten in the back by a shepherd dog about 2 months ago. Presently, he has back pain and is paraparetic with upper motor neuron signs to the pelvic limbs.

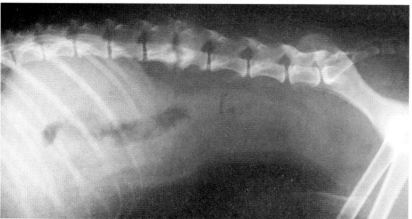

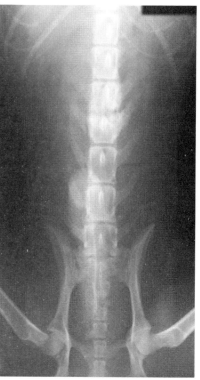

Radiographic Findings

The radiographs show end plate destruction at L3-4 with disc space collapse. The destruction has resulted in shortening of the vertebrae, poorly organized reactive new bone, and ventral displacement and rotation of the spine caudal to the affected disc space. Note that the pedicles and true vertebral joints are involved in the destructive process as well (see arrows on the enlarged lateral view below). The fractures of the transverse processes on the right are best seen on the enlarged ventrodorsal view (arrows). The diagnosis is a discospondylitis and vertebral fractures, secondary to a bite wound.

Comments

"Prancer" is a different case from "J-J" in that "Prancer's" radiographic changes are severe dorsally as well as ventrally and are focused on a single disc space. For that reason, the lesion is more likely the result of a puncture wound rather than grass-awn migration. Another less-likely possibility in "Prancer's" case is hematogenous discospondylitis, and microbial culture of the blood and urine is recommended.

Tissue obtained at the time of surgical decompression was submitted for histological examination with a diagnosis of reactive bone with no evidence of the cause. Because the dog produces so much reactive bone around an inflammatory lesion, submission of tissue for histological examination should include tissue obtained from the depth of the lesion as well as the surrounding reactive tissue.

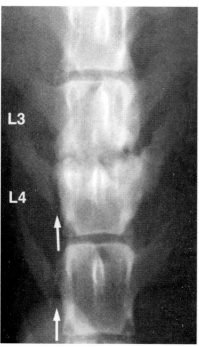

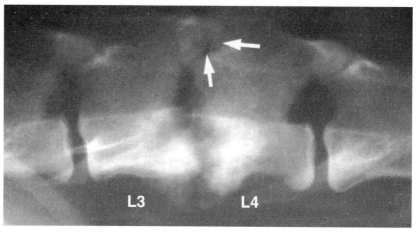

Case Description

"Lassie" is a 10-year-old male terrier who has been depressed and showing pain on movement of the head for the past 10 days. Lateral views of the spine were made following anesthesia. When questioned about the dog's immediate past history, the owner admitted that the dog was absent from home for several days 2 weeks ago.

Radiographic Findings

The radiographs show: (1) malalignment of T12-13 vertebrae, (2) end plate fracture of T12 (black arrow), (3) separation of the facets of the vertebral joints (white arrow), and (4) narrowing of L1-2 disc space with minimal spondylosis deformans. In addition there is narrowing of C4-5 disc space. Fourteen thoracic-type vertebrae are identified. The diagnosis is a fracture-luxation of T12-13 with vertebral malalignment. The fracture (black arrow) and joint luxation (white arrow) are best seen on the enlarged view (below).

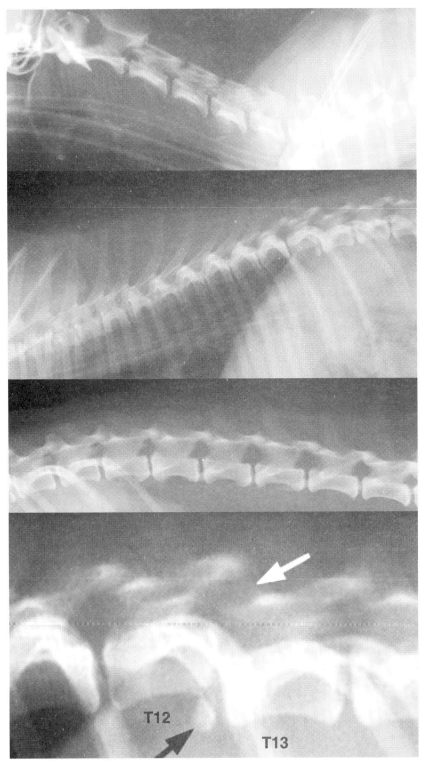

Comments

The fracture-luxation is probably the cause of the acute clinical signs. The narrowed cervical disc space in an older dog is probably indicative of chronic disc degeneration without nuclear herniation, but the possibility of associated disc protrusion must be considered.

Often with a history that is nonspecific, lateral radiographs of the spine are made as a type of survey study. If a lesion is detected, spot films as well as a ventrodorsal view of the area of interest should be made to provide additional information concerning the lesion.

It is always important to carefully study the first cervical vertebra because of the frequency of congenital anomalies at this site in smaller breeds of dogs. Often the display of neurologic signs relative to these congenital anomalies is delayed because of the manner in which they are protected during their life.

Evaluation of Calcified Discs in Four Dogs

The presence of calcified material within intervertebral discs in chondrodystrophic dogs may make radiographic diagnosis of herniated discs easier. However, calcified herniated disc tissue may spread out within the vertebral canal so that radiographic identification on noncontrast radiographs is virtually impossible. Another problem is that all the discs may have a calcified nucleus and all discs may have a Type II protrusion, which is just a "bulging" of the anulus fibrosus with less importance clinically. Thus, it may be possible for calcified tissue to appear within the vertebral canal and not be of immediate clinical importance. Examine the following cases and make a assessment regarding the probable clinical importance of the abnormal discs.

The following rules are generally of value:
1. An empty disc space adjacent to discs with calcified nuclei may indicate a recent extravasation of nuclear material.
2. A narrowed disc space without end plate sclerosis or spondylosis deformans may suggest a recent narrowing of potential clinical importance.
3. Calcified tissue within the vertebral canal may suggest extravasation of nuclear tissue, but does not suggest when this happened.

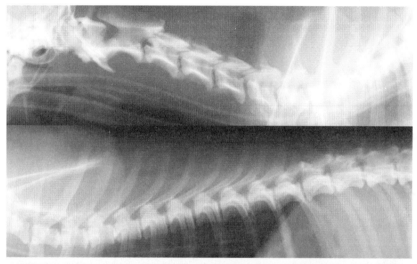

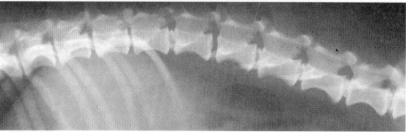

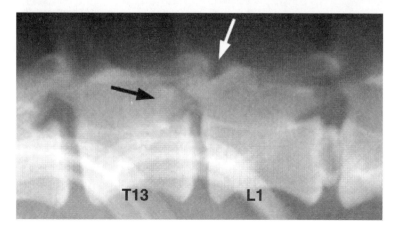

Case Description

"Toby" is a 4-year-old male dachshund with paraparesis. Lateral noncontrast radiographs of the entire spine are shown

.

Radiographic Findings

The disc space at T13-L1 is narrowed, a pattern of calcified tissue is present in the vertebral canal over the disc as seen more clearly on the enlarged view (black arrow), and narrowing is present in the width of the interarcuate space dorsal to this disc (white arrow).

The radiographic findings also include minimal to moderate calcification of the nucleus pulposus of C3-4, C6-T1, T1-T5, T8-9, L1-2, and LS discs without evidence of nuclear herniation. The disc space at T10-11 is narrowed; however, this is near the anticlinal segment and the minimal change in width is probably normal. Note the general absence of any spondylosis deformans.

Comments

This study suggests that T13-L1 is the clinically important disc.

Case Description

"**Samantha**" is an 8-year-old female cocker spaniel cross with a 2-week history of lethargy and reluctance to move.

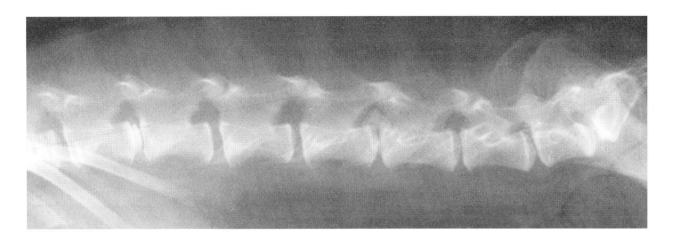

Radiographic Findings

The lateral radiograph shows a completely calcified disc at L4-5 that has herniated dorsally into the vertebral canal, a disc at L1-2 that is calcified but has not herniated, and a disc at L6-7 that has partially herniated. Note on the enlarged ventrodorsal view that the herniated discal tissue at L4-5 (circle) is on the midline and therefore within the vertebral canal.

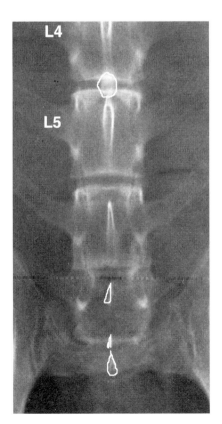

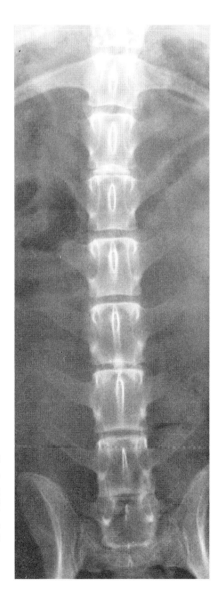

Comments

Several congenital anomalies are present, including a transitional TL vertebra with failure of segmentation of the last ribs, a hypoplastic arch of L7 with a small spinous process (ring), and hypoplastic sacral spinous processes (rings).

Case Description

"**Dinky**" is a 5-year-old female dachshund with mild pain and tenderness over the TL junction. A slight proprioceptive deficit is present in the left pelvic limb.

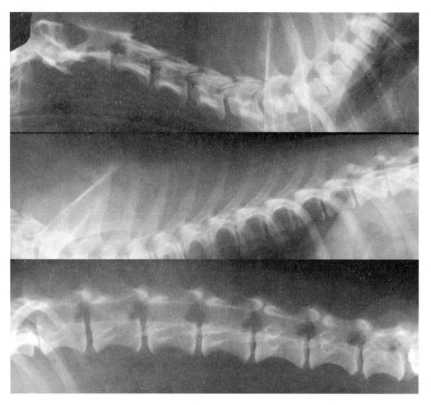

Radiographic Findings

The lateral radiographs show calcified disc tissue in the vertebral canal over the body of L2. The disc material is difficult to see because it is between the vertebral laminae. It is indicated on the enlarged lateral view (white arrows). On the enlargement of the ventrodorsal view, the calcified tissue is on the midline but blends with the shadow of the spinous process (black arrows). Note the number of discs that are calcified: C2-3, C4-5, C7-T1, T11-12, and T12-13.

Comments

Often the severity of the clinical signs does not match the apparent size of the herniated disc tissue.

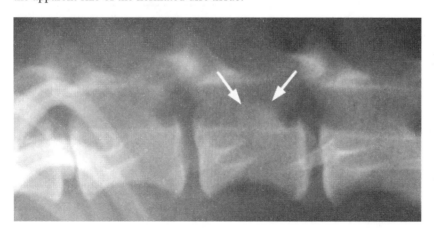

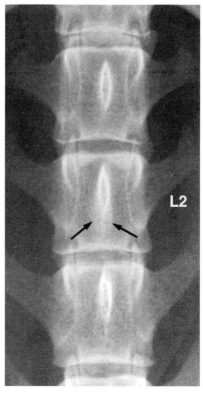

Case Description

"**Daisy**" is a 5-year-old female dachshund with a history of left pelvic limb lameness and pain on being handled. Lumbar hyperesthesia is present.

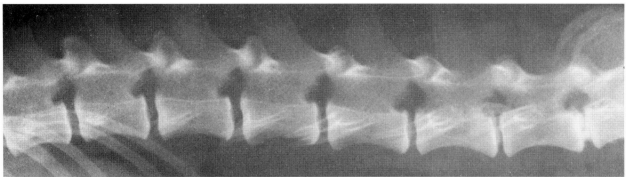

Radiographic Findings

The disc space at L5-6 is narrowed with calcified tissue dorsal to the disc space. If the positioning of the patient is good, it is possible to evaluate the width and contents of the disc spaces. Use the width of the disc spaces immediately cranial and caudal to the one in question to determine if narrowing has occurred. Also check the vertebral end plates for sclerosis to determine acute or chronic disc disease. The L6-7 disc has calcified but not herniated. These findings are more easily identified on the enlarged view. The L5-6 disc herniation is the cause of the clinical findings.

Comments

Two of the cases in this group had UMN signs while two of the cases had LMN signs in the pelvic limbs.

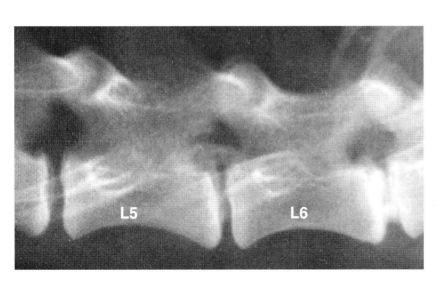

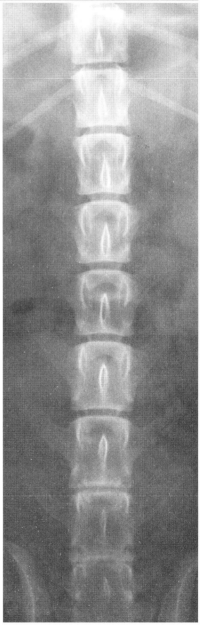

Suspect Cauda Equina Syndrome in Four Large Dogs

One of the causes of cauda equina syndrome is stenosis (narrowing) of the lumbosacral vertebral canal. Note the variety of radiographic changes in this group of dogs with lumbosacral stenosis. In some patients the specific cause of the stenosis can be identified while in others a summation of changes results in a stenotic lesion with congenital/developmental, inflammatory, and degenerative lesions all having played a role.

Case Description

"**Kim**" is an 11-year-old male collie who is painful around the tail and anal region especially if the tail is moved from side to side.

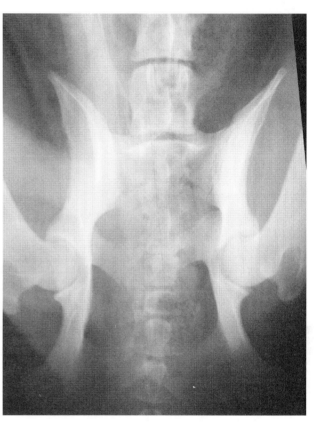

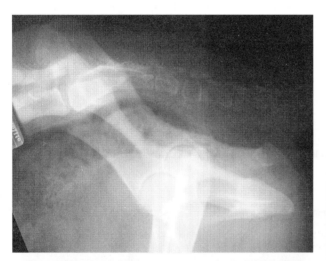

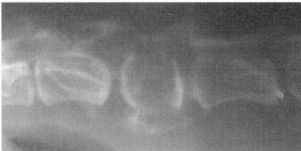

Radiographic Findings

Pelvic radiographs show destruction and collapse of the body of second caudal segment with some new bone production. The differential diagnoses include an: (1) infectious, (2) neoplastic, or (3) post-traumatic lesion. A chronic osteomyelitis was diagnosed by biopsy of the lesion. The changes are seen more easily on the enlarged view.

Comment

The preservation of the end plates suggests that the lesion originated within the vertebral body and is expanding outward. The vertebral collapse is due to a pathologic fracture. These radiographic features are really not specific for a particular diagnosis.

Note that if you examine the ventrodorsal view carefully you can identify the shortened segment.

Treatment of a lesion such as this, regardless of cause probably requires surgical removal of the tail and the diagnosis can be made at that time by histopathologic examination.

"Kim" was placed in this group because he had clinical signs that were suggestive of a cauda equina syndrome. Actually his lesion is in a caudal segment and should not be treated as a CES.

Case Description

"Baron" is an 8-year-old male shepherd with hind limb lameness for 3 months.

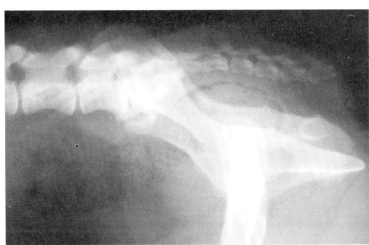

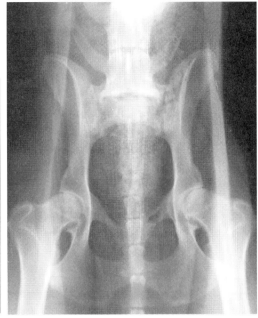

Radiographic Findings

The radiographs show a pattern of changes including:
1. collapse LS disc space
2. end plate sclerosis LS disc space
3. spondylosis deformans LS disc space
4. destruction of the cranial end plate of the sacrum
5. arthrosis of both hip joints secondary to hip dysplasia
6. prostatic enlargement
7. 4 sacral vertebrae

The radiographs do not show:
1. instability at LS disc
2. malalignment at LS disc
3. vertebral canal stenosis

"Baron's" radiographic features are unusual in that they consist of both destructive and productive patterns. Neither a congenital or developmental disease is suggested. The destructive changes in the end plates are best identified on the enlarged ventrodorsal view (arrows) and suggest chronic discospondylitis. However, the pattern of secondary changes suggest repair of an old disease and not an active inflammatory process at this time.

"Baron" is a typical older patient, with the summation of several lesions all of which may be contributing to the LS lesion at this time. "Baron" is thought to have a LS discospondylitis but the stage of activity is not evident from the radiographs.

Comments

Depending on the status of the patient you can learn more concerning the LS junction by performing:
1. a physical examination to determine if the LS junction has instability and is painful on motion
2. stress radiographs to record any LS instability
3. a contrast study to detect a lumbosacral vertebral canal mass

In addition, the status of the hips and stifle joints can be determined by performing:
1. palpation of the hip joints using care not to stress the LS junction
2. an anesthetic block of the hip joints to determine pain at that site
3. radiographs of the hips and stifle joints

"Baron" was released with a diagnosis of arthrosis secondary to hip dysplasia and possible CES requiring further workup. Another confusing patient.

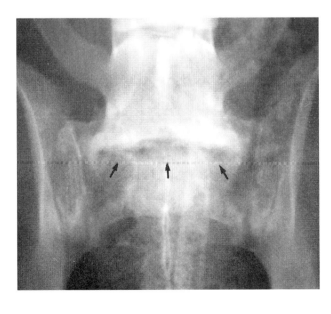

Case Description

"**Zeus**" is a 10-year-old male shepherd with history of lumbosacral pain that has been present for an unknown period of time.

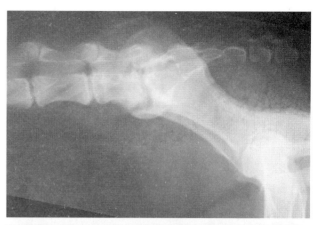

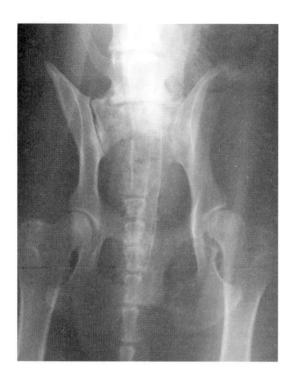

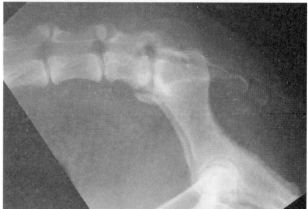

Radiographic Findings

The radiographs show a transititional LS segment with a malpositioned sacrum causing a lack of symmetry in the sacroiliac joints. Note the abbreviated transverse process from the transitional segment on the left. Marked sacral canal stenosis is present at the level of the transitional segment (lines). Disc degeneration with end plate sclerosis and secondary spondylosis deformans are also present.

Compare the two lateral views (below) made with "Zeus's" hind limbs in a neutral position and in flexion to see the degree of LS instability and the congenital vertebral canal stenosis.

Comments

"Zeus" has a commonly occurring LS transitional vertebra with resulting vertebral malalignment, LS instability, sacral canal stenosis causing cauda equina syndrome plus pelvic rotation that influences the manner in which the osteoarthrosis secondary to hip dysplasia has developed. It is more accurate to classify the stenotic lesion as a congenital/developmental lesion. Careful physical examination is required to determine what is causing the back pain.

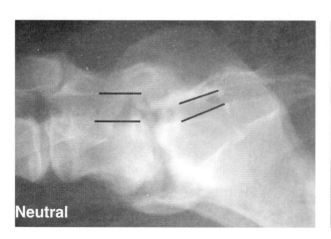

Neutral

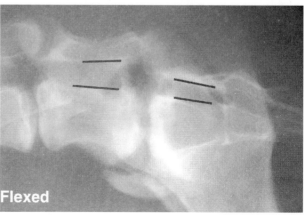

Flexed

Case Description

"Schwartz" is a 7-year-old male shepherd with a chronic history of fecal incontinence. There seems to be a loss of voluntary movement of the tail. A loss of tone of the anal sphincter is noted on neurological examination. Compare the lateral views made in flexion and extension.

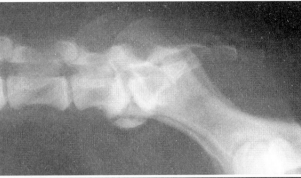

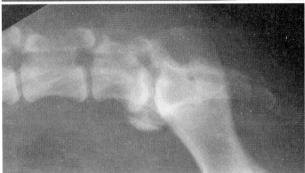

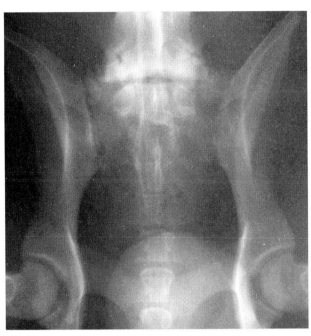

Radiographic Findings

Pelvic radiographs show a transitional LS segment with ventral displacement of the sacrum. LS spondylosis deformans and end plate sclerosis suggest chronicity. The LS vertebral canal stenosis is identified on the enlarged views (lines). Instability is proven on comparison of the extended and flexed views.

The diagnosis is a degenerated LS disc with vertebral malalignment, vertebral instability, and canal stenosis causing a cauda equina syndrome.

Comments

We assume that malalignment at the LS junction in the presence of a transitional LS segment is associated with the congenital lesion. Note the resulting separation of the articular facets at the LS junction. In addition, the attachment of the pelvis is at an oblique angle because of the transitional segment.

We can classify this cauda equina lesion as having a congenital etiology as long as we understand that the secondary changes contribute to the progression of the clinical signs.

In a patient with this type of lesion, surgery may need to accomplish decompression as well as achieve stabilization.

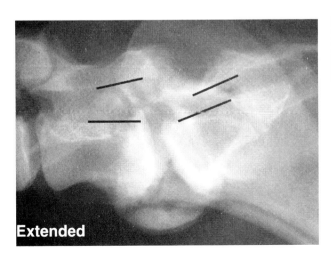

Extended

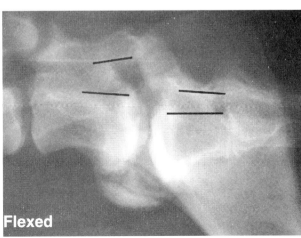

Flexed

General Comments

Note the similarity in radiographic appearance in "Baron", "Zeus", and "Schwartz". Note that all 3 are older shepherds with a chronic clinical history.

Examination of the end plates can show areas of destruction that suggest the possibility that a discospondylitis has been present earlier causing weakness, LS instability, and progression of the LS disease. It is also possible that the converse is true and discospondylitis can be secondary to chronic disc disease.

"Baron", "Zeus", or "Schwartz" can all have sacral osteochondrosis as a primary lesion causing LS instability with resulting secondary change that preclude the diagnosis of the primary lesion. Osteochondrosis of the sacrum is an inherited disease that occurs frequently in shepherds.

In many patients the etiology of the canal stenosis is specific and rather easy to determine. Primary stenosis is the result of a congenital malformation or a developmental disorder which creates a vertebral canal of less than normal dimensions (see outline on this page). Secondary or acquired stenosis implies that the vertebral canal developed normally, but then became narrowed because of an acquired disorder.

The most common type of spinal stenosis causing clinical problems in the dog is lumbosacral stenosis secondary to degenerative changes of the spine. These secondary changes can include disc protrusion into the vertebral canal, hypertrophy of the ligamentum flavum, hypertrophy of the joint capsules of the true vertebral joints, arthrosis of the true vertebral joints, and malalignment/instability at the lumbosacral disc space. The intervertebral foramina can become stenotic as well as the vertebral canal itself.

Classification of Primary Vertebral Canal Stenosis

1. Primary stenosis produced by the bony arch due to
   a. congenital stenosis at the site of
      1. congenital vertebral block
      2. congenital hemivertebra (wedge)
         a. with normal articular processes
         b. with hypotrophic articular processes
         c. with hyperplastic articular processes
      3. "butterfly" vertebrae
      4. transitional vertebral vertebrae
         a. with normal articular processes
         b. with hyperplastic articular processes
      5. primary kyphosis, lordosis, or scoliosis
   b. vertebral malalignment
      1. at the OAA region
      2. with cervical spondylopathy
      3. at the LS junction
   c. vertebral instability
      1. with congenital absence of dens
      2. with cervical spondylopathy
   d. idiopathic stenosis at T4-5 in the Doberman Pinscher
   e. intervertebral foraminal stenosis
   f. hyperplastic articular processes

2. Developmental stenosis due to inborn errors of skeletal growth
   a. achondroplasia
   b. hereditary multiple exostosis (multiple osteochondromatosis)
   c. Disseminated Idiopathic Skeletal Hyperostosis (DISH)
   d. mucopolysaccharidosis (VII)
   e. malalignment due to cervical osteochondrosis
   f. canal stenosis due to overnutrition
   g. osteochondrosis of
      1. cervical articular processes
      2. body of cervical vertebrae
      3. sacral body
   h. prenatal and perinatal malnutrition
3. Idiopathic stenosis
   a. with conjoining cord lesion (benign tumors)
   b. without conjoining cord lesion
4. Primary stenosis produced by the nonosseous components of the walls of the vertebral canal.
   a. periarticular cysts
   b. soft tissue developmental tumor (teratoma)

Transitional Lumbosacral Vertebral Anomaly in the Dog

At the junction of the major divisions of the spine, a single vertebra may assume characteristics typical of either division. With a lumbosacral transitional vertebra (LSTS), the dorsal laminae and transverse processes are affected to the greatest degree, with lesser alteration in the shape of the vertebral body. A unique feature of a LSTS is that a new disc space may be created between the normally fused first and second sacral vertebrae.

The presence of LSTS in dogs is common. First descriptions suggested that they were of little clinical importance, however, later they were described as a predisposing cause of cauda equina syndrome (CES) in German Shepherd Dogs (GSD) and were thought to be probably familiar in their occurrence. Recently LSTS was reported to be inherited in the Labrador retriever.

Radiographic features

On the lateral view, the anomaly is typically characterized by the separation of what normally are the first and second sacral vertebrae causing an apparent caudal shifting of the last lumbar vertebra or "lumbarization of the first sacral vertebra". The disc space between the last lumbar vertebra and the now-separated anomalous vertebra is usually well-defined and the end plates are usually of normal width and density.

The newly created disc space between the anomalous vertebra and the newly formed first sacral vertebra varies in width and can appear with partial fusion with only a narrow to slit-like disc space and thin vertebral end plate or may have a width more like that found in the lumbar spine. Malalignment and instability of either disc space are uncommon.

The height of the vertebral canal may narrow abruptly at the anomalous vertebra often to one-half of the height of the lumbar canal. Angulation of the floor of the vertebral canal at the junction of the last normal lumbar vertebra and the anomalous vertebra remains similar to that seen on the radiograph of the dog with a normal LS junction.

The junction of the last sacral and the first coccygeal vertebrae varies creating a sacrum characterized by: (1) 3 fused vertebrae indicating that what was the first coccygeal segment has now fused to the sacrum, (2) an intermediate pattern characterized by partial fusion of the last sacral and the first coccygeal vertebrae with a narrow to slit-like disc space and thin vertebral end plates, or (3) only 2 fused vertebrae indicating that the first coccygeal vertebra remains separated.

On the VD view, the most helpful radiographic finding is the separation of the fused spinous processes of the sacrum that are normally seen as three round to oblong connected radiodense shadows. With an anomalous LS vertebra, the most cranial of these shadows is separated and displaced cranially regardless of the number of vertebrae in the sacrum. The caudal two shadows remain connected or are joined by the shadow representing the spinous process of the first coccygeal vertebra dependent on whether the sacrum is formed by 2 or 3 fused vertebrae.

The appearance of the body and transverse processes of the anomalous vertebra on the VD view can be divided into patterns in which: (1) the lateral processes appear as symmetrical wings with a persistent ilial attachment bilaterally without pelvic angulation or rotation, (2) cranially directed transverse processes on both sides of the anomalous vertebra more similar to that seen normally on the lumbar vertebra with weakened sacroiliac joints, or (3) the transverse processes show marked asymmetry with one side characterized by a large wing-like process that fuses with the ilium and the other side characterized by a long, thin process similar to that of a transverse process of a lumbar vertebra with a weakened sacroiliac joint. The influence of the anomalous vertebra on the strength of the sacroiliac joints is thought to be important in the loss of the strength of the LS disc.

Many of the dogs with a transitional vertebra have concurrent hip dysplasia. If the pelvic attachment in these dogs caused angulation and/or pelvic rotation, an asymmetrical arthrosis results. The resulting degree of femoral head subluxation and secondary osteoarthrosis is greater in the hip in which the dorsal acetabular coverage is decreased.

Transitional vertebrae in the cat are frequent and have a similar appearance to what is seen in the dog, however, they rarely are associated with a clinical problem. This may be the result of the cat's small size or may relate to their physical activities.

"Hit By a Car"

Differences in culture determine the frequency of automobile accidents. Unfortunately many owners permit dogs to run without any restraint so both young and old dogs are affected. These patients may present immediately after the injury or may remain at home for some time before the owner brings the dog for treatment.

Case Description

"Rinty" is a 6-year-old female crossed-breed shepherd presented to your clinic by the police after a suspected motor accident. She presented with a distended abdomen and was ataxic and had hyper-reflexive patellas.

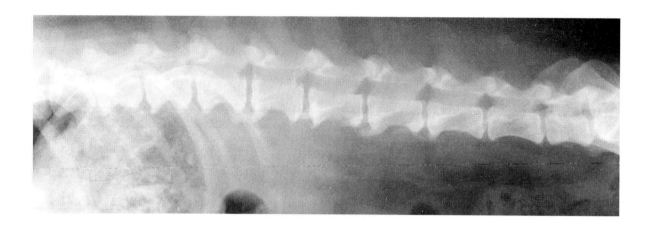

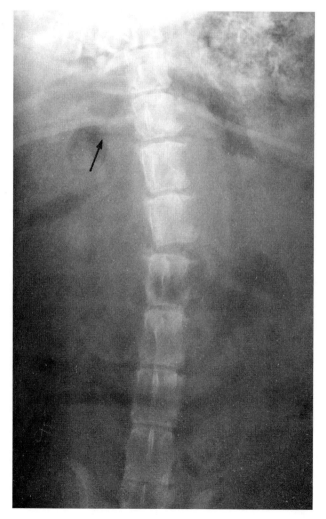

Radiographic Findings

The noncontrast radiographs show a fracture-luxation of L2-3 and a fracture of the right 13th rib (arrow). Remember that the extent of spinal injury often does not correspond with the neurological signs.

This case introduces a new concept, that of ambulatory paraparesis. Sometimes the patient is ambulatory immediately after injury, then becomes non-ambulatory later. This happens because the spine probably is unstable permitting additional injury to the spinal cord or hemorrhage is occurring within the vertebral canal and an extradural mass is increasing slowly.

Comments

It is interesting that the interarcuate space around the spinous processes is narrow at L3-4, but this is one segment caudal to the injury.

Question #1

Would you have found the injury if you had used lateral views only?

Case Description

"**Nanook**" is a 6-months-old female shepherd who was run over by a car. The dog was dyspneic with a low PCV. Both urination and defecation were normal. (Continue on the next page.)

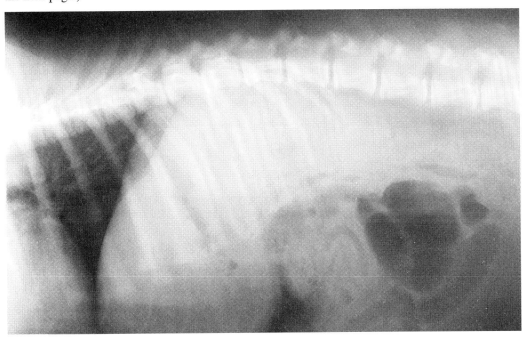

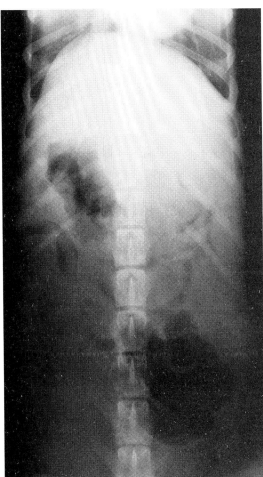

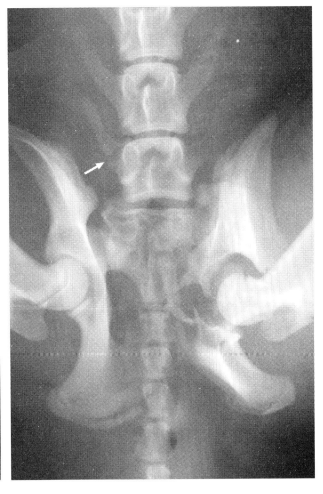

Radiographic Findings (at the time of injury)

The radiographs show a series of injuries including:

1. right sacroiliac separation
2. left acetabular fracture
3. left pubic fracture
4. left ischial fracture
5. fracture right transverse process on L7 (arrow)

Unfortunately we missed the more clinically important lesion. Take another look at the first study before you examine the study made 1 month later.

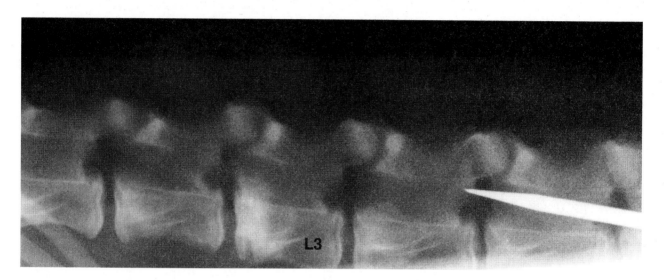

Radiographic Findings (one month later)

Radiographs made one month later (above) show callus forming around the cranial physeal fracture of the body of L3.

There is evidence of trauma supported by the owner and by the first radiographic study. The clinical signs seem to be more related to the pelvic injury. The follow-up radiographs were made to evaluate a continued hesitancy to walk normally.

Question #2

Can the IM pin really be within the vertebral canal as it appears on the lateral view?

Question #3

If the pin was positioned as a DeVita pin to stabilize the pelvic fractures, how did it move?

Question #4

What is the role of myelography in this patient 1 month after the trauma?

Case Description
"**Joaquin**" is a 7-year-old male Weimeraner who was hit by a car and had caudal paralysis.

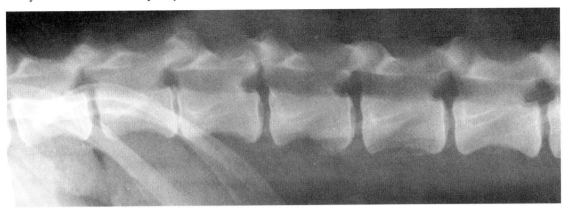

Radiographic Findings
The radiographs show an L1-2 spinal fracture-luxation. Detection of the rotational deformity on the VD view suggests the potential severity of the injury.

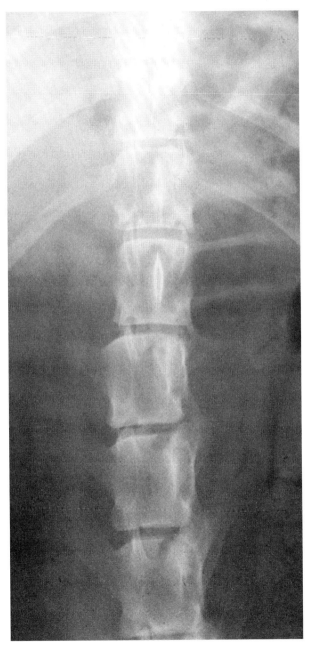

Comments
It is difficult to know the exact site of injury in a trauma case and impossible to know if a second or third lesion is present. For these reasons, a complete spinal series is often made in a trauma case using only lateral views. After evaluation of those radiographs, VD views of specific portions of the spine can be made. A second lesion can "hide" most easily at the cervicothoracic junction or within the thoracic region. However, any lesion can hide on the lateral view if the vertebral displacement is lateral. These patients require a complete physical and neurological examination as well.

Case Description

"**Randy**" is a 2-year-old female mixed breed with paraplegia and was radiographed following a motor accident. Upper motor neuron signs were noted in the pelvic limbs with an absence of deep pain perception in the pelvic limbs. A survey study was made using only lateral views.

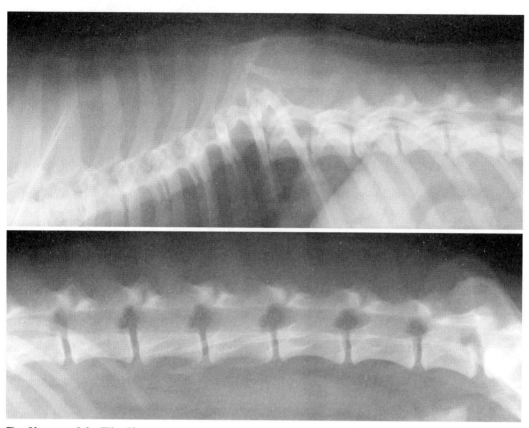

Radiographic Findings

Radiographs show a fracture-luxation at T8 with dorsal displacement of the body of T8 and fracture of the spinous processes of T7 and T8 (arrows). The changes are better identified on the enlarged view.

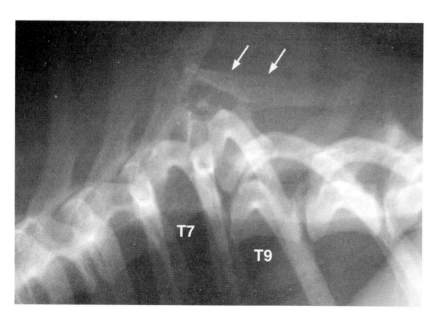

Comments

Gas filled loops of bowel were seen in the abdominal radiographs and suggested a paralytic ileus secondary to the trauma.

Because of the potential injury to the spinal cord and nerve roots, special attention needs be given to the trauma patient.

Question #5

What is the importance of the absence of deep pain perception in the pelvic limbs?

Answer #1

Probably not. "Rinty" presents a problem of having to risk VD positioning to obtain a second radiographic view or to try to obtain a complete evaluation from the lateral radiograph only. However, in this case use of the lateral view alone might have caused a false negative study of the lumbar spine.

Answer #2

No. It is within the soft tissues lateral to the spine. The second orthogonal view makes absolute localization possible.

Answer #3

Because of muscle action it is common for a linear foreign body to "move" within the soft tissues. A threaded pin moves rather quickly.

Answer #4

The myelogram isn't needed at this time to make the diagnosis but would provide additional information concerning the presence of cord compression. A good neurological examination may provide more information than the myelogram at this time.

Answer #5

The absence of deep pain sensation tell you of severe cord injury or possible cord transection. It is interesting that a "Schiff Sherrington" sign isn't present in this severe injury.

"Four Poodles with Cervical Pain"

These are four poodle dogs that have acute cervical pain. Examine the radiographs and see if you can identify the cause of the pain. The questions are answered following the case presentations.

Case Description

"CR" was an 11-year-old female poodle who was radiographed because of pain noted on palpation of her neck. She was suspected to have an esophageal foreign body.

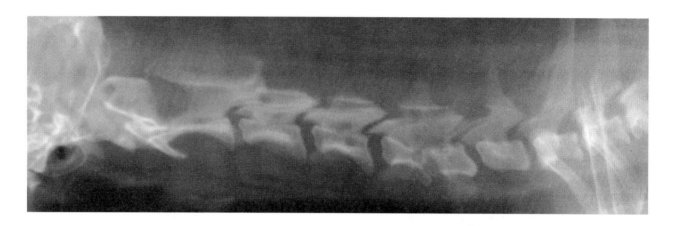

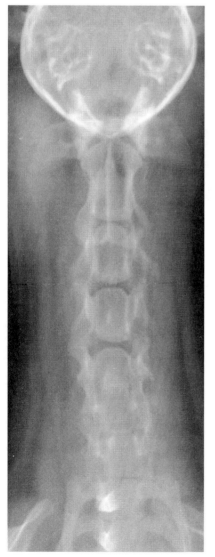

Radiographic Findings

The radiographs show a congenital block vertebrae at C5-6 with a single dorsal arch.

Comment

Congenital lesions need to be evaluated for the possibility of instability, malalignment, or vertebral canal stenosis any of which can lead to cord pressure. None of these were present, in fact, the canal at C5-6 appears to have an increase in height with the width of the canal appearing unchanged.

Block vertebrae usually do not cause clinical problems. Therefore, this dog's cervical pain can be investigated further with a cerebellomedullary CSF analysis. Myelography can follow if the results of CSF analysis are normal or non-diagnostic. Further questioning of the owner produced the information that "CR's" history included a soft tissue injury in the neck. Examination of the soft tissues revealed an infected lesion.

Block vertebrae may involve only the vertebral body or may involve the arch as well. Hemivertebrae are the most common congenital vertebral anomaly to cause spinal cord compression. Hemivertebrae occur most frequently in the screw-tailed breeds, and in the thoracic region, not the cervical region.

Question #1

Name two diseases that "CR" could have which could cause cervical pain and would not be evident on noncontrast cervical radiographs.

Case Description

"**Pepe**" is a 7-year-old male miniature poodle who had cervical pain for 2 months.

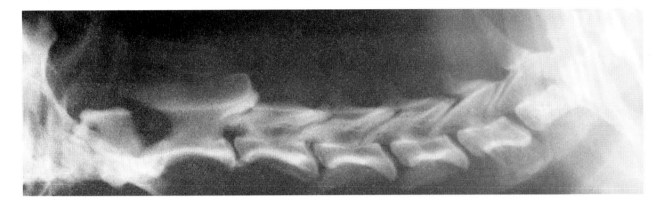

Radiographic Findings

The radiographic studies show the disc spaces at C2-3, C3-4, C5-6, and C6-7 are more narrow than expected. A calcified fragmented disc at C3-4 plus calcified tissue on the midline dorsal to C3-4 is supportive of a diagnosis of a calcified nuclear herniation that was proven at surgery. The herniated calcified C3-4 disc is seen on the midline on the VD view.

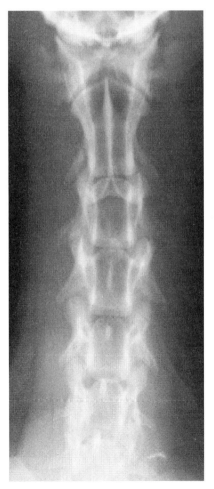

Comments

Identification of the roof of the cervical vertebral canal is relatively easy on the well positioned lateral radiograph. Note how the heads of the first ribs cover the C7-T1 disc space making evaluation of disc disease at this site difficult.

Case Description

"**Count**" is a 4-year-old male poodle who was attacked by a larger dog 1-week ago and is now showing cervical pain.

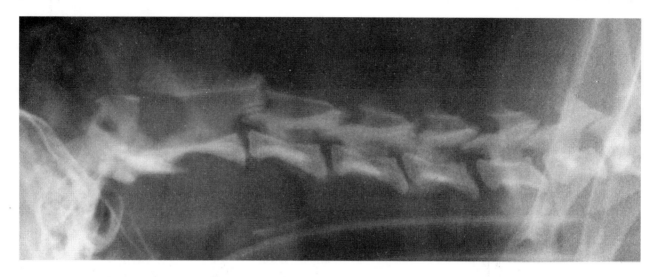

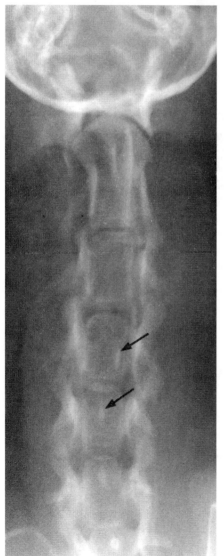

Radiographic Findings

The radiographs show collapse of C4-5 disc space with minimal dorsal displacement of C5 and a fracture of an articular process of C5. The displacement causes a break in the line identifying the roof of the vertebral canal. It is helpful in reaching your diagnosis to note the malalignment of the spinous processes on the VD view (arrows). The diagnosis is a fracture-luxation of C4-5.

Comments

The clinical history is important in this patient in reaching a diagnosis of trauma. The narrow disc space might mistakenly have been interpreted as an acute disc herniation. However, the fracture and the malalignment of the vertebrae are indicative of trauma.

Case Description

"**Monte**" is a 14-year-old male standard poodle with progressive cervical pain for 1 month that has become severe in the past few days. On physical examination, the prostate gland was enlarged.

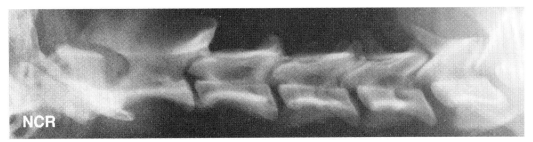

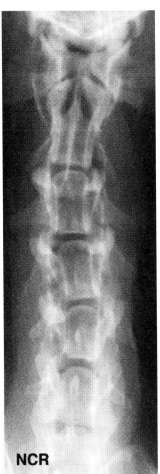

Radiographic Findings

Noncontrast radiographs of the cervical spine (above and to the left) show scoliosis with concavity to the left centering on C2-4 and concavity to the right centering on C4-5. The disc space at C2-3 is slightly narrow. The tentative diagnosis was a herniated C2-3 disc.

Question #2

What are the top 3 diseases on your list of differential diagnoses, in order of decreasing probability?

Question #3

Is the scoliosis an important radiographic finding?

Myelographic Findings

The myelogram (below and to the right) shows a large left-sided extradural mass at C4-5 with a shifting of the cord to the right resulting in collapse of the subarachnoid columns (black arrows). The mass causes a shifting of the spinal cord causing a narrowing of both the dorsal and ventral subarachnoid space (white arrow). The mass was removed at surgery and was surprisingly reported to be a hemangiosarcoma. Note the small dorsally protrusion of the C2-3 disc.

Question #4.

What are your top 3 differentials after performing the myelogram in "Monte", in order of decreasing probability?

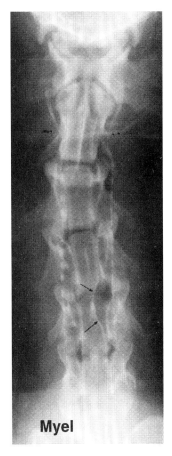

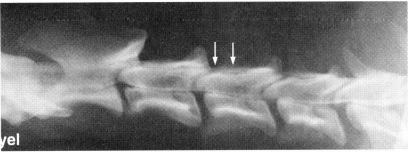

Question #5

If not already done as part of the minimum data base collection, what additional radiographic study should be done at this point?

Question #6

Why should spinal radiography and myelography include the entire spinal column?

Comments

Mass lesions of this type that center on an intervertebral foramina and are laterally located are often nerve sheath tumors.

The absence of any positive radiographic signs of disc disease and the location of the lesion (lateral rather than ventral or ventrolateral) should make you suspicious that the mass is something other than herniated disc material.

Bony change is difficult to see on these noncontrast studies; however, the mass has expanded laterally causing an expansion of the vertebral canal visible on the VD view of the myelogram causing an "opening" of the intervertebral foramina.

The value of the VD view is appreciated on this case. Additional shadows seen on the VD view are not always helpful and include the curvilinear shadow cast by the pedicles and the segmented shadows cast by the tracheal rings. If an endotracheal tube is position, this creates additional shadows. All of these confuse the interpretation of the linear shadows casts by the contrast columns in the myelogram.

Answer #1

Granulomatous meningoencephalomyelitis and steroid-responsive meningitis

Answer #2

Granulomatous meningoencephalomyelitis, steroid-responsive meningitis, meningeal or nerve root neoplasia, and Type II disc protrusion.

Answer #3

Scoliosis is an abnormal lateral curvature of the spine with concavity directed to one side or the other. It is tempting to use a scoliosis to indicate a site of muscle spasm due to irritation secondary to a spinal lesion. In "Monte", the scoliosis, with left-sided convexity, is at the tumor site and may be the result of loss of muscle tone (lower motor neuron sign) in the muscles innervated by the spinal cord segments and nerve roots affected by the mass.

Answer #4

Neoplasia, herniated disc, or granuloma.

Answer #5

Because the mass is likely to be neoplastic, thoracic radiographs should be made to look for metastatic lung lesions. The thoracic studies in this patient showed multiple pulmonary nodules.

Answer #6

There are 2 reasons the entire spinal column should be examined. First, some spinal diseases are commonly multifocal, e.g., intervertebral disc disease, infectious inflammatory diseases, and trauma. Secondly, the clinical signs caused by a spinal lesion may be "hidden" or masked by the signs of an additional spinal lesion. For example, if a dog has two lesions compressing the spinal cord, one at C3-4 and another at T13-L1, upper motor neurons signs caused by the TL lesion could be masked by upper motor neuron signs caused by the cervical lesion.

Cervical Pain Due to Spinal Column or Neural Disease

Cervical pain may be the result of disease of any of the tissues or structures in the neck region. These tissues and structures include all the extraspinal soft tissues (e.g., muscles, connective tissue, esophagus, lymph nodes, peripheral nerves), as well as the components of the spinal column and the intraspinal neural tissues. The classic neural sources of pain are disease of the meninges (meningopathy) and disease of the nerve roots (radiculopathy). The spinal cord itself does not have pain receptors.

Cervical pain with a neural cause may also be associated with diseases that are not localized in the neck. Two common examples of this phenomenon are cervical pain associated with brain disease (generally neoplasia or inflammation) and cervical pain accompanying cranial thoracic spinal disease such as trauma or neoplasia.

Differential diagnoses for cervical pain

1. Degenerative disease
   a. intervertebral disc disease
2. Congenital anomalies
   a. cervical spondylopathy
   b. deformities of the dens resulting in atlanto-axial luxation or meningeal/nerve root irritation
3. Metabolic disease
   a. hypervitaminosis A
   b. pathologic fracture secondary to metabolic bone disease
4. Neoplasia
   a. bone
   b. cartilage
   c. meningeal
   d. nerve root
   e. extraspinal soft tissue neoplasia invading spinal tissues
5. Inflammation - Infectious
   a. bacterial infection
   b. fungal infection
   c. protozoal infection
   d. rickettsial infection
   e. viral infection
6. Inflammation - Noninfectious
   a. aseptic meningitis (e.g., after myelography or subarachnoid hemorrhage)
   b. granulomatous meningoencephalomyelitis
   c. meningeal and/or nerve root inflammation caused by herniated disc material
   d. polyarthritis
   e. steroid-responsive meningitis
   f. vasculitis and meningitis, a.k.a. canine pain syndrome
7. Trauma
   a. brachial plexus/nerve root trauma
   b. spinal fracture-luxation
   c. traumatic disc protrusion

Diagnostic plan for cervical pain.

1. VD and lateral, noncontrast radiographs of the entire spinal column, taken with the dog under general anesthesia. The signalment, history, or findings on the cervical noncontrast studies may suggest positional films. For example, a 6-month-old Maltese should have oblique lateral films of the atlanto-axial joint to ascertain the presence and shape of the dens.
2. Analysis of cerebrospinal fluid aspirated from the cerebellomedullary cistern. This procedure should be done if the noncontrast films are not diagnostic, and always before a myelogram is performed. Dogs with Type II disc protrusion, steroid responsive meningitis, granulomatous meningoencephalomyelitis, or cervical neoplasia may all have the same clinical signs, including the same neurologic abnormalities. Cerebellomedullary cistern CSF is preferred to lumbar subarachnoid space CSF because CSF closest to the lesion may reflect the disease process more accurately.
3. Myelography of the entire spinal subarachnoid space.
4. CT or MRI may be of value to clarify radiographic abnormalities identified on the noncontrast studies or myelogram.

"Big Dogs with a Big Pain in the Neck"

A group of dogs with cervical pain are presented for your consideration. Noncontrast studies are offered for your evaluation. Myelograms are included for some of the patients. What do you think is the cause of the cervical pain in each dog?

Case Description

"**Freckles**" is a 9-year-old female Dalmatian with neck pain and a stiff gait. She has pain on flexion of her neck.

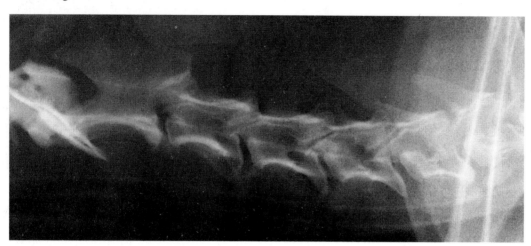

Radiographic Findings

The radiographs show narrowing of the C4-5 disc and a calcified mass in the vertebral canal dorsal to the C4-5 space. The diagnosis is a calcified herniated cervical disc.

Comments

Although nonchondrodystrophic dogs typically do not calcify the intervertebral discs, calcified discs may be seen, particularly in Doberman Pinschers.

Note the mineralized clavicular bones on the VD view.

Question #1

As the spinal cord itself does not have pain receptors, what might be the source of "Freckles" pain?

Case Description

"**Skippy**" is a 7-year-old male cocker spaniel with neck pain especially when the head is elevated.

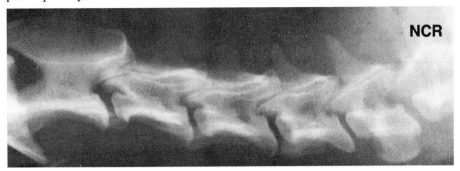

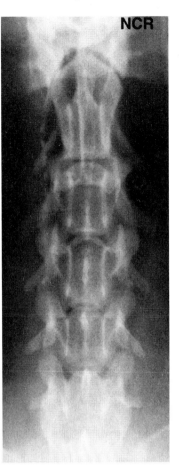

Radiographic Findings

The radiographic findings include narrowing of the C3-6 disc spaces with no calcified tissue within the discs and no spondylosis deformans or end plate sclerosis. The noncontrast study (above and to the right) does not identify the lesion site.

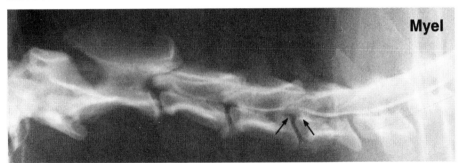

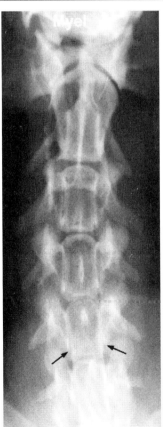

Myelographic Findings

The myelographic findings include a ventral extradural mass (arrows), most likely a C4-5 Type II disc protrusion, causing dorsal elevation of the spinal cord and compression of the subarachnoid spaces. The contrast columns on the VD view terminate at C5 (arrows) and it is not possible to determine laterality of the mass.

Comments

Dorsal extension of the head increased the amount of disc protrusion and exaggerated the extent of the spinal cord compression explaining why "Skippy" did not like to elevate his head.

Tension placed on the head during the lateral views caused a widening of the width of the cervical disc spaces as the disc protrusion was reduced.

The ventral decompression surgical procedure is the preferred method for removing protruded cervical disc material that is located immediately dorsal to the intervertebral disc (the most common location). The disadvantage of the procedure is the potential for hemorrhage from the adjacent internal vertebral venous plexus, and the inability to remove laterally located disc material.

Case Description

"Soirée" is a 1-year-old male Doberman Pinscher with acute cervical pain. The tentative diagnosis based on physical and neurological examination is a cervical fracture-luxation.

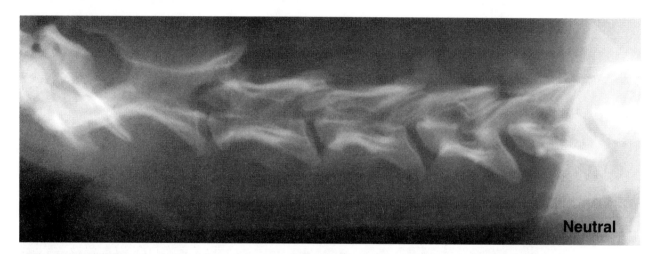

Neutral

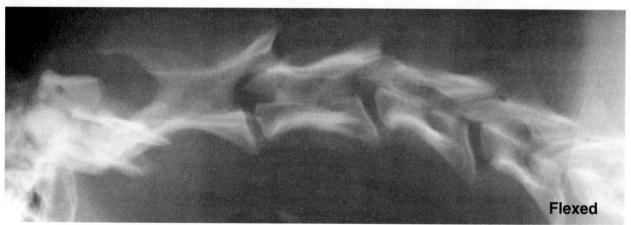

Flexed

Radiographic Findings

The noncontrast radiographs made in a neutral position shows marked subluxation of C2-3. On a radiograph made in ventral flexion of the head, the instability shifts to C3-4. The diagnosis is cervical spondylopathy.

Comments

The instability resulting in the cervical subluxation seen in "Soirée" is a part of the developmental syndrome, called cervical spondylopathy, seen in the cervical spine of many Doberman Pinschers. It is interesting that the cervical instability as seen on the radiograph varies in location depending on positioning of the head.

The subluxation and subsequent excessive motion of the cervical vertebrae probably stretch and compress the adjacent meninges and nerve roots, producing the pain and resistance to flexion of the neck seen in the dog.

Note the dense scars in the vertebral bodies that are the result of closure of the growth plates that separate the vertebral end plates.

"Soirée" was treated successfully by fusion at C3-4. Two years later, he had recurrent cervical pain and was diagnosed as having a C6-7 subluxation. This was treated by an extension of the fusion from C3 through C7 by use of a ventrally placed bone graft. Later, he ran into a fence and was diagnosed with malalignment of C2-3. "Soirée" remained painful throughout the remainder of his life. He is an example of the "domino" effect seen following vertebral fusion.

Case Description

"**Tuff**" is a 10-year-old female mixed breed dog with cervical pain and quadriparesis that has been present for 1 month.

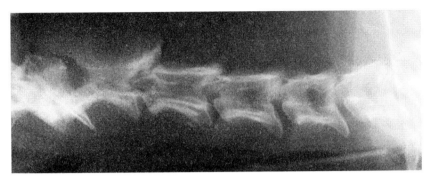

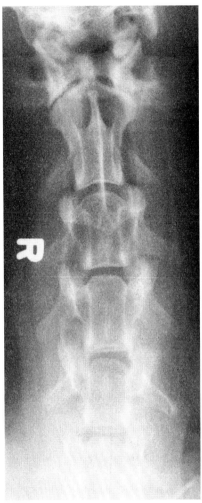

Radiographic Findings

The noncontrast cervical radiographs show a well-marginated destructive pattern within the arch of C1. The diagnosis is most likely a malignant primary bone tumor. A hemangiosarcoma was diagnosed at biopsy. The lesion is better seen in the detail view (arrow).

Comments

The pattern of destruction is referred to as a geographic pattern suggesting a rather slow expansion of the tumor. Note the break in the cortex which supports a diagnosis of malignant tumor (arrow). The lesion in the dorsal arch is not identified on the VD view.

A second set of radiographs was made 4 months after the first set and showed a progressive nature of the lesion.

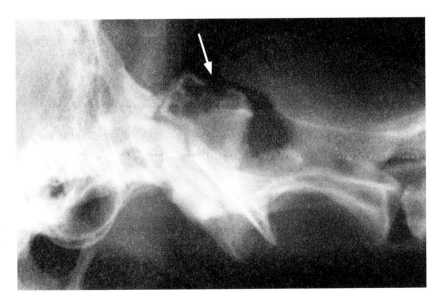

Answer #1

"Skippy's" pain may be due to stretching of the meninges and nerve roots by the mass of herniated disc material. Pain receptor fibers have also been identified within intervertebral discs and the process of disc degeneration and collapse may stimulate these fibers resulting in pain.

"Small Dogs with a Big Pain in the Neck"

A group of four dogs with cervical pain are presented. Only noncontrast studies were made.

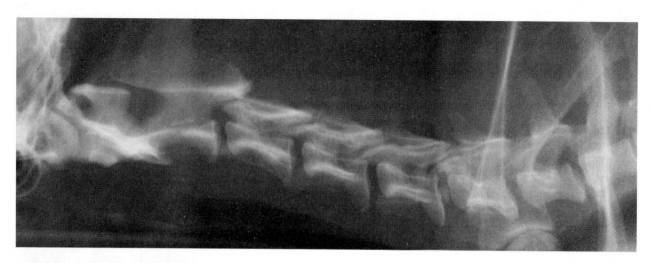

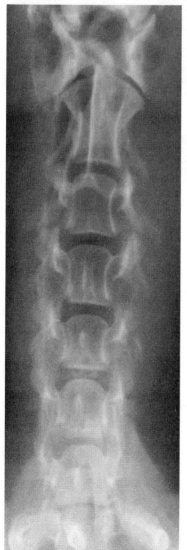

Case Description

"**Little Red**" is a 5-year-old male dachshund who had cervical pain for 1 week.

Radiographic Findings

The radiographs show a calcified disc at C5-6 with a trail of calcified tissue that leads dorsally into a calcified mass in the vertebral canal. The calcified nuclear tissue is seen on both views to have spread cranially and caudally to the affected disc space. The diagnosis is a Type 1 calcified herniated disc.

Case Description

"**Tina**" is a 6-year-old female toy fox terrier with a 2-day history of screaming in pain when jumping off objects. She is reluctant to move her head, preferring to keep her neck rigid. She had an episode of neck pain 16 months ago, which was diagnosed as caused by cervical disc herniation. A ventral decompression at C2-3 and fenestration of the C3-4, C4-5, and C5-6 discs was performed and her pain resolved until 2 days ago.

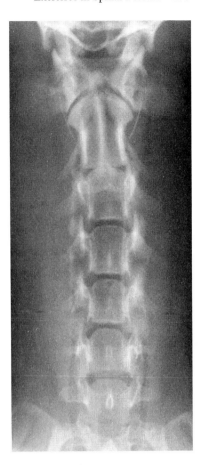

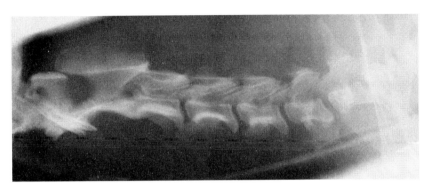

Radiographic Findings (today's studies)

Radiographs made today show a fusion of the vertebral bodies of C2-3 subsequent to the ventral decompression. No evidence of an active process is evident at that site. No cause for the current cervical pain was found.

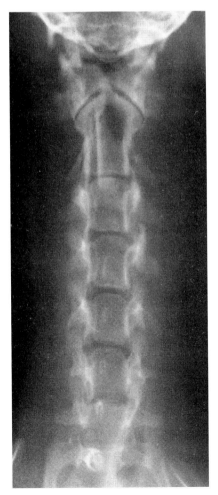

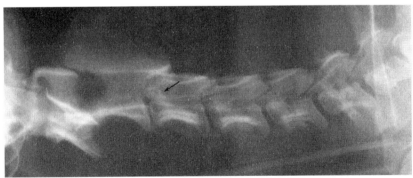

Radiographic Findings (16 months ago)

The earlier radiographs that were made 16 months ago were evaluated and showed the calcified herniated disc at C2-3 (arrow). Postoperative radiographs were made immediately after surgery and demonstrated the slot that was cut at C2-3 with the removal of most of the calcified disc material.

Comment

The final diagnosis on today's radiographs is a bony fusion of C2-3 following a ventral decompression performed 16 months earlier. Based solely on the radiographic appearance today, the differential diagnosis for the C2-3 vertebral abnormality would include a congenital block vertebra.

"Tina" was noted to favor her right pelvic limb at the time of the later admission. She had radiographic signs of an arthrosis in the right stifle joint that were thought to explain her resistance in jumping recently noticed by the owner.

Case Description

"**Butterfly**" is a 12-months-old female Shih Tzu with periodic bouts of cervical pain since she was 4 months of age. She is hyperesthetic in the cranial cervical region.

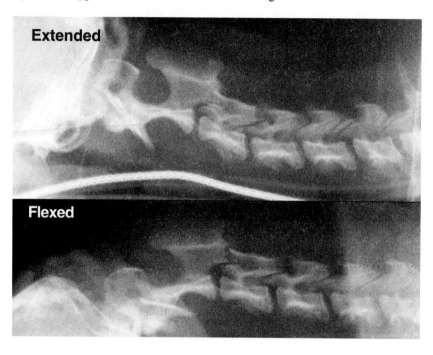

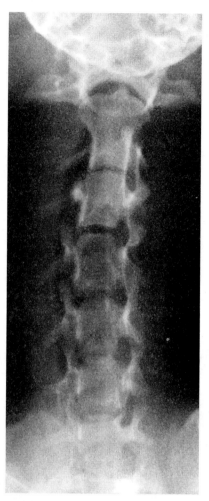

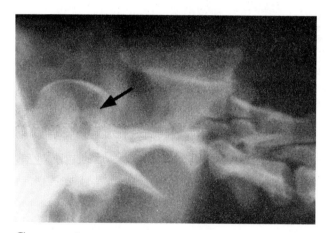

Radiographic Findings

The radiographs show a probable atlanto-axial instability with the odontoid process angled dorsally causing it to project into the vertebral canal (arrow). This malposition is accentuated by flexion of the head. The diagnosis is a congenital malformation of the odontoid process causing spinal cord compression.

Comments

Dorsal angulation of the odontoid process is an uncommon malformation. Hypoplasia or aplasia is more common. Odontoid process malformations are often associated with complex malformations of the atlas, axis and occipital bone, particularly in toy breed dogs (e.g., toy poodle or Maltese).

Cases of atlanto-axial congenital anomaly often require stress views and rotational views in addition to conventional views to permit visualization of the odontoid process. Unfortunately, the atlanto-axial joint is often unstable in these dogs; therefore, positioning the dog for these views carries substantial risk for additional compression and trauma to the spinal cord.

The most efficacious treatment for the malformed odontoid process is an odontoidectomy via a ventral approach and stabilization of the atlanto-axial joint with Steinman pins or K wires embedded in polymethylmethacrylate.

Note how "Butterfly" is badly positioned causing the VD view to be obliqued with the spinous process of C2 incorrectly appearing to cause a bony fusion on the left side of C2-3.

Case Description

"**Holly**" is a 4-year-old female dachshund with recurrent cervical pain. She has been to the clinic repeatedly with the same complaint. Radiographs were made at the time of the initial episode, and again 7 months later when the cervical pain recurred.

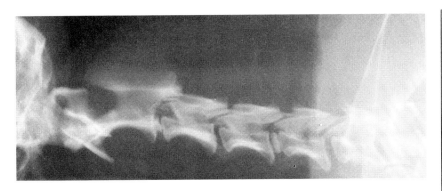

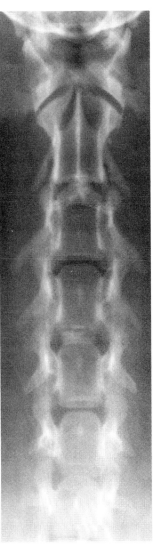

Radiographic Findings (initial study)

The initial radiographs show a calcified herniated disc at C2-3 and another calcified nucleus at C4-5 that appears to be contained within the center of the disc. "Holly" was treated with a ventral decompression at C2-3 and fenestration of the remaining cervical discs.

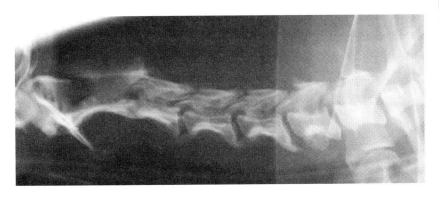

Radiographic Findings (7 months later)

The cervical radiographs made 7 months post-operatively demonstrate a postsurgical ankylosis at C2-3. Vertebral osteophytes have formed at C4-5 and C5-6 secondary to the fenestration. The cause of "Holly's" cervical pain is not evident on the radiographic studies.

Comments

This case shows the value of a complete physical examination and the error in assuming the original cause of the neck pain might be associated with the cause of the clinical signs today.

Question #1

What are your differential diagnoses for the cause of "Holly's" current pain?

Answer #1

Meningeal irritation/inflammation, meningeal or nerve root neoplasia, and herniated intervertebral disc. A discospondylitis at the site of the ventral decompression could be added to the list.

Congenital Occipito-atlanto-axial Lesions in the Dog

Congenital occipito-atlanto-axial lesions may present in several ways. They may be characterized by an occipital bone that has hypoplastic occipital condyles, an enlarged foramen magnum that is "key hole" shaped, and a shortened hypoplastic axis. The thickness of the cortex of the occipital bone is reduced as seen on the lateral view. In other dogs, the occipital condyles may be fused with the atlas creating rigidity. In others the odontoid process is malformed, hypoplastic, or missing resulting in instability between the vertebrae.

Atlanto-axial developmental lesions cause an instability of the atlanto-axial joint that allows excessive flexion of the joint. During this excessive flexion, the dens moves dorsally into the vertebral canal and compresses the spinal cord. The odontoid process of the axis may be normal in size and shape, be attached so as to protrude into the vertebral canal, or be hypoplastic or aplastic. In addition, the first cervical segment is often shortened and hypoplastic in appearance. Atlanto-axial subluxation is usually due to a congenital lesion but it can be the result of trauma.

This group of congenital occipito-atlanto-axial lesions occur primarily in toy and miniature breeds and the most common lesion causes instability and is due to agenesis or hypoplasia of the dens or to nonunion of the dens with the axis. Typically, the clinical signs appear during the first year of life and they may develop acutely or slowly over several months; they may even be intermittent. The signs vary from cervical pain and rigidity to complete, irreversible, upper motor neuron quadriplegia. Occasionally, a dog with this congenital lesion shows no clinical signs until sometime during adult life when an abnormal stress occurs, perhaps a trauma that would be insignificant to a normal dog, and subluxation occurs with unexpected clinical consequences.

Radiographic features of instability are noted on lateral views taken with the dog's head in slight flexion. The open mouth view of the skull may show agenesis, nonunion, or fracture of the dens and shows the nature of the foramen magnum. A lateral view of the cervical spine with the head slightly obliqued creates a window between the shadows cast by the lateral processes of the atlas and enables the odontoid process to be clearly identified.

Radiographic features of occipito-atlanto-axial lesions

1. Occipito-atlantal region
   a. fusion of atlanto-occipital joint
   b. large foramen magnum
   c. hypoplastic occipital condyles
   d. hypoplastic occipital bone
   e. shortened hypoplastic atlas
2. Atlanto-axial region
   a. ununited ossified odontoid process
   b. fractured ossified odontoid process
   c. nonvisualized odontoid process (agenesis/ cartilaginous)
   d. atlanto-axial instability
   e. tearing of atlanto-axial ligament
   f. hypoplastic atlas

Sacral Osteochondrosis

The pathophysiology of osteochondrosis of the sacrum is similar in appearance to osteochondrosis lesions found throughout the body except that this lesion is in a joint characterized by an intervertebral disc instead of a true joint and by the time it is identified it has assumed the form of an osteochondritis dessicans. It is comparable to the irregular cartilage proliferation including degenerative changes and fissure formation noted in osteochondrosis in other sites. Cartilage retention is followed by necrosis in the deepest layers of the lesion. The lesions vary from the more commonly noted osteochondrosis in that the resulting displaced cartilage mass originating from the sacrum has a bony center. The resulting injury to the end plate leads to a faulty attachment of the dorsal anular fibers and increased mechanical stress on the LS intervertebral disc precipitating disc degeneration. Rupture of the disc in the area of the end plate defect leads to protrusion of disc material between the detached fragment and the sacrum. Eventually ventral slippage of the sacrum occurs because of the weakened anular tissue. Thus, the osteochondrosis lesion predisposes LS disc degeneration and this, plus the resulting malalignment of the sacrum, leads to canal stenosis and becomes a common cause for cauda equina syndrome. Radiographically it resembles an avulsion fracture from the dorsocranial corner of the sacrum, however, histologically, the resulting cartilaginous mass found on the floor of the vertebral canal originates from disturbed endochondral ossification in the dorsal part of the growth cartilage of the sacral end plate.

The radiographic diagnosis is based on the detection of the osteochondral fragment that originates from the dorsal lip of the sacrum on lateral and ventrodorsal survey radiographs with the resulting osseous fragment(s) lying free on the floor of the vertebral canal. Usually the surrounding bone that forms the fragment bed has become sclerotic. In the more chronic lesion, a bony lip suggests that the previously free chondral fragment has reattached to the sacral lip. Changes at the LS disc are secondary to the resulting instability and include early disc space narrowing, end plate sclerosis, minimal spondylosis deformans, and secondary change involving the dorsal articular processes. However, detection of a mass on the floor of the vertebral canal at this site does not permit distinguishing between disc degeneration caused by an osteochondrosis lesion and an uncomplicated disc disease. Epidurography or discography may be helpful in determining the extent of nuclear degeneration and the nature of the resulting epidural mass.

Sacral OCD can cause spinal stenosis in two ways. First, the disc degeneration may permit sacral displacement and second, the osseous fragment or the lip of new bone or dorsal protrusion of the LS annulus may create an epidural mass.

Genetic predisposition is suggested by the unusually high frequency within the German Shepherd Dog breed as well as finding affected littermates where it causes clinical signs in males at a ratio of 4.5 :1. The condition can be present without clinical signs.

Two Puppies with Soft Tissue Masses in the Neck

These puppies both have soft tissues masses in the neck that were detected at the time of grooming. They were hard and adherent to the underlying structures, were not painful on palpation, and caused the puppies minimal discomfort. The owners were highly concerned about the lesions.

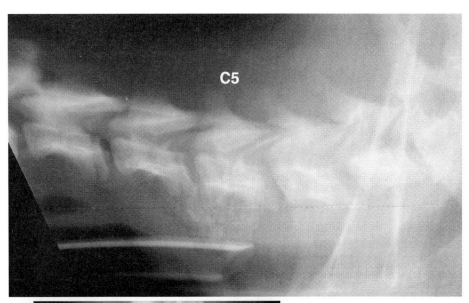

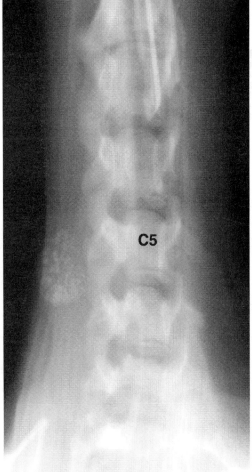

Case Description

"Cheer" is a 4-months-old female English setter with a cervical mass that appeared to attach to C5 on the right side. The owner thought that she had "neck pain".

Radiographic Findings

The radiographs clearly identify the well marginated lesion to contain multiple flocculated densities typical of calcified tissue. It was contained within the perivertebral soft tissues and not attached to a vertebra. The histological characteristics were typical of a granulomatous reaction.

Case Description
"**Deb**" is a 6-month-old male German Shepherd Dog with bilateral swellings noted on the neck at the region of C5. He was ataxic and had cervical stiffness.

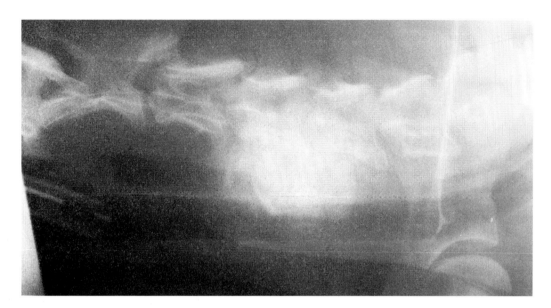

Radiographic Findings
The radiographs showed the lesions to be bilateral and with a pattern typical of calcified tissue. They did not attach to the adjacent vertebrae. The lesions were removed surgically and were noted to be firm, multilobular, with evidence of calcification in pockets containing "pus".

Comments
These soft tissue mineralized masses may be associated with von Willebrand's disease which is a disorder that is due to a deficiency or abnormality of a plasma factor that is required for the stabilization of Factor VIII in the circulation for the normal adherence of platelets to sites of vascular injury. The absence of this factor may be associated with a severe hemorrhagic disorder or an asymptomatic condition that is only a laboratory curiosity. In many patients, the hemorrhagic tendency usually becomes evident only with trauma, surgery, or dental extractions. It is thought with the trauma of puppies playing or with the trauma of intramuscular injections that the bleeding occurs. Later the resulting lesion heals with mineralization. The lesions usually have multiple foci that appear as calcified tissue and are frequently noted in the cervical region and adjacent to the hip joints.

While both of these dogs were thought to have cervical pain, the lesions are not associated with the cervical spine.

Hemiplegia or paraplegia has been reported to be associated with heterotrophic bone formation occurring near the hip joints and pelvis.

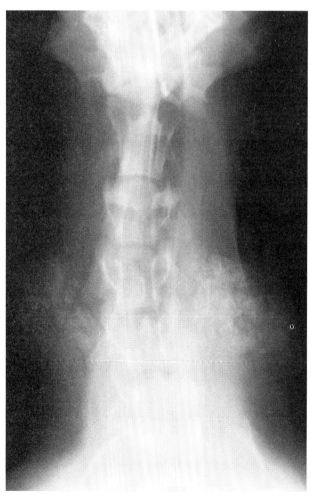

Hind Limb Lameness

Case Description

"**Murphy**" is a 2-year-old male mixed-breed shepherd with a 6-week history of right hind limb lameness. No neurological deficits are present. Pain is elicited on extension of the right hip joint.

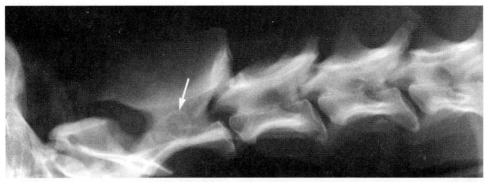

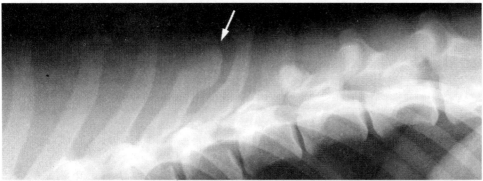

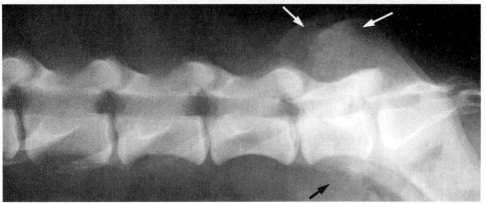

Radiographic Findings

Several focal, expansile, smoothly marginated lesions arise from the arches of C2 and C4 (arrows), the thoracic spinous processes (arrows), and the lumbar transverse processes (arrows). A mixed productive/destructive lesion is present at the lumbosacral region on the right and is seen on both VD and lateral views of the pelvis (arrows). The productive element originates at the sacroiliac joint while the destructive element involves the transverse process of L7.

This pattern, plus the soft tissue mineralization, suggests a malignant process, probably a primary bone tumor in contrast to the focal, expansile lesions with intact cortical borders that are benign in appearance. The radiographic diagnosis is multiple osteochondromatosis with malignant transformation of the lesion at the LS region. Most malignant transformations are interpreted histologically as chondrosarcomas.

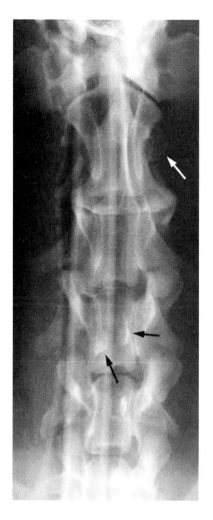
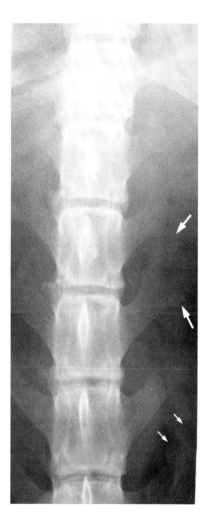
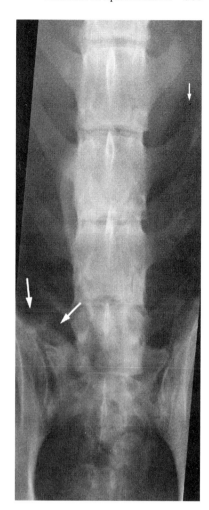

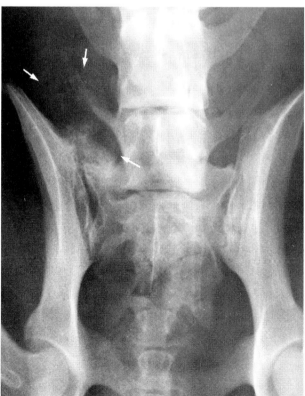

Comments

The pathology report of the biopsy specimen was a chondrosarcoma supporting the radiographic diagnosis

The detection of the multiple, benign-appearing, bony lesions is of value in this dog in reaching the diagnosis. Multiple osteochondromatosis is of clinical importance in two situations, one when the benign lesions encroach on the spinal cord causing a transverse myelopathy. The other situation is when a lesion undergoes malignant transformation as in "Murphy".

"Joshua"

Case Description

"Joshua" is a 9-year-old male Dalmatian with a 3-year history of LS pain and cauda equina deficits with pelvic limb paresis. He also has caudal thoracic pain, perhaps indicating a TL myelopathy which could contribute to the paresis. In addition, he has had abdominal surgery at 3 different times for removal of cystic calculi, and currently has renal calcification, somewhat confusing the evaluation of the LS pain.

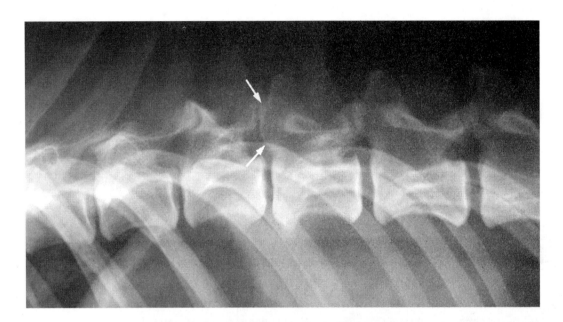

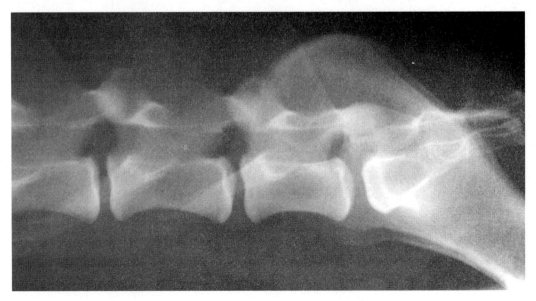

Noncontrast Radiographic Findings

Malformed articular processes with secondary degenerative changes are present at T11-L1. The interposed intervertebral foramina have an abnormal contour suggesting malformation of the laminae as well. In addition, the disc space at T11-12 is narrowed with spondylosis deformans.

No radiographic changes are detected at the LS junction.

In order to assess the effect of the TL developmental anomalies on the spinal cord, myelography was done. Studies of the LS region were scheduled as well because of the clinical signs.

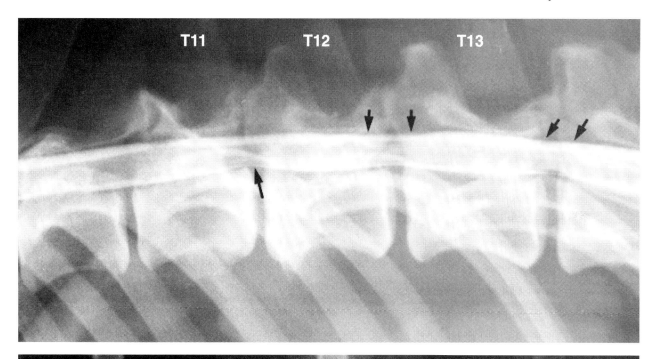

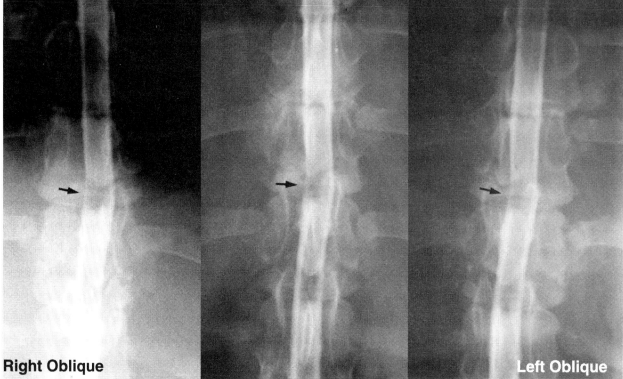

Right Oblique

Left Oblique

Myelographic Findings

Thinning of the ventral contrast column is seen at T11-12 (arrow), T12-13, and T13-L1. A more prominent ventral displacement of the dorsal contrast column is seen at T12-13 and T13-L1 (arrows). A prominent shift of the spinal cord to the left (arrows) at T11-T12 is associated with thinning of the contrast column on the right.

See next page

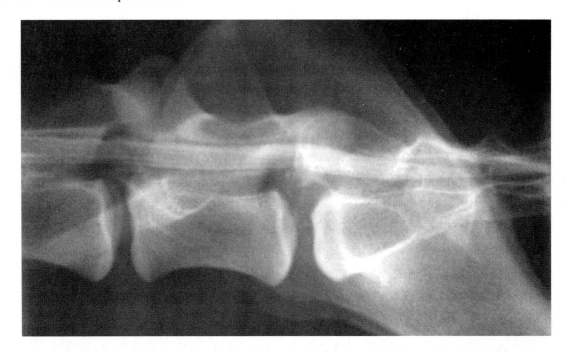

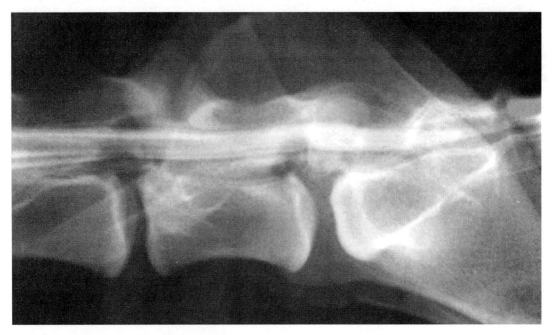

LS Myelodiscographic Findings

The myelogram shows slight dorsal deviation of the conus medullaris at L7-S1. Because of this finding, a discogram and epidurogram were performed. Only a small amount of contrast agent could be injected directly into the LS disc but this appeared to concentrate more dorsally than expected (2 views shown).

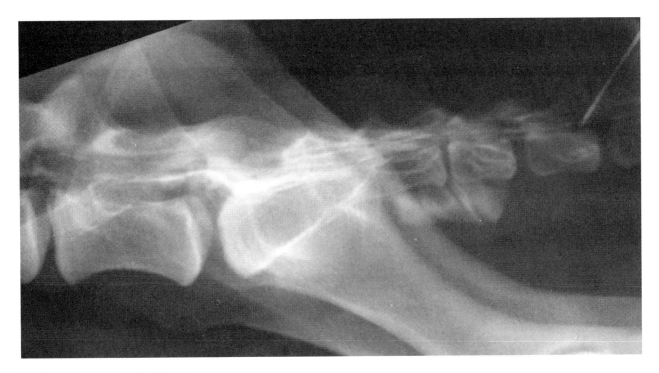

LS Epidurographic Findings

The epidurographic study more clearly shows the discal protrusion causing dorsal displacement of the contrast agent. Compression of the conus medullaris was best seen on the extended projection while the degree of compression was reduced on flexion. Note the spinal needle in position in a caudal vertebra for the epidurogram. A small amount of contrast agent leaked from the vertebral canal ventral to the sacrocaudal junction.

Comments

The malformation of the articular processes from T11-L1 causes a laterally located extradural mass. A prominent joint capsule and ligamentum flavum may contribute in part to the mass effect. The protruding LS disc is a potential cause of the lumbosacral pain.

This is a patient with two definite lesions, one probably developmental and one degenerative. Neither caused the dog sufficient clinical signs for the owner to request treatment.

"Abby"

Case Description

"Abby" is a 10-year-old female Pug with ataxia that began in the right pelvic limb 5 months ago, and has progressed to involve other limbs. The owners think she is slow in going up the stairs. They feel that she is uncomfortable but not painful. The physical examination was as expected for a dog of this age.

The neurologic examination showed ataxia and proprioceptive deficits in all 4 limbs. The spinal reflexes were normal. The conclusion was a C1-5 myelopathy (UMN signs in all 4 limbs).

Thoracic Radiographic Findings

Radiographs are typical for an older member of this breed with incomplete inspiration at the time of exposure. Marked widening of the cranial mediastinum is associated with obesity. The kyphosis of the thoracic spine is prominent. No active pulmonary disease is noted.

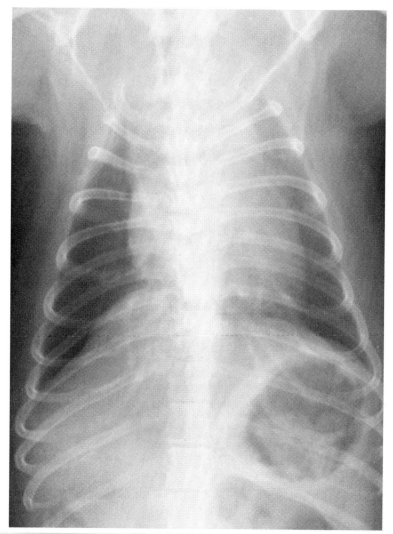

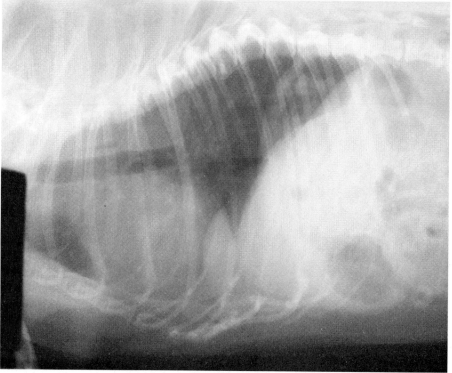

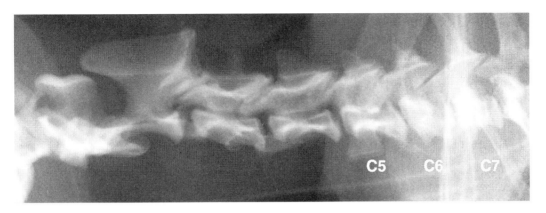

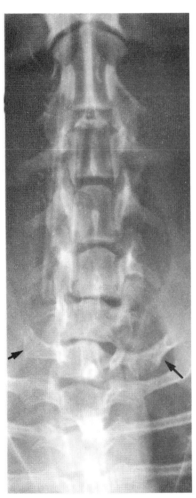

Noncontrast Radiographic Findings

The C7 vertebra is a transitional segment, with a malformed transverse process on the right and a rib on the left (arrows). C5-6 and C6-T1 disc spaces were narrowed with spondylosis deformans. There are only 12 thoracic vertebrae. Marked wedging of T8 was noted with associated spondylosis deformans. Note the disc space collapse and vertebral malalignment at T12-L1, the result of hypoplastic articular processes. A myelographic study was ordered.

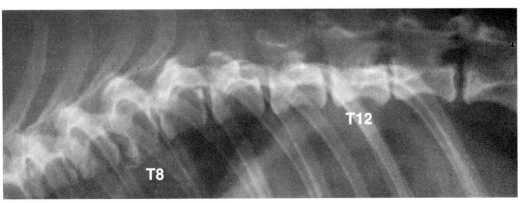

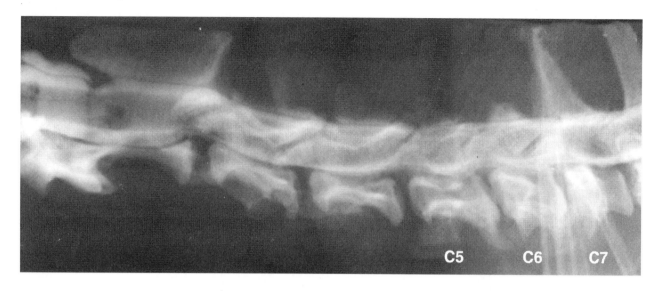

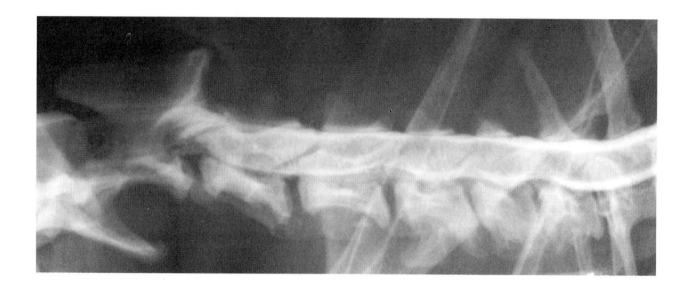

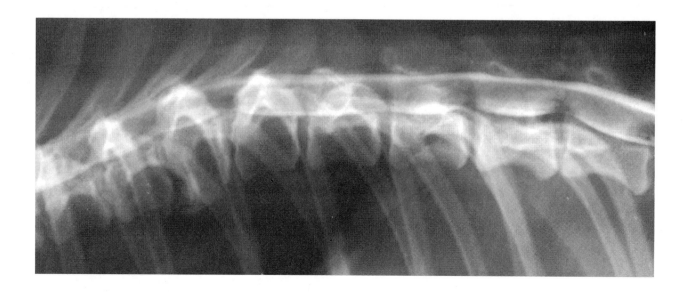

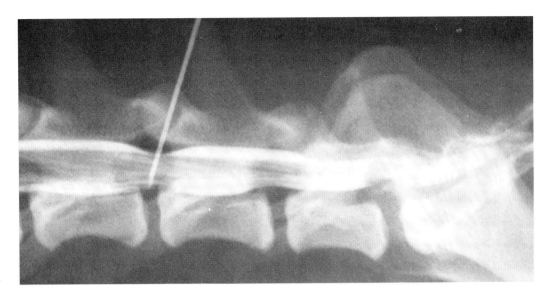

Myelographic Findings

Dorsal displacement of the ventral contrast column is present at several sites in the cervical and thoracic spine associated with chronic Type II disc disease. The most suggestive sites clinically are C4-5 and C5-6 where dorsal displacement of the cord is sufficient to cause narrowing of the dorsal contrast column. The cord narrowing at T7-9 is minimal. A dorsal LS disc protrusion is clearly seen the result of the pooling of contrast agent caudally.

Comments

It is difficult to determine the specific site of the lesion causing the clinical signs. The protruding cervical discs may all contribute to the neurologic signs. The wedging of T8 is probably developmental and has been present throughout the life of the dog, although a progressive narrowing of the vertebral canal could occur. The contribution of the hemivertebra and the L-S disc protrusion to the manifestations of the initial signs in the right pelvic limb is interesting to consider.

Because of the chronic nature of the disc disease, the good ambulation of the dog, and the absence of pain as observed by the owner, they chose to treat "Abby" with rest and confinement. If further vertebral stabilization occurs via the spondylosis deformans at C5-7, the possibility exists of further disc protrusion at C4-5 due to a "domino" effect.

Surgery or Neurology Service?

Certain patients have clinical signs characterized by shoulder or neck pain and are thought to represent musculoskeletal disease. After a more thorough examination, certain neurologic deficits are noted and the cases are subsequently worked up as cases with neurologic disease. Here are two such cases.

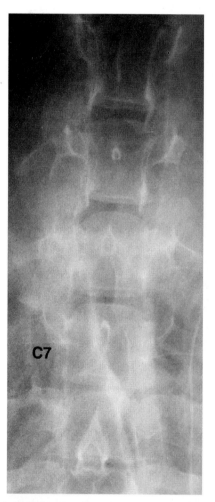

Case Description

"**Schultz**" is a 6-year-old male Weimaraner who presented with a 3-month history of right forelimb lameness. The owners added that during this time, cervical stiffness and lumbosacral pain had also been noted and "Schultz" had developed a short, choppy gait in both forelimbs. He had been treated with 5cc of dexamethasone subcutaneously and started on 20 mg prednisone per-os once daily. He returned to his veterinarian 5 days ago with a painful cranial abdomen. Abdominal radiographs showed a food distended stomach and a fecal filled colon that was thought to be due to "Schultz" having difficulty assuming a defecating position.

On physical examination, mild, right-thoracic-limb muscle atrophy was noted. The abdomen was tense with no organomegaly or masses palpated. Because of the history, the dog was referred to the neurology service where a neurological examination found a hypometric gait in the thoracic limbs and a weak, ataxic gait in the pelvic limbs. Placing reactions were mildly diminished in both thoracic limbs and markedly diminished in both pelvic limbs. The cutaneus trunci reflex was weak bilaterally to bilateral stimulation. The lesion was localized to the cervicothoracic region of the spinal cord.

The differential diagnosis at this time included: (1) caudal cervical spondylopathy, (2) granulomatous meningoencephalomyelitis, (3) discospondylitis of varying causes, (4) traumatic disc protrusion, (5) primary spinal tumor. Radiography of the spine was ordered.

Radiographic Findings

Loss of the lamina of C7 was noted on the right side. The cause of the lesion was further explored by myelography.

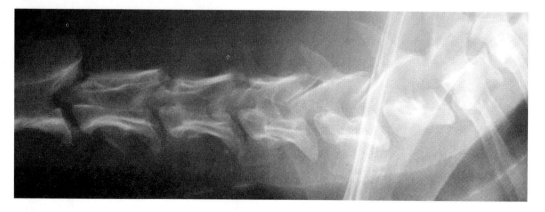

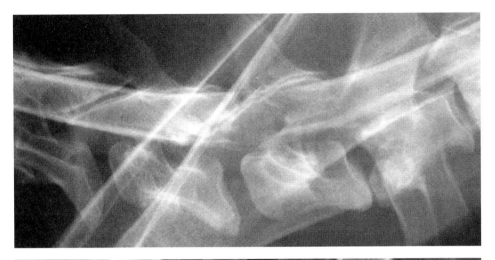

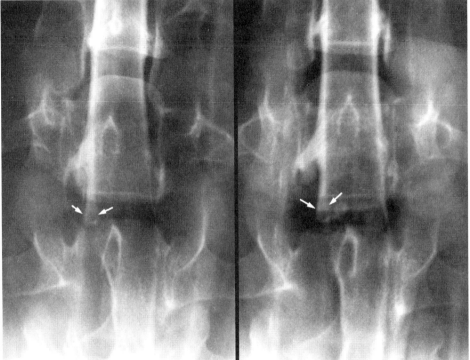

Myelographic Findings

The myelogram was performed following insertion of the spinal needle into the subarachnoid space at the cisterna magna and contrast medium was injected to achieve filling to the level of the cauda equina. Axial deviation of the contrast column on the right extends from the midbody of C7 to the midbody of T2. Irregularity is noted in the width of the contrast columns at this site and a "tee" sign is present on the right at the cranial aspect of C6 (arrows). Just caudal to the "tee" sign, contrast material appears to be pooling around a soft tissue mass that is within the intervertebral foramen. Attentuation of the contrast column on the left is present as well. A filling defect is present over the cranial aspect of C7 on the lateral view. The radiographic findings are typical for an intradural-extramedullary lesion at C7 with associated bony destruction of the right lamina. A nerve sheath tumor was suspected.

Comments

The owners agreed to a surgical biopsy. The tumor involving the nerve root of C8 was exposed after a right hemilaminectomy. Due to the invasive nature of the tumor the owners elected to euthanize "Schultz" on the OR table. A malignant peripheral nerve sheath tumor causing secondary axonal degeneration was found on necropsy.

Case Description

"**Casey**" is a 10-year-old male golden retriever with atrophy of the shoulder muscles and bilateral thoracic limb weakness. He has a 1-year history of progressive weakness and lethargy with an increased progressions of signs the past 3 weeks.

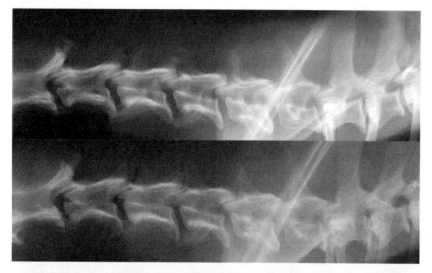

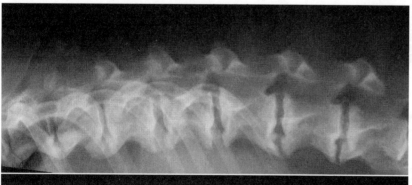

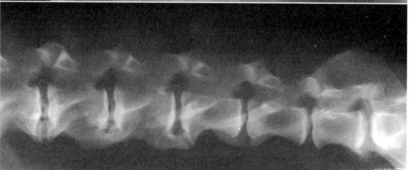

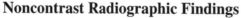

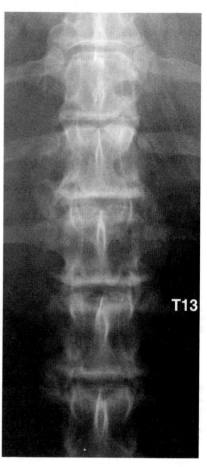

Noncontrast Radiographic Findings

Destruction of bone was noted within the body of C7 and the left pedicle and transverse process of T13. Prominent spondylosis deformans, typical for age, was present throughout the spine with only minimal disc space narrowing.

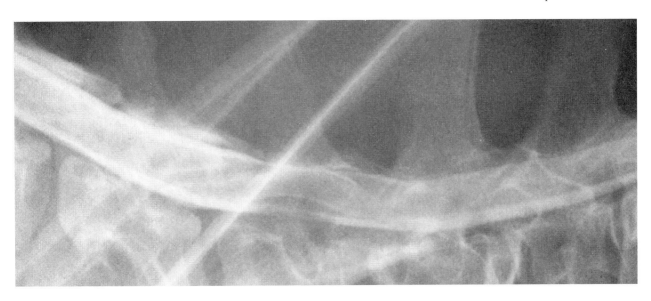

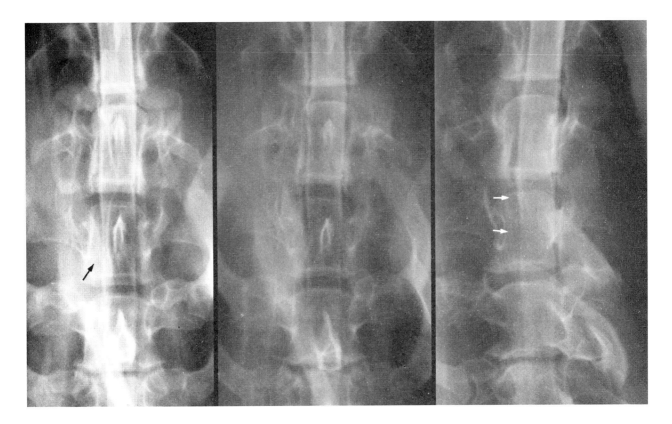

Cervical Myelographic Findings

A broad based area of elevation of the ventral contrast column is present over the body of C7 with slight displacement of the cord to the left on the VD view (arrow). The destruction in the left pedicle remains evident.

see next page

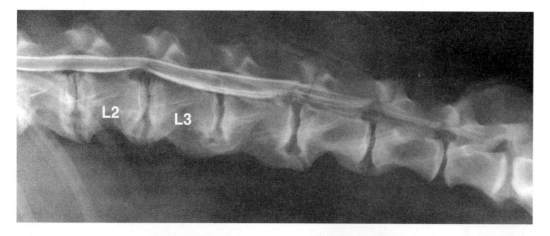

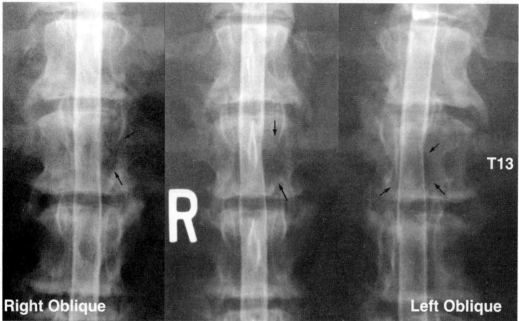

Thoracolumbar Myelographic Findings

The cord is elevated at L2-3 due to a suspect disc protrusion. Disruption of the contrast columns from L4-S1 is thought to be due to a large extradural mass. Axial deviation of the left contrast column is seen in the midbody of T13 at the site of bony destruction.

A suspect malignant process involves C7 and T13 with an extradural cord compression more prominent at C7. In addition, the tumor probably occupies much of the caudal lumbar extradural space.

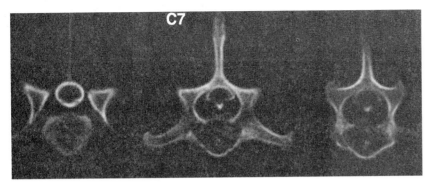

C7

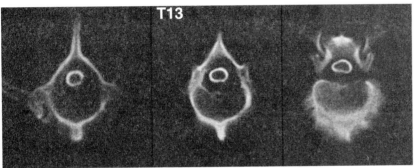

T13

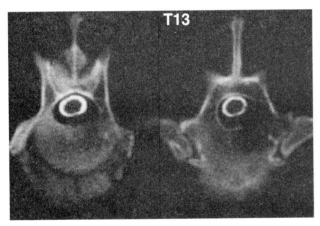

T13

CT Myelographic Findings

Destruction of bone is apparent within the vertebral bodies at C7 and T13 with extension of the tumor mass into the vertebral canal causing compression of the overlying spinal cord. Note how the destructive process involves the new bone of the spondylosis deformans as well. In the L5 section, the mass displaces the elements of the cauda equina dorsally away from the floor of the vertebral canal.

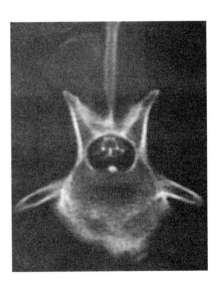

Comments

Malignant changes in more than one site throughout the spine are strongly suggestive of metastatic disease. The absence of any reactive appearing periosteal new bone tends to rule out an inflammatory process. The diagnosis for "Casey" was a metastatic plasmacytoma.

Three Dogs with T3-L3 Lesions

These dogs were of varying ages, 6 months, 3 years, and 10 years, but the clinical signs were all chronic. **"Mikey"** had pelvic limb ataxia, paresis and an abnormal posture, **"Maggie"** had pelvic limb ataxia, paresis and an abnormal posture, and **"Ritter"** had a short, choppy gait in the thoracic limbs. Each owner admitted that signs had been present for at least 1 month and probably longer. Each dog was thought to have T3-L3 lesion. The cases were worked up in a standard manner with physical examination followed by a neurological examination, noncontrast radiographs, and myelography.

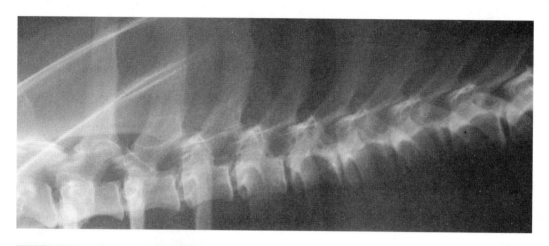

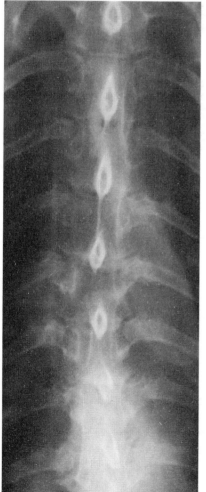

Case Description

"**Ritter**" is a 10-year-old male golden retriever with a chronic history of difficulty in rising. Placing reactions were decreased in the pelvic limbs. Spinal reflexes were normal except for crossed-extension of the right pelvic limb. The thoracic limbs were neurologically normal. The lesions was localized to T3-L3. Radiographs of the pelvis showed normal hip joints.

Radiographic Findings

No spinal lesions were noted except for slight kyphosis at T2-3. Spondylosis deformans was noted in the lumbar spine.

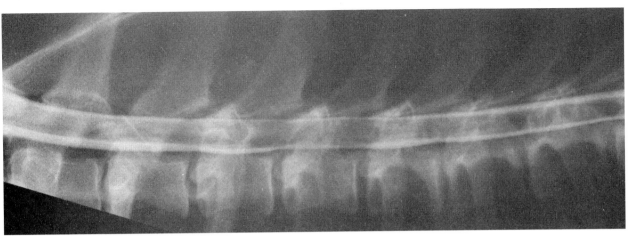

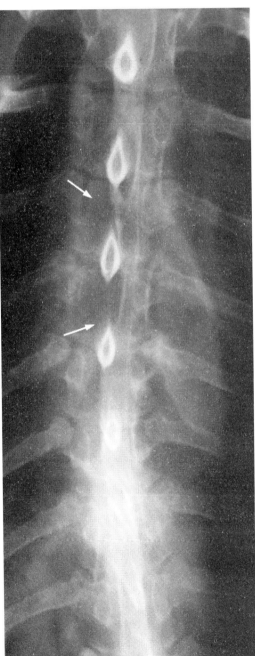

Myelographic Findings

Thinning of the contrast columns was seen dorsally and ventrally at T4 with axial deviation of the right column from T3 to T5 (arrows). A "tee" sign is present at the cranial portion of the mass on the right (arrows). Caudally the mass appears to be on the right with pooling of the contrast agent. The right-sided extradural mass was thought to be a nerve sheath tumor. No bone destruction was noted.

Comments

Exploratory surgery revealed a T3 dorsal nerve sheath tumor that invaded the spinal cord. The tumor was reported to be a malignant mesenchymal tumor. The owner opted to euthanize the dog at surgery.

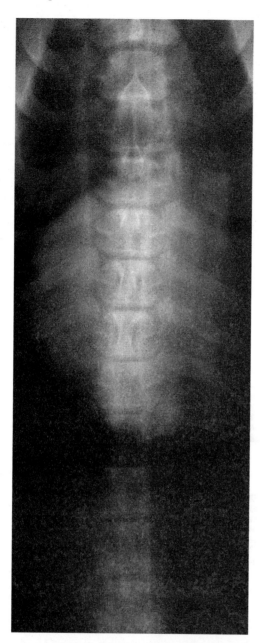

Case Description

"**Mikey**" is a 6-month-old large male mixed-breed dog with a 1-month history of pelvic limb ataxia, paresis, and abnormal posture. He has no history of trauma and is otherwise a healthy patient. His neurologic lesion was localized to T3-L3.

Radiographic Findings

The vertebral arches of T4-T6 appear subtely malformed and shortened (craniocaudal dimension). The intervertebral foramina appear smaller than normal. Disc spaces are of normal width. End plates are open as expected for the age of the dog. The suspected lesions have no secondary bony response and suggest a congenital/developmental etiology.

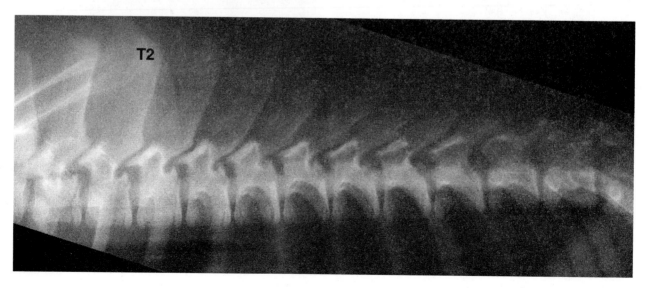

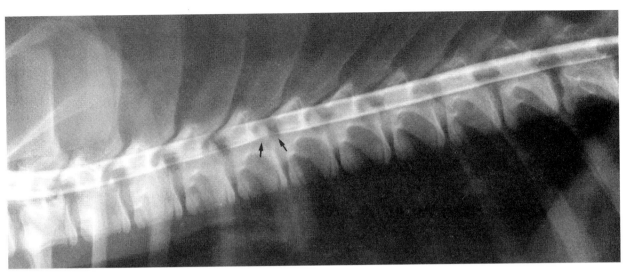

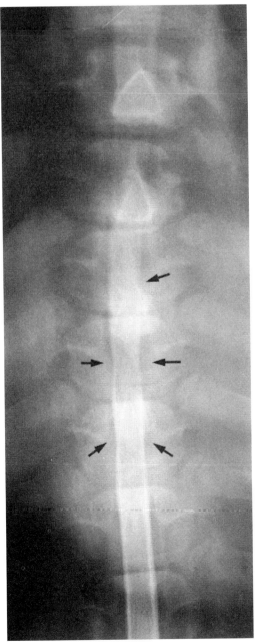

Myelographic Findings

Thinning of the contrast columns is present on both lateral and VD views from T4-T6 (arrows). In addition, a decrease in the size of the spinal cord is especially evident on the VD view. The diagnosis is a congenital/developmental vertebral canal stenosis.

Comments

"Mikey" had an extensive hemilaminectomy to decompress the spinal cord. Unfortunately, a spinal scoliosis developed subsequently causing a persistent canal stenosis.

Case Description

"**Maggie**" is a 3-year-old female Labrador retriever with back pain who is undergoing treatment for a discospondylitis at L1-2. On neurologic examination she has decreased to absent proprioceptive placing in the pelvic limbs. The patellar reflexes are increased in both limbs. The cutaneus trunci reflex is decreased on the right in the lumbar region. Pain can be elicited in the back at L1-2.

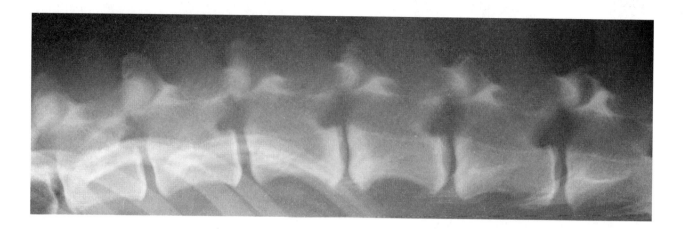

Radiographic Findings

Chronic changes are present on the noncontrast radiographs at L1-2 and consist of disc space narrowing, end plate sclerosis, and spondylosis deformans. It is interesting that this is the only site of disc disease and that it is so advanced for a dog of her age. These changes are not indicative of a discospondylitis.

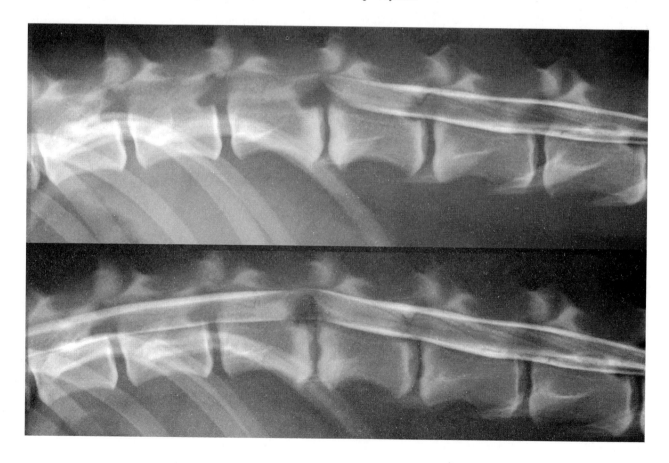

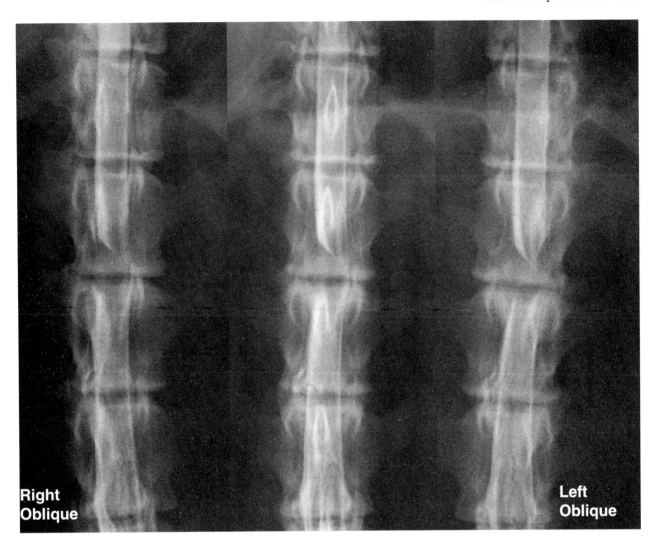

Right
Oblique

Left
Oblique

Myelographic Findings

A focal axial deviation of the right contrast column at L1-2 is evident on the VD view. Note the "bending" of the right contrast column medially. Also, note how contrast agent pools cranial and caudal to the mass lesion on the lateral view (opposite page). The height of the spinal cord is increased with attenuation of the contrast columns (bottom figure). Certainly, it is an operable lesion.

The fluid dynamics of myelography are shown on the lateral views. Note the incomplete filling of the subarachnoid space on the first view of the myelogram made after a trial injection. On the second view made following further injection, the contrast agent has flowed cranially past the lesion causing a more complete filling that permits identification of the lesion.

All of the VD views were made after removal of the needle following complete injection of the contrast agent.

The radiographic changes are most compatible with a tumor mass. The location and the changes in the disc space and end plate force the consideration of disc protrusion.

Comments

A hemilaminectomy was performed at L1-2 and a pea-sized mass that was adherent to the dura was removed. The unique appearance of the extradural mass made its identification from the gross examination impossible. It was sent for histological examination and was reported to be consistent with intervertebral disc tissue with no evidence of neoplasia or inflammation.

The exact nature of the mass could not be determined radiographically because changes consistent with both a tumor and a disc protrusion were present. The original diagnosis was that of a Type I disc disease suggesting an acute lesion, however, this does not agree with the radiographic patterns since the lack of cord swelling and the focal nature of the lesion suggest a chronic disc lesion or even a tumor mass. If a disc lesion is present, it might be better thought of as a Type III disc lesion.

"Spencer"

Case Description

"**Spencer**" is a 6-year-old male wolfhound with a long history of occasional pain noted by the owners when he walked or played. He was referred with a tentative diagnosis of cauda equina syndrome.

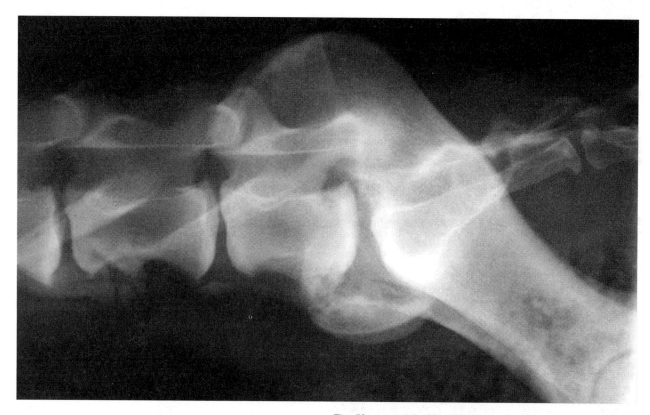

Radiographic Findings

Today's noncontrast radiographs demonstrate disc space narrowing, end plate sclerosis, spondylosis deformans, and malalignment resulting in a "stair-step" deformity at the LS junction similar to that seen on referral radiographs made 2 weeks earlier.

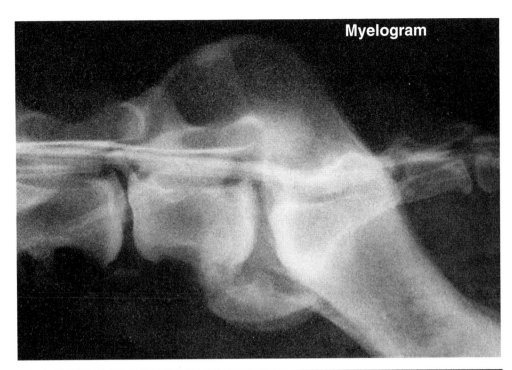

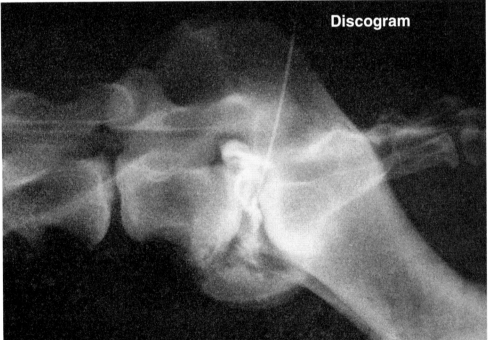

Contrast Radiographic Findings

The noncontrast study and myelogram show the malalignment at the LS junction. The myelogram does not identify the massive LS disc protrusion that is seen on the discogram where the large contrast-filled cavity in the central portion of the LS disc has only a thin outer anulus fibrosus remaining. The needle remains in position on the radiograph of the discogram.

Comments

The noncontrast study is diagnostic of marked malalignment and suspected instability at the LS junction. The myelogram does not clearly show the disc lesion that is easily seen on the discogram. Perhaps the protruding disc material is lateral to the conus medullaris in the region of the intervertebral foramina and does not have an effect on the myelogram. This patient clearly demonstrates the value of the use of more than one diagnostic techniques while searching for the one that best demonstrates the lesion.

Index of Diseases